Clinical Immunobiology

Edited by

VOLUME 3

FRITZ H. BACH, M.D.

IMMUNOBIOLOGY RESEARCH CENTER
DEPARTMENTS OF MEDICAL GENETICS
AND SURGERY
UNIVERSITY OF WISCONSIN
MADISON, WISCONSIN

ROBERT A. GOOD, Ph.D., M.D.

MEMORIAL SLOAN-KETTERING
CANCER CENTER
NEW YORK, NEW YORK

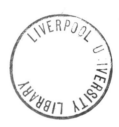

ACADEMIC PRESS   New York   San Francisco   London   1976
A Subsidiary of Harcourt Brace Jovanovich, Publishers

ACADEMIC PRESS, INC.
111 Fifth Avenue, New York, New York 10003

United Kingdom Edition published by
ACADEMIC PRESS, INC. (LONDON) LTD.
24/28 Oval Road, London NW1

LIBRARY OF CONGRESS CATALOG CARD NUMBER: 72-77356

ISBN 0-12-070003-4

PRINTED IN THE UNITED STATES OF AMERICA

Contents

Evaluation of the Immunoglobulins

Richard Hong

Electrophoresis and Immunoelectrophoresis in the Evaluation of Homogeneous Immunoglobulin Components

Edward C. Franklin

Leukocyte Aggregation Test for Evaluating Cell-Mediated Immunity

Baldwin H. Tom and Barry D. Kahan

The HLA System: Serologically Defined Antigens

Ekkehard D. Albert

Mixed Leukocyte Cultures: A Cellular Approach to Histocompatibility Testing

Fritz H. Bach

The Reticuloendothelial System

W. F. Cunningham-Rundles

Complement

Harvey R. Colten and Chester A. Alper

Detection of Tumor-Associated Antigens in Plasma or Serum

Morton K. Schwartz

Neutrophil Function

Michael E. Miller

List of Contributors

Numbers in parentheses indicate the pages on which the authors' contributions begin.

N. FRANKLIN ADKINSON, JR., Division of Clinical Immunology, Department of Medicine of the Johns Hopkins University School of Medicine at The Good Samaritan Hospital, Baltimore, Maryland (305)

EKKEHARD D. ALBERT, Kinderpoliklinik der Universität München, Munich, Germany (237)

CHESTER A. ALPER, Allergy Division, Department of Medicine, Children's Hospital Medical Center, The Center for Blood Research, and the Department of Pediatrics, Harvard Medical School, Boston, Massachusetts (387)

FRITZ H. BACH, Immunobiology Research Center and Departments of Medical Genetics and Surgery, The University of Wisconsin, Madison, Wisconsin (273)

SILVIO BARANDUN, Institute for Clinical and Experimental Cancer Research, Tiefenau Hospital, Berne, Switzerland (37,57)

HARVEY R. COLTEN, Allergy Division, Department of Medicine, Children's Hospital Medical Center, The Center for Blood Research, and the Department of Pediatrics, Harvard Medical School, Boston, Massachusetts (387)

SUSANNA CUNNINGHAM-RUNDLES, Clinical Immunology Laboratory, Memorial Sloan-Kettering Cancer Center, New York, New York (151)

W. F. CUNNINGHAM-RUNDLES, Memorial Sloan-Kettering Cancer Center, New York, New York (289)

BO DUPONT, Clinical Immunology Laboratory, Memorial Sloan-Kettering Cancer Center, New York, New York (151)

C. P. ENGELFRIET, Central Laboratory of the Netherlands, Red Cross Blood Transfusion Service, Amsterdam, The Netherlands (345)

EDWARD C. FRANKLIN, Irvington House Institute and the Rheumatic Diseases Study Group, New York University Medical Center, New York, New York (21)

JOHN A. HANSEN, Clinical Immunology Laboratory, Memorial Sloan-Kettering Cancer Center, New York, New York (151)

RICHARD HONG, Department of Pediatrics, University of Wisconsin, Madison, Wisconsin (1)

HUGO E. JASIN, Department of Internal Medicine, The University of Texas, Southwestern Medical School, Dallas, Texas (365)

BARRY D. KAHAN, Laboratory of Surgical Immunology, Departments of Surgery and Physiology, Northwestern University Medical Center, and the Veterans Administration Lakeside Hospital, Chicago, Illinois (221)

LAWRENCE M. LICHTENSTEIN, Division of Clinical Immunology, Department of Medicine of the Johns Hopkins University School of Medicine at The Good Samaritan Hospital, Baltimore, Maryland (305)

MICHAEL E. MILLER, Department of Pediatrics, University of California, Los Angeles, School of Medicine at the Harbor General Hospital, Los Angeles, California (427)

ANDREAS MORELL, Institute for Clinical and Experimental Cancer Research, Tiefenau Hospital, Berne, Switzerland (37,57)

PETER PERLMANN, Department of Immunology, Wenner-Gren Institute, University of Stockholm, Stockholm, Sweden (107)

CARL M. PINSKY, Memorial Sloan-Kettering Cancer Center, New York, New York (97)

ROSS E. ROCKLIN, Department of Medicine, Robert B. Brigham Hospital, Harvard Medical School, Boston, Massachusetts (195)

MORTON K. SCHWARTZ, Laboratory of Applied and Diagnostic Biochemistry, Memorial Sloan-Kettering Cancer Center, New York, New York (405)

FRANTISEK SKVARIL, Institute for Clinical and Experimental Cancer Research, Tiefenau Hospital, Berne, Switzerland (37, 57)

J. DONALD SMILEY, Department of Internal Medicine, The University of Texas, Southwestern Medical School, Dallas, Texas (365)

WARREN STROBER, Metabolism Branch, National Cancer Institute, NIH, Bethesda, Maryland (71)

NORMAN TALAL, Department of Medicine, University of California, San Francisco, California (375)

BALDWIN H. TOM, Laboratory of Surgical Immunology, Departments of Surgery and Physiology, Northwestern University Medical Center, and the Veterans Administration Lakeside Hospital, Chicago, Illinois (221)

THOMAS A. WALDMANN, Metabolism Branch, National Cancer Institute, NIH, Bethesda, Maryland (71)

J. WUNDERLICH, Immunology Branch, National Cancer Institute, NIH, Bethesda, Maryland (133)

Preface

Physicians, these days, are being continually bombarded with new information from the burgeoning science of immunobiology. Some of this must be translated into the pragmatic analysis of sick patients; the physician must use and interpret immunological tests that are new and sometimes confusing. Since many of the methods used in evaluation of a patient's immunological status have been described only recently in a scientific and clinical literature that is highly dispersed, the student or physician may not understand these new tools as well as he would like. We have attempted in this volume to provide some of the essential information that can help in the elucidation of immunological mechanisms that are of importance in a wide variety of diseases and that have focused attention on methodological requirements for careful analysis of immunocompetence in the patient. This is a complex and difficult subject. It is this need that has persuaded us, in this third volume of *Clinical Immunobiology*, to depart somewhat from the format of the first two volumes. Rather than cover exhaustively a few areas of current interest in clinical immunobiology, we have asked a larger number of contributors to discuss a variety of methods used for assaying the immune status of an individual.

The emphasis we intended was to attempt to provide the reader, first, with something of a background of the issue to which the clinical test would be applied; second, to give in broad outline the methodological procedures used in the analyses without stressing cookbook-like details; third, to give some examples of the kinds of data that can be generated with the procedures used and thus to provide guidelines for interpretation of the tests; and, fourth, to present a discussion of the value of the immunological test procedures in differential diagnosis and analysis of diseases; further, to discuss where possible the usefulness of these procedures in prognosis of disease and the consequences of immunological manipulation undertaken for treatment or prevention of disease.

Whereas it would have been desirable to describe in this one volume all the immunological test procedures currently in clinical use, two factors made this impossible. First, to avoid inordinately long delays for contributors of some of the articles included in this volume, we felt we should go to press even though not every article we had solicited had been submitted. Further, certain test procedures have not yet been established as routine for the clinical laboratory, and we felt that these were better presented in a subsequent volume of *Clinical Immunobiology* following our usual format of having two or more articles discussing the same general topic in order to give sufficiently broad consideration. An example of the latter need is the study of the enormously important area of enumeration of the different classes and subclasses of lymphocytes. We felt that this area deserved a series of articles dealing with various methods of identification and their interpretation. Another subject which could have been included in greater detail in this volume is histocompatibility typing. We have promised in prior volumes to treat this subject at an early date. Advances in this field, especially the association of histocompatibility with disease, are exceedingly important and are becoming a major concern to the physician. This subject will be dealt with in broad context in Volume 4.

We hope and expect that a consideration of the several techniques presented here will aid the student of medicine, the practitioner as well as the basic immunologist, in formulating further questions of both basic and clinical interest in the context of immunobiological disturbances in disease. Methods used to quantitate both normal and pathologic immunoglobulins and their subclasses and metabolism, the means used to test cell-mediated immunity *in vitro* and *in vivo,* and analyses of the products of activated lymphocytes are areas which already must be faced by many clinicians almost every day. So it is also with the assessment of allergic states, the need to consider the quantitation of IgE, and the measurement of allergen-specific IgE antibody. Analyses of autoantibodies and rheumatoid factors, especially in lupus, rheumatoid arthritis, and hematologic disorders, require methods that must be understood by most general practitioners, internists, and pediatricians. Quantitation of complement and the components of the complement system becomes ever more important in clinical medicine as the complement system and its primary and secondary deficiencies are being defined. These are all addressed in the present volume. The chapters on evaluation of neutrophils and their function, and an introduction to means of assessing the major histocompatibility system in man should be of increasing importance. Although they have not yet reached the point of definitive diagnostic value, studies of tumor-associated antigens are of importance in following the results of cancer therapy and in detecting at an early stage recurrences of certain malignancies.

Thus, in this volume, we present a discussion of many methods and attempt to evaluate the clinical usefulness of a wide range of immunological methodologies. We hope and trust that this volume will help medical students, internists, pediatricians, and surgeons to understand the immunological methodologies they must call upon with increasing frequency. By understanding these methods and by recognizing their values and limitations, we anticipate that their use can be increased and their applications made most appropriate to needs. We must hope that this volume, focused on immunological methodologies, will fill a need for all students of medicine and encourage the continuing expansion of the already great contributions of immunology to clinical discourse.

FRITZ H. BACH
ROBERT A. GOOD

Contents of Previous Volumes

Volume 2

Evaluation of the Immunoglobulins

RICHARD HONG

Department of Pediatrics, University of Wisconsin, Madison, Wisconsin

I. Introduction

In the initial assessment of immunoglobulins (Igs), one is usually concerned with the extent of heterogeneity (judged by electrophoretic characteristics) and the quantitative levels in serum. Heterogeneity implies an ability to express an immune response to many diverse stimuli by many Ig-producing cell lines—termed a polyclonal response. Monoclonal or homogeneous increases may serve as markers of malignancies directly involving the lymphoid system (myeloma) or may be associated with nonlymphoid tumors; sometimes no associated disease is detectable.

Quantitatively, lower than normal values are seen in the large heterogeneous groups of immunoglobulin-deficiency syndromes, where recurrent life-threatening infections may cause early demise. Since the immunoglobulins reflect the environmental experience of the individual, they increase with age and in any age group may show a broad range of

1

"normal" values. Five major classes are known; of these, IgG, IgA, and IgM are routinely studied. IgE can be readily quantitated with special reagents, but little is known of IgD values in health and disease.

Both quantitative and qualitative approaches are employed in assessment of immunoglobulins, especially when evaluating immunodeficiency. Immunodeficiency syndromes usually involve hypogammaglobulinemia of all three major classes. Less commonly, normal or even elevated immunoglobulin levels are found. In these cases, however, the elevation usually involves only IgG or IgM, and there is reciprocal deficiency of the other Igs. Unusual electrophoretic mobility patterns are often found (see Fig. 4). In such situations a qualitative assessment of the functional capability of the Ig proteins or examination of certain physiochemical parameters allows more precise judgment of the protective capability of the Igs present, irrespective of the amounts detected.

II. Techniques

In qualitative evaluation of the immunoglobulins, two measures of functionality are studied—electrophoretic characteristics and ability to bind antigen. For study of electrophoretic characteristics, the serum is applied to a support medium, usually cellulose acetate, although thin layers of agarose may also be employed. At the pH of the usual buffer systems (8.2–8.6), all serum proteins, save IgG, are negatively charged and migrate toward the anode. IgG remains at the origin or may migrate cathodally. The latter phenomenon is, in actuality, an artifact due to electroendosmosis wherein the migrating proteins are "swept cathodally" as hydrated positive ions are attracted to the negative electrode during electrophoresis. After the separation, a protein-binding dye, e.g., amido black or Ponceau S, is applied and the five separated groups are visualized as bands. A semiquantitative assessment is made by measuring optically the amount of dye bound to each band and expressing it as a percentage. Each group percentage is then multiplied by the total serum protein value (determined by another method) giving values for albumin, α_1-, α_2-, β-, and γ-globulin groups. An assumption in quantitation by this method is that dye-binding is essentially equal among all proteins. This is not strictly true. Further, since there are at least 95 serum proteins, each "band" represents a large number of different entities, so the term "α_2" has little functional or biological meaning. The γ-globulin area, however, is relatively pure and contains only minor amounts of the two other major Ig classes. By inspection, monoclonal peaks (or "M spikes") can be readily discerned from study of protein electrophoretic patterns (Figs. 1, 3, and 4).

Finer separation can be obtained by using media of greater resolving power, which separate by size as well as charge. Starch gel or acrylamide polymers have superior resolving capability, and upwards of twenty serum fractions are easily detected. Unfortunately, these techniques have not added much to the clinical assessment of the γ-globulins and are primarily of help in demonstrating genetic variants and isozyme patterns of other serum proteins (Fig. 3).

Further discrimination of electrophoretically separated proteins is accomplished by adding the exquisite sensitivity and specificity of immunological precipitation. The technique of immunoelectrophoretic analysis, first described by Grabar and Williams, then subsequently modified by Scheiddegger for microscope slides, is today a routine laboratory procedure. After electrophoresis in agar or on cellulose acetate, a polyvalent antiserum usually capable of reacting with 20 or more serum proteins is allowed to diffuse at right angles to the line of electrophoretic migration. A series of precipitin lines appears after overnight incubation (Fig. 2). Arcs developed in agar can be viewed directly by indirect lighting. The use of a properly constructed view box and slight magnification with binocular loupes (7.5×) is essential for full appreciation of

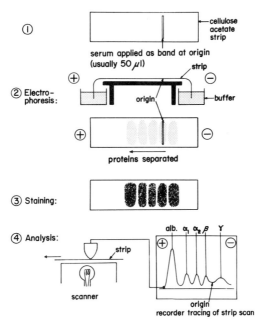

Fig. 1. Technique of serum electrophoresis on cellulose acetate. For actual patterns, see Fig. 3A,B. Abbreviations: alb. = albumin; α_1, α_2, β, γ = the corresponding globulins.

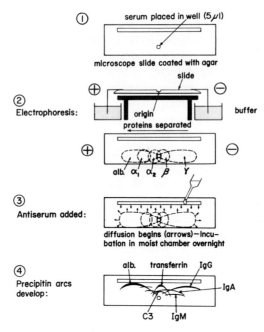

Fig. 2. Technique of immunoelectrophoretic analysis. For actual patterns, see Figs. 4C and 5.

the pattern. Staining is required to visualize patterns developed on cellulose and may be alternatively used with agar patterns.

In another variation, the finer resolution of thin-layer agarose electrophoresis is combined with immunological precipitation performed in an

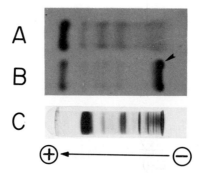

Fig. 3. Comparison of cellulose acetate and acrylamide electrophoresis. (A) normal serum pattern. (B) γG myeloma; the thin monoclonal IgG band (arrow) contrasts with the broad heterogeneous normal IgG peak of (A). (C) Acrylamide electrophoresis: resolution into many serum components is apparent.

electric field. Electrophoresis is performed in two directions at right angles to each other ("crossed electrophoresis"). The first run separates the proteins in the usual manner, but into more than five groups. The strip of agar containing the separated fractions is then cut out and placed in apposition to another strip containing antibody. Electrophoresis is restarted at right angles to the original electrophoretic axis, and the proteins now migrate out of the original agarose strip into the antibody containing gels. Precipitation occurs during the second electrophoresis and the proteins are visualized as "mountains." This technique enhances the minor variations seen in heterogeneous populations and demonstrates subgroups or genetic variants in a striking way (Fig. 4).

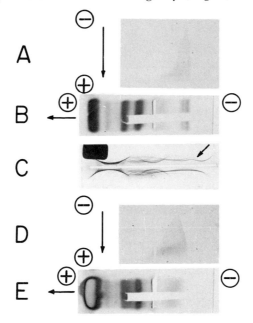

Fig. 4. Comparison of agarose (B and E), agarose crossed-electrophoresis technique (A and D), and immunoelectrophoretic analysis (C). The electrophoretic axes for the crossed technique are shown. B is from a patient with immunodeficiency but normal levels of IgG (980 mg/dl). Note the two thin bands of IgG as compared to the broad "smear" of normal IgG seen in pattern E. The defect in the gel shows the portion removed (before staining) and then applied to the antibody (anti-IgG)-containing gel in pattern A. After a second electrophoresis, the IgG precipitated and could be shown by staining as narrow peaks (A). The same technique utilized for a normal serum sample (D and E) shows a broad heterogeneous IgG peak. Panel C shows the patient's serum assessed by immunoelectrophoretic analysis. The biclonal nature of the IgG arc (arrow) is again apparent. The study shows that, even with normal levels of IgG, patients with congenital immunodeficiency have obvious electrophoretic abnormalities.

Through the use of selected antisera, specific immunoglobulins or immunoglobulin subunits can be identified and characterized (Fig. 5). When only one Ig is studied, immunoelectrophoretic analysis may not be necessary, and specific antisera can be used in Ouchterlony double-diffusion analysis. In some cases of immunodeficiency, subunits not ordinarily found in the serum, such as free light chains or monomeric IgM (7 S IgM), occur. Detection of free light chains requires special

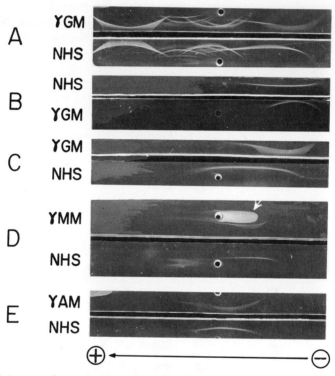

Fig. 5. Immunoelectrophoretic analysis showing use of specific antisera. (A) Normal serum (NHS) below and IgG myeloma (γGM) above reacted against antiserum to all serum proteins. In the patterns of this figure the elevated levels of myeloma are apparent from the thickness of the arcs. The lesser density of the precipitin arcs is due in part to the high levels, but it may also be caused by lack of some antigenic determinants in the myeloma, as compared to normal, populations. (B) NHS above and γGM below reacted against anti-γ chain. (C) γGM above and NHS below reacted against anti-κ chain. Reaction against anti-λ antiserum showed no reaction with γGM, but the same broad reaction versus NHS as that shown by anti-κ. Therefore, the myeloma is of the kappa type. (D) Macroglobulinemia of Waldenström (γMM) above and NHS below reacted with anti-μ. In addition to limited heterogeneity, the macroglobulinemic serum shows spontaneous precipitation in agar (arrow) common in this disorder and in some cases of cryoglobulinemia. (E) IgA myeloma (γAM) above and NHS below.

antisera, which are not generally available. Monomeric IgM can be detected by its ability to permeate media that restrict the diffusion of the pentamer. Four percent acrylamide or an 8% gelatin–1% agar mixture rather than the usual medium of 1–1.5% agar can be used in Ouchterlony double-diffusion analyses. Pentameric IgM usually will not produce a precipitin arc under these circumstances whereas monomeric will. If an arc is seen with the pentamer, it is extremely close to the antigen well and shows marked curving toward the antigen side typical of high-molecular-weight reactants. Monomeric IgM precipitates approximately midway between the antigen and antibody wells as a straight precipitin line.

The ultimate clinical evaluation of the immunoglobulin involves demonstration of its ability to bind antigen. In terms of biological significance and importance to the host, this represents the key test. Here one measures the specific antibody response to known antigens. Antigens can be those to which the patient is assumed to have had natural exposure, those known to have been given in the past, or those that are purposefully given for study of the antibody response. (The administration of antigen may also be given to stimulate lymph nodes so that their morphology can be assessed.) Suitable antigens for immunization and assessment are given in a World Health Organization report on immunodeficiency disorders. Additional information can be derived from using the nonpathogenic virus ϕX174.[1] Measurement of functional antibody capacity involves standard agglutination, complement fixation, and virus neutralization techniques.

It should be emphasized that, except for ϕX174, live-virus vaccines are contraindicated in assessment of immunodeficiency syndromes, as fatal infection can result.

Scant attention has been given to determining the antibody class of Ig involved in host responses. Older methods used the loss of reactivity following reduction by 2-mercaptoethanol as presumptive evidence that the antibody was IgM. Later separation of the antibody by size, using ultracentrifugation or gel filtration, was used. These methods are too tedious and limited in capability for large-scale clinical studies. An individual class response can be determined by the radio allergosorbent test (RAST), which was devised to measure the amount of specific IgE antibody directed against an allergen. The antigen, insolubilized on a plastic surface or solid particles, is incubated with the test serum. Antibodies are absorbed onto the antigen. A radiolabeled antibody directed against IgE is then added, and the amount of radioactivity which

[1] Obtainable from Dr. Ralph Wedgwood, Department of Pediatrics, University of Washington Medical School, Seattle, Washington 98195.

adheres is a measure of the specific IgE directed against the antigen. Slight modifications would permit determinations of antibodies of the other Ig classes to many other antigens (Fig. 6).

It is now known that some B-cell defects may be related to faulty synthesis or secretion. B cells ostensibly capable of being "triggered" for these terminal events of antibody production are found in normal numbers in some variants of deficiency states. To further assess these functions, *in vitro* studies of B-lymphocyte immunoglobulin production can be performed. However, the techniques and interpretations of the results are best performed in specialized research laboratories. Abnormalities of *in vitro* biosynthesis have also been observed in autoimmune thrombocytopenic purpura, suggesting that ineffective or aberrant Ig assembly and secretion is associated with clinical forms of altered immunity other than deficiency.

QUANTITATIVE ASSESSMENT TECHNIQUES

The most widely employed techniques for Ig quantitation in use today utilize the Mancini single radial diffusion technique. The technique is simple, and prepared plates can be commercially purchased, eliminating the need for laboratories of limited resources to develop their own antisera and standards. The principle is based upon the quantitative precipitin reaction, in which an antigen reacting with constant amounts of the specific antibody yields an amount of precipitate that is proportional to the amount of antigen used. The reaction is not linear with all proportions of reactants—only where the amount of antibody is in moderate excess to the antigen. In the test as commonly employed, monospecific antiserum reacting only with the heavy chain of the immunoglobulin to be measured is incorporated into a flat agar sheet. Holes are carefully punched to receive the serum sample, which may or may not be diluted. Various conditions of time and temperature for the incubation are employed, and the diameter of the circle of precipitation is measured. Here again proper lighting and magnification is desirable, as the diameters are only millimeters in length. A standard curve is drawn based on precipitin rings generated by standards of known concentration.

Various methods of plotting the results are employed: the log of the concentration ($\log c$) versus the diameter (d) or the diameter squared (d^2) on semilog paper; the square of the diameter versus the concentration, or the area versus the concentration on linear scales. A number of methods are used to record the data because the time for the reaction to come to completion is not the same for all wells, being a matter of

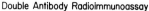

Double Antibody Radioimmunoassay

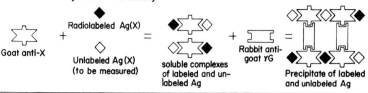

Radioimmunosorbent Test (RIST)

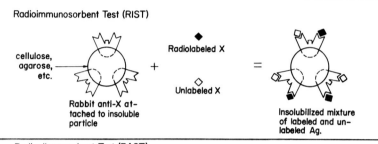

Radioallergosorbent Test (RAST)

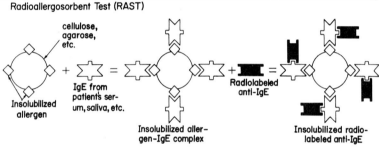

Fig. 6. Principles of radioimmunoassay techniques. In the double antibody and RIST techniques, the Ig to be measured is radiolabeled. Ig present in the sample to be quantitated is not radiolabeled and competes for the limited number of antibody sites. The more sample Ig present, the less labeled Ig is bound. A second antibody is added to precipitate the antibody-bound labeled Ig. Nonantibody bound radioactivity is removed by washing the precipitate. Alternatively, in the RIST technique the antibody is already insolubilized and the unbound label is readily washed away. In the double antibody and RIST techniques the amount of precipitated isotope varies *inversely* with the amount of Ig present in the sample, since it is a competitive assay. If the patient has antibodies directed against the species of origin of the anti-Ig antibody (e.g., antigoat γG antibodies), he may bind the anti-Ig and prevent precipitation of isotope. This will decrease the amount of precipitated radioactivity, giving rise to a falsely high value for the Ig being measured. If antibodies to the Ig (e.g., antihuman γA or antihuman γE) are present in the patient, they can also bind the label but will not come down with the insolubilized reagent. Noninsolubilized radioactivity will be washed away. The resultant decrease in insolubilized radioisotope is interpreted as a false high value of the Ig being measured.

The RAST technique measures specific antibodies of a particular class. The anti-Ig is radiolabeled and the antigen of interest is insolubilized. The isotope is precipitated only if an Ig from the added patient serum is attached to the insolubilized antigen. Here the amount of radioactivity precipitated is directly proportional to the amount of Ig present in the sample. In the example shown, IgE antibodies to "allergen" (ragweed) are shown. Using different antigens and different heavy-chain antibodies, other Ig class responses could be assessed.

hours at low antigen concentration but several days for the higher amounts of antigen or for slowly diffusing antigens (IgM). In clinical use, it is impractical to wait 4–6 days for an Ig determination. For clinical purposes, accuracy at low levels (0–300 mg of IgG per deciliter) is most important; whether a patient had IgG at 3000 instead of 2000 mg/dl is of little diagnostic import. If plates are measured early (after 5–11 hours of incubation at room temperature), straight lines are obtained with log c versus d or log c versus d^2. If the circles are measured after the reaction has gone to completion (usually 140 hours), d^2 versus c plots on linear scales should be used. In no event should one extrapolate beyond the points of lowest and highest antigen concentration actually used to determine the standard curve. The major disadvantage of short incubation periods is that precipitin rings are more difficult to measure accurately since the borders are indistinct. Suitable compromise can be obtained by an overnight incubation, accepting a slight curvature of the line. A plot of area versus concentration on linear scales is used by the author.

Although not in widespread use at the moment, automated methods based on nephelometry or inhibition of agglutination in continuous-flow systems may soon become readily available, permitting rapid determination of Igs. The methodology can be adapted to detect nanogram (10^{-6} mg) quantities.

Other methods of quantitation require either equipment or experience not as readily available as would be required for general widespread clinical use. However, sensitivity is greatly augmented. The "rocket" method of Laurell speeds the precipitation reaction by electrophoresing the antigen into antibody-containing agarose. As the antigen migrates in the antibody milieu, formation of soluble antigen–antibody complexes followed by precipitation occurs and will continue until the reaction is complete. The precipitation pattern resembles an arrowhead or rocket, and the length of the precipitate is proportional to the antigen concentration. Stained or unstained precipitates can be measured. Recently a marked increase in sensitivity has been accomplished by augmenting ordinarily nonvisible "rockets" with a second antibody conjugated to horseradish peroxidase followed by staining for this enzyme. This makes nanogram detection possible.

The quantitation of IgD, IgE, and 11 S IgA in the serum or of all Igs in fluids other than serum (CSF, urine, etc.) requires techniques other than the Mancini method, which measures conveniently only to levels of 1–10 μg/ml. Capability to detect nanograms is necessary, and radioimmunoassay techniques originally devised for hormone quantitation are suitable for this degree of sensitivity. These techniques require a continuously available source of pure radiolabeled Ig and thus are not convenient for general clinical use. The principle involved in these and related tests is shown schematically in Fig. 6. An augmented Mancini technique devised by Rowe uses a radiolabeled antibody directed against the γ-globulin of the antihuman Ig. This antibody adheres to an invisible precipitin ring produced by the traces of Ig and its specific antibody. After incubation and washing, a radioautograph is made and the circles on the exposed film are measured. The rings can also be augmented by a second antibody labeled with fluorescein and visualized under blue light.

Quantitation of Ig subgroups is possible with a variety of the above techniques, but the antisera are very difficult to produce and extreme care must be taken to assure specificity.

III. Results

A. QUALITATIVE ASSESSMENT

The first study of the immunoglobulins is often a view of the electrophoretic pattern. Immunoelectrophoretic analysis provides a rapid method of qualitatively assessing the three major classes of Igs. With monospecific antisera the broad heterogeneity characteristic of normal Ig populations is apparent. The slight charge differences of the individual molecules cause migration in an electric field to vary over a wide range (Figs. 1 and 2). This normal diverse response to antigenic stimulation is described as polyclonal. In most cases of immunodeficiency, because of hypogammaglobulinemia, the arcs are poorly visible and the heterogeneity cannot be assessed. A number of cases of normal to elevated levels of IgG or IgM have been observed, however, in congenital immunodeficiency. In these cases the immunoglobulin G arc is mono- or biclonal in character and resembles the pattern seen in multiple myeloma (Fig. 4). Often the proteins of restricted heterogeneity are also restricted to a single light-chain class and are therefore monoclonal. However, monoclonal proteins are more characteristic of multiple myeloma and the "benign monoclonal gammopathies." These entities are further considered in the chapter by Franklin.

Standard protein electrophoresis, which resolves serum proteins into five major groups, is of value in demonstration of limited heterogeneity (monoclonal peaks or M spikes) (Figs. 3 and 4). It should never be used to diagnose deficiency states since it is too insensitive. Quantitation of Igs is more appropriately accomplished by the immunological techniques described above.

More precise definition of immunoglobulin quality is obtained by demonstration of its functional capability. Functional assessment is especially important in establishing deficiency in the face of only modestly depressed normal or even elevated Ig levels. Recently ϕX174 has been utilized as an antigen. Six types of responses are noted, depending upon major Ig class response, rate of phage clearance, and presence or absence of a secondary response. These studies may have predictive value for anticipating response to γ-globulin therapy.

B. QUANTITATIVE ASSESSMENT

Normal Ig values vary greatly from individual to individual. Especially wide variation is seen with age. It is important to compare values in early years with values for appropriate age-matched controls. Buckley and Dorsey (1971) have devised a high-order polynomial expression that "erases" the effect of age and allows the ready comparison of different groups by comparing to $\log_e$ values of a common standard. Typical ranges for normal Ig values are shown in Table I.

When similar samples of serum are quantitated by different laboratories, marked variations in results are obtained, as much as 2- to 5-fold. The discrepancies are most likely due to the nature of the reagents employed. Since Igs have many antigenic groups, each antiserum raised will vary considerably in its range of reactivity. The variability of the antiserum reactivity is further confounded by the use of differing standards. In some cases myelomas are used as standards and often as the immunizing agent. Failure to detect certain antigens or the reaction of the antiserum with the individual specific (idiotypic) antigens of the immunizing protein further leads to variability. One approach has been to utilize international standards prepared by the World Health Organization. In these standards the values of IgG, IgA, and IgM are arbitrarily set at 100 units.[2] Local values are expressed in terms of the international standard as units. When this method is used the agreement between laboratories is very good, but between 17 and 30% variation still exists. Because the variability in general is so great, absolute values reported from different laboratories cannot be directly compared. The preceding

---

[2] The equivalence of international units to mass is as follows (μg/IU): IgG, 80.4; IgA, 14.2; IgM, 8.47 when the International Reference Preparation is used. (NCI Immunoglobulin Reference Center, 6715 Electronics Dr., Springfield, Virginia 22151.)

TABLE I
LEVELS OF IMMUNOGLOBULINS

	IgG (mg/ml)[a]	IgM (mg/ml)[a]	IgA (mg/ml)[a]	IgE (IU/ml)[b]
Serum				
Age				
Newborn	10.31 ± 2[c]	0.11 ± 0.05	0.02 ± 0.03	0–7.5
6 Months	4.27 ± 1.86	0.43 ± 0.17	0.28 ± 0.18	—
12 Months	6.61 ± 2.19	0.54 ± 0.23	0.37 ± 0.18	—
24 Months	7.62 ± 2.09	0.58 ± 0.23	0.50 ± 0.24	137 ± 47
8 Years	9.23 ± 2.56	0.65 ± 0.25	1.24 ± 0.45	251 ± 167
16 Years	9.46 ± 1.24	0.59 ± 0.20	1.48 ± 0.63	330 ± 212
Adult	11.58 ± 3.05	0.99 ± 0.27	2.00 ± 0.61	200[d]
Secretions[e]				
Colostrum	0.10	0.61	12.34	—
Stimulated parotid saliva	0.00036	0.00043	0.039	—
Unstimulated whole saliva	0.0486	0.0055	0.304	—
Jejunum	0.34	0.7	—	—
Seminal fluid[f]	5.1	0.9	1.16	—
Cerebrospinal fluid[g]				
Normal	0.03 ± 01	0	0.004 ± 0.005	—
Purulent infection	0.09	0.04	0.04	—
Viral infection	0.04	0.005	0.01	—

[a] Stiehm and Fudenberg, 1966.
[b] Berg and Johansson, 1969.
[c] Mean ± SD.
[d] Values up to 800 IU/ml are normal.
[e] Hanson and Brandtzaeg, 1973.
[f] Uehling, 1971.
[g] Smith et al., 1973.

considerations are of greater concern when elevated values are compared. Values in deficiency states are usually so low that minor variations are unimportant.

As far as immunodeficiency is concerned, levels of IgG below 200 mg/dl, as well as 25 mg/dl for IgA and IgM, in the absence of protein loss or hypercatabolism usually indicates congenital or acquired immunodeficiency if the patient is more than 6 months of age. Below this age such values can be normal, and levels of IgG less than 100 mg/dl and IgA and IgM less than 10–15 mg/dl are more often seen with immunodeficiency. Appropriate clinical findings are helpful. One expects to have an associated history of severe recurrent life-threatening infections and an absence of lymphoid tissue on physical examination. Lacking these one should be alert to the possibility of protein loss or hypercatabolism. Associated low albumin levels make protein loss virtually a certainty, for poor albumin synthesis due, for instance, to long-standing liver disease, would result not in hypo- but rather in hypergammaglobulinemia. Study of the gastrointestinal and genitourinary secretions by appropriate means will reveal the cause. Hypercatabolic states require special techniques and expertise, and their assessment is beyond the scope of most clinical laboratories. As mentioned previously, response of the patient to immunization helps to determine the significance of slightly low Ig levels. When immunoglobulins are low owing to excessive loss, increased susceptibility to infection is not associated, and antibody response is normal.

Some children with immunodeficiency may have disproportionately high levels of IgM. This is usually due to the presence of monomeric 7 S IgM, which diffuses much more rapidly than the normal pentameter, producing falsely high values.

Selective deficiencies primarily involve IgE and IgA. The significance of selective γE deficiency remains in doubt, as conflicting reports exist. In one study, γE deficiency associated with lymphopenia was associated with severe recurrent pulmonary disease resulting in death during adolescence in one patient and bronchiectasis in two others. In another, isolated γE deficiency was unassociated with disease and also seemed to be associated with a less severe clinical course when combined with IgA deficiency. Lymphocyte counts were not recorded in this study. IgA deficiency, the most common of all immunodeficiency states, is associated with autoimmunity, cancer, T-cell deficiency, pulmonary hemosiderosis, and ataxia-telangiectasia; often the individual is in good health.

Primary isolated IgM deficiency is extremely rare in children. Five cases have been described. No unique clinical syndrome was associated, but serious infections occurred. Hobbs observed 47 cases secondary to malignancy and 29 of unknown causes in a survey of 3000 patients. A high incidence of bacteremia and serious systemic infection was observed. Newborns have a transient IgM deficiency since they do not receive passive maternal protection. The increased efficiency of IgM in complement fixation and phagocytic mechanisms makes it of special importance in containing infectious agents upon initial exposure.

It is hazardous to attempt to predict a suitable Ig response to various infectious agents. Failure to demonstrate hyperimmunoglobulinemia following repeated infections is not sufficient grounds to render a diagnosis of "relative" hypogammaglobulinemia.

A special problem in quantitation exists in patients who have selective IgA deficiency. For reasons not fully understood, antibodies to bovine serum proteins are found in nearly 50% of the patients. These antibodies will cross-react with goat γ-globulin. When anti-gamma A antisera of goat origin are used in a Mancini diffusion assay, a precipitin ring will form, which can be mistakenly interpreted as indicating the presence of modest levels of IgA. In cases of suspected IgA deficiency, one must either use rabbit antiserum for the quantitation or confirm the absence of IgA and the presence of antigoat antibodies through the use of immuno-electrophoretic analysis. If normal goat serum is used instead of antibody, a precipitin arc will develop in the IgG position, representing patient IgG precipitating with normal goat proteins. Normals will show no arc under these circumstances.

It is theoretically possible that secretory IgA could be absent in an individual who possesses normal levels of serum IgA. Only one instance is known to the author, in a case of adenosine deaminase deficiency. The situation is further confounded because a bone marrow transplant was performed, which may have selectively populated only the non-secreting IgA system. In another case marked deficiency of secretory IgA with normal serum levels was found in a patient with chronic renal disease and intractable diarrhea. For practical purposes, it can be assumed that if serum gamma A levels are normal, secretory levels will be present in normal amounts. Yet the finding of fairly normal levels of secretory IgA in the face of nondetectable serum IgA does occur. The definition of "normal" levels of secretory IgA as measured in secretions is difficult to define. In the secretions there are varying percentages of 7 S IgA, polymeric IgA with and without bound secretory component, as well as free secretory component. A reliable estimate can be made by using a serum pool as a standard and converting its value into secretory IgA by increasing by a factor of 1.17 as shown by Brandtzaeg. Quantitation of IgA in the urine and in gastrointestinal fluids where fragmentation of the immunoglobulins have occurred may require even more specialized techniques. In addition, the rate of secretion affects the level and artifacts resulting from handling procedures, such as concentration, further add to the difficulty of accurate quantitation of IgA within secretions. Because of all the above technical problems, absolute IgA values are not generally available. Representative levels as determined by Brandtzaeg and Tomasi are shown in Table I.

IgE quantitation has resulted in much disparate data. Because of minimal quantity of available antigen, most antisera were originally prepared against a single myeloma, which was also employed as a standard. Later another myeloma became available. The use of antisera and standards of such limited reactivity resulted in widely differing results in data compared from different laboratories. Also, antisera raised in sheep or goats are known to yield false high values because of the high percentage of humans (normal as well as patients) who have antibodies to bovine γ-globulin. These antibodies cross-react with sheep or goat γ-globulin and prevent the combination of the sheep (goat) antisera with the radiolabeled standard in the RIST test (Fig. 6). The resulting decrease in precipitation of the standard is interpreted as a higher than true value of IgE. Similar erroneous results occur when antibodies to IgE exist in a patient who in actuality has absence of IgE (Fig. 6). IgE levels determined by the RIST technique appear to be erroneously high when extremely low values are studied. At the present the preferred method would seem to be a double antibody radioimmunoassay employing rabbit anti-IgE antisera. An international standard has been developed for IgE in an attempt to minimize interlaboratory variation.

In diffusion analyses, molecular size heterogeneity may introduce significant variation. Mention has been made of the difficulties encountered in IgA quantitation. IgM can also produce confusing results when a substantial portion is monomeric. The smaller size results in a larger precipitin ring than would result from an equal amount of antigen present as 19 S IgM. Significant amounts of monomeric IgM occur in systemic lupus, Waldenström's macroglobulinemia and immunodeficiency with hyper IgM (dysgammaglobulinemia).

Polyclonal elevation of immunoglobulins usually means that chronic stimulation from inflammation or infection has occurred. Collagen diseases, liver disease, and chronic granulomata are the commonest causes. Usually, all three major classes are involved. When a single class is disproportionately elevated, one thinks of benign monoclonal gammapathy or multiple myeloma (see chapter by Franklin). Elevations of single classes of immunoglobulins have limited diagnostic import; some recorded observations are shown in Table II.

Limited data are available on immunoglobulin quantitation and assessment in fluids other than the serum. The degree of transudation compared to the amount of local production, if any, makes the interpretation of Ig levels in nonserum samples of limited value. As mentioned previously, there is no convincing evidence that localized deficiency of immunoglobulins can exist and cause significant disease if serum levels are detected in normal amounts. Except for secretory IgA, it is not clear that an immune response can be localized to a fluid collection independent from serum responses. Examination of gastrointestinal secretions in a number of disorders have led to variable results and, except for defining specific roles in local autoimmune destructive reactions, their measurement has not provided much useful clinical information. Some values for Igs in various secretions are shown in Table I.

TABLE II

DISPROPORTIONATE ELEVATIONS OF SINGLE IG CLASSES OR SUBUNITS

IgM
    Benign monoclonal
    Early hepatitis
    Neonatal or intrauterine infection
    Recent viral infection
    Waldenström's macroglobulinemia
7 S IgM
    Ataxia-telangiectasia
    Immunodeficiency with hyper IgM
    Leprosy
    Liver disease
    Lupus
    Waldenström's macroglobulinemia
    Normal cord blood
    Rheumatoid arthritis
7 S IgA
    Aldrich syndrome (associated with low IgM)
    Ataxia-telangiectasia
    Benign monoclonal
    Early cirrhosis
    Familial thrombocytopenia
    Gluten-sensitive enteropathy
    Heavy drinking
    Hereditary sensory neuropathy
    Myeloma
    Persistent neutropenia
11 S IgA (in serum)
    Bowel disease
    Fever, undetermined origin
    Lactating women
IgG
    Benign monoclonal
    Myeloma
IgE
    Aldrich syndrome (may have elevated IgA also)
    Associated with undue susceptibility to infection ("Buckley syndrome")
    Asthma
    Other atopic states
    Parasitic infestation
Free light chains
    Renal disease
    Myeloma (low Ig form)
Heavy chains
    Alpha chain disease
    Gamma chain disease (Franklin's disease)
    Mu chain disease

In spinal fluid assessments, four basic patterns are seen. These are:
(1) the extracerebrospinal fluid pattern, (2) the capillary permeability
pattern, (3) the degenerative pattern, and (4) the γ-globulin pattern.
The first represents simple transfer of a component present in excessive
amounts in the serum (e.g., a myeloma protein). The second is due
to inflammatory meningeal changes resulting in increased capillary
permeability and resembling a dilute serum pattern. It can be seen in
inflammation, neoplasia, and cerebroarterial disease. The third pattern
is unrelated to immunoglobulins and shows an increase primarily of
"slow" transferrin. The fourth pattern represents a marked increase in Ig
which is disproportionate to the serum level. Production by lymphoid
tissue contiguous to or part of the central nervous system is implied.
Multiple sclerosis and subacute sclerosing panencephalitis can result in
striking elevations of IgG. The Ig levels in the latter may be associated
with an extreme specific antibody response to measles antigen. In proteinuria, the pattern seen is a net result of glomerular filtration and
tubular reabsorption. Serum proteins are selectively filtered through the
glomerulus according to their molecular size. If a plot is made of the
amount of protein cleared versus increasing molecular weight, a smooth
line of negative slope is produced. A lesser slope (more horizontal line)
is seen with more chronic glomerular lesions. IgM is among the largest
of the serum proteins, and hence its clearance in appreciable amounts
implies prolonged disease. IgG is of the medium molecular weight range.
As the "pore size" of the glomerular filter enlarges owing to long-standing
renal disease, proportionately more of the heavier serum components
are seen. This pattern is denoted nonselective proteinuria.

The kidney, especially the renal tubule, plays a major role in metabolism and reabsorption of immunoglobulin fragments, such as light chains
and a small portion of the Fc_γ fragment known as β_2 microglobulin.
These proteins are of less than 25,000 molecular weight. When renal
tubular disease is significant these components are elevated in serum and
urine. Normally, free L chains are present in urine in amounts up to
approximately 5 mg/day. In the serum of normals, levels of 0.005–0.008
μg/ml are recorded. Slight elevations during pregnancy are seen (0.016
μg/ml). Most patients with systemic lupus erythematosus, even without
clinically detectable renal disease, show elevations of the order of
0.08 μg/ml. In renal disease confined to the glomeruli, β_2 microglobulin
urine levels are less than 17 μg/ml. Primary tubular disorders (e.g.,
Fanconi's syndrome, hypokalemic nephropathy) are associated with
levels greater than this, with a mean of 58 μg/ml. Urine assay for β_2
microglobulin levels may provide a good index of primary renal tubular
dysfunction.

IV. Summary

Appropriate evaluation of immunoglobulins requires a combination of quantitative and qualitative approaches interpreted within the framework of the patient's symptomatology. They are primarily of interest in the study of deficiency syndromes and monoclonal disorders.

References

Berg, T., and Johansson, S. G. O. (1969). *Acta Paediat. Scand.* **58,** 513.

Berne, B. H. (1974). Differing methodology and equations used in quantitating immunoglobulins by radial immunodiffusion. A comparative evaluation of reported and commercial techniques. *Clin. Chem.* **20,** 61–69.

British Medical Bulletin. (1974). Radioimmunoassay and saturation analysis. **30** (1).

Buckley, C. E., III, and Dorsey, F. C. (1971). *Ann. Intern. Med.* **75,** 673.

Fudenberg, H., Good, R. A., Goodman, H. C., Hitzig, W., Kunkel, H. G., Roitt, I. M., Rosen, F. S., Rowe, D. S., Seligmann, M., and Soothill, J. R. (1971). Primary immunodeficiencies. Report of a World Health Organization Committee. *Pediatrics* **47,** 927–946.

Grabar, P., and Burtin, P., eds. (1964). "Immunoelectrophoretic Analysis." Elsevier, Amsterdam.

Hanson, L. A., and Brandtzaeg, P. (1973). *In* "Immunologic Disorders in Infants and Children," Chapter 8. Saunders, Philadelphia, Pennsylvania.

Joachim, G. R., Cameron, J. S., Schwartz, M., and Becker, E. L. (1964). Selectivity of protein excretion in patients with the nephrotic syndrome. *J. Clin. Invest.* **43,** 2332–2346.

Laurell, C. B. (1972). Electrophoretic and electroimmunochemical analysis of proteins. *Scand. J. Clin. Lab. Invest.* **29,** Suppl 124.

Mancini, G., Carbonara, A. O., and Heremans, J. F. (1965). Immunochemical quantitation of antigens by single radial diffusion. *Immunochemistry* **2,** 235.

Markowitz, H., and Tschida, A. R. (1972). Automated quantitative immunochemical analysis of human immunoglobulins. *Clin. Chem.* **18,** 1364–1367.

Smith, H., Bannister, B., and O'Shea, M. J. (1973). *Lancet* **2,** 591.

Stiehm, E. R., and Fudenberg, H. H. (1966). *Pediatrics* **37,** 715.

Uehling, D. (1971). *Fert. Steril.* **22,** 769.

Electrophoresis and Immunoelectrophoresis in the Evaluation of Homogeneous Immunoglobulin Components[1]

EDWARD C. FRANKLIN

Irvington House Institute and the Rheumatic Diseases Study Group, New York University Medical Center, New York, New York

I. Introduction

There are few if any cells in the body that lend themselves as readily to precise biochemical analysis as the plasma cells and lymphocytes. This favored position is largely due to the fact that each clone of cells secretes a single homogeneous protein, which constitutes often more than 20% of its total synthetic product, and that the type of protein pro-

[1] This work was supported by USPHS Grants #AM 02594 and AM 01431 and the Helen and Michael Schaffer Fund.

TABLE I

The Major Immunoglobulin Classes and Subclasses and Those
Currently Identifiable with Commercially Available Antisera

Ig class	Heavy-chain class[a]	Subclass[b]	Variable region subclass	Light-chain class[a]	Variable region subclasses
IgG	γ	γ1,2,3,4		κ and λ	
IgM	μ	Several?		κ and λ	V_κ 1–4
IgA	α	α1 and 2	V_H 1–4	κ and λ	and
IgD	δ	1, 2		κ and λ	V_λ 1–5
IgE	ϵ	?		κ and λ	

[a] Reagents to test for constant regions are commercially available.
[b] Reagents to these subclasses are often used in specialized situations.

duced generally remains constant for long periods of time. Since there exist more than 40 known classes and subclasses of heavy chains, at least nine subclasses of light chains, and many thousands of heavy and light chains different in their primary structure, it will ultimately be possible to identify and follow the fate of virtually every clone biochemically by examining the secreted immunoglobulin (Gally and Edelman, 1972).[2]

Table I lists the currently recognized classes and subclasses of immunoglobulins and their constituent polypeptide chains, and identifies those that can be recognized with currently available commercial antisera. Each immunoglobulin consists of two types of polypeptide chains, known as heavy (H) and light (L). The H chains, denoted by the Greek letter corresponding to the class, are different for each class or subclass. The two types of L chains known as κ and λ are common to all classes of immunoglobulins. Each immunoglobulin polypeptide chain is divisible into two regions. One, known as the variable region, is involved in antigen binding and specificity. The other, the constant region, is unique for each class or subclass. There are four variable region subclasses common to all types of H chains, and four variable regions for the κ and five for the λ L chains, respectively. It should be emphasized that all the commercially available antisera at this time are directed to determinants on the constant region, and cannot recognize the variable regions. Ultimately, it seems likely that it will be possible to recognize serologically all the classes and subclasses of H and L chains.

The techniques available to study these molecules are largely based on

[2] A review of the field is included in a series of papers in *Seminars in Hematology* (Franklin, 1973).

their charge, size, antigenic properties, or a combination of several of these (Scheidegger, 1955; Williams and Chase, 1970). In practical terms, preliminary screening is generally performed by zone electrophoresis, most commonly employing cellulose acetate. Precise identification of the immunoglobulin fraction is carried out by immunoelectrophoretic analysis, and, if necessary, quantitation of individual components can be carried out by a variety of techniques, most commonly radial immunodiffusion. During the past few years a number of more sophisticated automated techniques have come into wide use for quantitation, especially in situations where large numbers of samples have to be examined. As the immunological techniques have become more precise and simple, the need to carry out ultracentrifugal analyses to determine the molecular size and shape has become ever more rare and is now reserved for unusual instances when discrepancies are noted in some of the immunological studies, or when there is a desire, usually for research purposes, but at times to clarify a clinical situation, to more clearly define the size or state of polymerization or aggregation of an immunoglobulin molecule.

II. Homogeneous Proteins in Disease States

Since there is a general increase in many different immunoglobulins in diseases associated with a diffuse state of hypergammaglobulinemia—as for example in chronic infections, cirrhosis of the liver, systemic lupus erythematosus, rheumatoid arthritis, and a host of other diseases—electrophoresis and immunoelectrophoresis and also immunoglobulin quantitation cannot be expected to detect specific changes in immunoglobulins and are consequently generally of little value diagnostically in these instances. In contrast, these techniques are very useful in those situations where a single clone of plasma cells or lymphocytes proliferates to produce large amounts of a homogeneous immunoglobulin or immunoglobulin fragment, which is readily detectable as a narrow band on ordinary serum electrophoresis. Such homogeneous immunoglobulin components are generally encountered in malignant diseases of plasma cells or lymphocytes. Occasionally they are also seen in what appears to be a benign disorder in which there is a clonal but not uncontrolled proliferation of immunoglobulin-producing cells, perhaps the result of an unusual antigenic stimulus or antigenic stimulation of an individual with a genetic predisposition to such limited immune response.

Disorders where monoclonal proteins are most often encountered include the following ones:

1. Multiple myeloma (including L-chain disease)
2. Macroglobulinemia: (a) malignant form, (b) benign form. (These probably represent a broad spectrum and often progress from the benign to the malignant form.)
3. H-chain diseases (γ, α, μ)
4. Benign monoclonal gammopathy—nonlymphomatous
5. Others (lymphomas and rare instances of monoclonal proteins in other diseases)

The homogeneous proteins present in the serum or urine of these patients are sometimes unexpectedly discovered during routine electrophoretic analyses, but generally they are encountered as a result of biochemical and immunological studies initiated in a patient suspected of having one of these disorders. The initial test performed is usually zone electrophoresis. Unfortunately, the concentration, mobility, or appearance of an electrophoretic spike on paper or cellulose acetate electrophoresis rarely if ever permits a more precise classification of the type of protein present. This limitation is due to the fact that the appearance and mobility of homogeneous spikes is not class or subclass specific, so that it is generally not possible to distinguish different types of proteins one from the other, with the possible exception of the broad spike often seen in IgA myelomas and some of the abnormal proteins seen in γ H-chain disease. Hence, it is necessary to employ other techniques, especially those relying on the antigenic features of these molecules, if one wishes more precise characterization of the proteins produced.

It is obviously not possible to study these molecules biochemically in terms of amino acid sequence for ordinary clinical use. The amount of work involved would be far in excess of the possible benefits to be derived. In the past 20 years we have learned to take advantage of the fact that the amino acid sequence differences are reflected in the antigenic properties of the molecules. By using homogeneous proteins belonging to the various classes and subclasses as antigens in immunizing a variety of animals, and then making the antisera specific by simple absorption with fractions devoid of the protein in question, it is possible to make antisera specific for each of the known immunoglobulin classes and subclasses of the constant regions of the H and L chains, and in the case of the L chains also for some of the variable region subclasses (Solomon and McLaughlin, 1973). To date it has not been possible to make similar antisera specific for H-chain variable regions. In certain instances, the differences between them are so subtle that it is necessary to produce antisera in primates or animals rendered tolerant to the common antigenic determinants of immunoglobulins. In general, the antisera are rendered specific by absorption with cord sera (devoid of IgM and IgA), agammaglobulinemic sera which are virtually devoid of all immunoglobulins, or purified myeloma proteins, macroglobulins, or κ or λ Bence-Jones proteins of a different type than the antigen used for immunization.

For most purposes in clinical practice, use of antisera specific for the five classes of H chains and κ and λ L chains is sufficient to permit classification of homogeneous proteins. Perhaps in the near future H-chain subclasses-specific antisera can be added to this list. It should be remembered, however, that every myeloma protein differs from almost every other myeloma protein, and that these differences can be recognized in their so-called "idiotypic" antigenic determinants. As a result, it is theoretically possible to make specific antibodies to virtually every myeloma protein and thus ultimately to recognize and classify every protein produced in disease. On the basis of experiments with murine plasma cell tumors and certain selected human antibodies, these idiotypic antisera may be directed to the antibody-binding site and hence react with all molecules having the same antibody specificity (Potter and Lieberman, 1970).

It is obvious that such precise classification is of little general value in clinical practice but is of great importance in increasing our understanding of antibody structure. To accurately classify the type of plasma cellular or lymphocyte neoplasm, a goal that can generally not be achieved either on the basis of the clinical or pathologic features, it is generally sufficient to determine only the H- and L-chain class immunologically. If reagents are available, determination of the H-chain subclass may also be of great potential clinical value since, with increasing experience, it has become apparent that certain features, such as hyperviscosity and cryoglobulinemia, are more frequent with certain subclasses of IgG than others and that amyloidosis is most often associated with $\lambda 1$ L chains. It seems likely that other clinical correlations may be noted as a result of careful immunological classifications in the future.

A detailed biochemical and immunological approach to the diagnosis and classification of plasma cell and lymphocyte neoplasms is of value for the following reasons: (1) It allows precise classification of the type of disorder, which is not always possible on clinical or pathological grounds. In certain instances, such as macroglobulinemia, H-chain diseases or L-chain production, this classification correlates with the clinical features of the disease, and on occasion also with the prognosis. In many instances, the type of protein produced and the amount present may influence the type of therapy to be used, i.e., choice of chemotherapy, plasmapheresis, etc. (2) It permits clear-cut insights into the biosynthetic processes occurring in normal and also in pathological neoplastic cells and hence significantly increases our understanding of factors controlling immunoglobulin synthesis. (3) It may ultimately lead to clinical and biochemical correlations of which we are not yet aware on the basis of our still limited biochemical analyses. (4) In practical terms, quantitation is at times of help in distinguishing a benign from a malignant form of one of these diseases, and in following the course of the disease and the response of the patient to therapy. (5) On the academic side, careful characterization and detailed studies of the products of these cells have provided clear insights into normal biochemistry and physiology of plasma cells and lymphocytes and have in the last 10 years been directly responsible for virtually all the important advances in immunochemistry that have taken place.

Great progress has been made in the last 30 years in the tools available to the clinician in achieving these goals. Initially only free electrophoresis combined with ultracentrifugation were available. This allowed the differentiation of a 7 S from a 19 S immunoglobulin. Each of these tests was complicated and time-consuming and not practical for routine clinical use. The introduction of electrophoresis on paper or other solid supporting media, such as cellulose acetate, which is the most widely used medium at the present time, made the detection of homogeneous proteins easier, but did not aid significantly in their precise identification. Only with the introduction of immunoelectrophoresis using specific antisera for classes and subclasses of immunoglobulins has it been possible to develop simple tests that can be applied in every clinical laboratory. Basically they require the availability of specific antisera, which permit the necessary typing and classification of immunoglobulins. As a result of the widespread use of this technique, the recognition, and hence the incidence of diseases with homogeneous proteins, has significantly increased and several new entities like the group of heavy-chain diseases have been discovered. In addition, the combination of paper or cellulose acetate electrophoresis combined with initial characterization of the type of protein produced by immunoelectrophoresis is in general equally as effective in quantitating the amount of an immunoglobulin fraction as is immunoglobulin quantitation and hence is of great value in following the course of a patient or his response to therapy. This is due to the fact that in most patients more than 90% of the protein associated with the spike consists of the homogeneous component in question. Nevertheless, quantitation of all the immunoglobulins, especially the so-called "normal background fractions" which are not part of the homogeneous component, is often necessary at the time of diagnosis, and perhaps occasionally during the course of the disease. This is particularly true, if a patient with a homogeneous spike suffers from recurrent infections or if on clinical grounds there is some question whether the patient has myeloma or benign monoclonal gammopathy. In general, normal or only slightly depressed levels of the other immunoglobulin fractions are more often seen in the benign form and give support to that diagnosis if the clinical and bone marrow picture point in that direction.

III. Techniques for Characterization and Quantitation of Homogeneous Immunoglobulin Components

Before going on to describe the immunological workup of an individual suspected of having a monoclonal protein, let us briefly consider the methods available and a general description of the techniques employed. Detailed descriptions of these are available in a variety of books and pamphlets and many of the reagents needed to perform these tests are commercially available (Williams and Chase, 1970).

A. ELECTROPHORESIS

Serum and, if indicated, urine electrophoresis (either on native or concentrated urine) are most often carried out on cellulose acetate membranes and less often on paper. Many commercially available power supplies, electrophoresis cells, and membranes are available, and the buffers and dyes needed for staining can be purchased from a number of suppliers. After electrophoretic separation, the strips are stained (most often with Ponceau S stain) and inspected visually for the presence of a homogeneous protein spike. After this, photometric scanning of the stained strips, together with quantitation of the total serum protein concentration, permits an accurate estimate of the concentration of the five major serum protein fractions (γ-, β-, $\alpha2$-, and $\alpha1$-globulins and albumin). In this group of diseases, the γ- and β-globulins are particularly informative. It should be pointed out that visual inspection is of particular value in the detection of homogeneous spikes, which are often difficult to appreciate on the densitometer scan and are clinically significant regardless of size or mobility. Since serum electrophoresis detects virtually all homogeneous spikes, it is usually not necessary to do additional studies if the results are negative. However, if the clinical picture warrants, and there is a strong suspicion of a plasma cell or lymphocyte neoplasm, the more sensitive immunological tests described below should be carried out, since they may detect an abnormal protein, even in the face of a normal electrophoretic pattern.

Since electrophoresis does not allow precise characterization and quantitation of the homogeneous component, immunoelectrophoresis is generally performed as the next step to clearly identify individual immunoglobulin fractions, and a variety of techniques, the simplest of which is radial immunodiffusion can be used for quantitation of individual immunoglobulins. If the homogeneous protein makes up the major fraction of the immunoglobulins and there is little residual normal immunoglobulin present, microzone electrophoresis can be used to quantitate the homogeneous spike, and the additional radial immunodiffusion step can be omitted.

B. Immunoelectrophoresis

The procedure is generally carried out on slides covered with 1% agar or agarose. They can easily be prepared, or they can be purchased ready for use from several commercial sources. After completion of the electrophoretic separation, specific antisera are added to the wells parallel to the axis of electrophoresis and allowed to react with the individual protein components. For routine analysis, antisera to whole serum, γ, α, μ, κ, and λ chains are used and identify virtually homogeneous components. Because of the rarity of IgD and IgE myelomas, these antisera need not be used in the initial screening, but they should be employed in the rare event that an expected homogeneous arc is not noted with the six antisera used. Homogeneous components are most often detected as a localized bulge on a normal precipitin line or as a homogeneous component of abnormal mobility with little normal residual immunoglobulin. It is advisable to include a normal serum in each run and to examine the slides unstained. For a permanent record, they can be stained or photographed. Although further classification of H-chain subclasses is sometimes desirable, it is not required in routine clinical practice.

C. Radial Immunodiffusion

Since an antigen that has diffused into an agar gel containing a monospecific antiserum forms a precipitin ring around the well whose diameter is logarithmically related to its concentration, it is possible to use such a system for quantitation, provided appropriate reagents and defined standard proteins are available. Such plates, containing a variety of specific antisera are commercially available. The concentration of the unknown is determined by comparing it to the standard curve obtained with a normal standard. One of the difficulties in accurately quantitating certain homogeneous proteins is that the ring diameter is markedly influenced by unusual physical properties of these molecules so that aggregated or polymer forms of proteins or incomplete molecules may introduce significant errors and give falsely low or elevated values, respectively. Normal values by this technique are as follows (mg/100 ml): IgG, 1200 (700–1700); IgA, 210 (70–350); IgM, 140 (70–210); IgD, 3 (0–40). The concentration of IgE is generally too low to be obtained by this technique and is best done by a radioimmunoassay. The normal level for IgE is 300 ng/ml (10–1000). It should be mentioned that a number of automated techniques for quantitating immunoglobulins and other proteins are coming into widespread use, especially in situations where a large volume of work is carried out. A description of these is beyond the scope of this chapter; suffice it to say that all of them are based on direct or indirect measurements of the amount of antigen antibody precipitate formed under well defined conditions.

D. Other Tests

Examination for urinary abnormalities can generally be carried out on unconcentrated urines since significant amounts of Bence-Jones proteins (BJPs) are usually excreted, but occasionally a concentrating step is necessary. It is important to remember that many BJPs do not react with the Albustix so that the absence of protein by this technique does not exclude the presence of a BJP. A rough screening test can be done by the classical heat test at pH 4.5–6, looking for the appearance of a precipitate at 56°–60°C. Since many of these proteins either do not go back in solution on boiling or their resolution is often masked by the concomitant presence of other proteins, it is not necessary to expend a great deal of effort in trying to demonstrate this property. Instead, reactivity on immunoelectrophoresis with antisera to κ or λ chains, but not antisera to H chains, definitively demonstrates the presence of a BJP. The technique of immunoelectrophoresis is the same as that employed for serum analysis. It is generally quite easy to distinguish clinically significant BJPs from the small amounts of heterogeneous L chains sometimes encountered normally or in other diseases because these are generally present in small amounts and consist of both κ and λ chains.

In addition to these standard tests, several additional procedures are sometimes indicated. The Sia water test, which detects water-insoluble proteins by the addition of 10 volumes of distilled water to the serum, was formerly used as a screening test for macroglobulinemia; it is no longer used owing to its lack of specificity. A search for cryoglobulins is often indicated. This can be most easily accomplished by carefully examining the serum after removal from the refrigerator after storage. If a precipitate that goes back in solution on warming at 37°C is present, further studies are indicated. The amount of cryoglobulin can be determined in a variety of ways. The easiest is to do a "cryocrit," with the precipitate expressed as percentage of the total volume. More accurate quantitation and characterization can be carried out by quantitation of protein, immunoelectrophoresis, or radial immunodiffusion of the purified precipitate obtained by several washings with cold saline until the supernatant is free of protein. It is important to emphasize that cryoglobulins can be lost if the blood is kept cold before separation of the serum or if they are not looked for prior to the performance of other tests. Pyroglobulins (proteins that precipitate at 56°C) are rarely looked for and usually are accidentally discovered during heat inactivation of serum for other serological tests. Cold agglutinins should be searched for, especially in patients with macroglobulinemia. In certain clinical states, measurement of the serum viscosity using a simple Ostwald viscosimeter is indicated and easily performed.

IV. Evaluation of Test Results

In evaluating the results of the tests described above, the following points should be kept in mind: (1) The diagnosis of a plasma cellular lymphocytic neoplasm is a morphological one; abnormalities of serum and urine proteins can only support the diagnosis. (2) The important thing to look for is a homogeneous spike—the quantity is less important. (3) In differentiating the malignant condition from the benign variant (benign monoclonal gammopathy), the findings in the marrow are of paramount importance. If the concentration of the homogeneous protein is less than 2 gm/100 ml, if there are near normal concentrations of the uninvolved immunoglobulins, if there is no Bence-Jones protein, and if the concentration of the spike remains constant for long periods of time, the diagnosis of a benign variant is more likely than if the contrary situations pertain.

Characterization of the type of immunoglobulin is essential for understanding the precise nature of a plasma cell and lymphocyte neoplasm and should be undertaken in all cases. Quantitation of immunoglobulins is of help in differentiating the benign from the malignant form of the disease and in following its course and the results of therapy.

Let us first consider the workup of an individual suspected of having a plasma cell or lymphocyte neoplasm or inadvertently found to have a homogeneous protein spike on routine electrophoresis. We shall limit ourselves in the discussion to individuals whose sera contain homogeneous immunoglobulins, polypeptide chains, or fragments. The best screening test is obviously paper or cellulose acetate electrophoresis. If a homogeneous band is found, one generally cannot classify it precisely, and hence immunoelectrophoresis with antisera for H and L chains is the next logical step. If the ordinary electrophoretic analysis is negative, one is not likely to find significant amounts of a homogeneous protein on immunoelectrophoresis with the exception of certain patients with γ, α, and μ H-chain diseases or some individuals with L chains in the serum. Because of the not infrequent occurrence of these entities and the great interest in discovering them, it is now generally felt that if the clinical state warrants it, even a negative electrophoretic serum analysis should not deter one from a further search for an abnormal protein by immunoelectrophoresis.

Let us next look at some practical illustrations of the use of immunoelectrophoresis in clinical medicine. Figures 1–3 summarize the major types of patterns one encounters in clinical practice. In the most common type of disorder, namely the patient who produces an intact immunoglobulin, the pattern will show a prominent precipitin arc whose appearance is the same when tested with an antiserum to an H-chain class or subclass and an antiserum to either κ or λ L chain (for example, IgG4 κ, IgA1 λ, or IgM λ). In rare instances, especially in the case of IgA myeloma proteins, the light chains may be hidden and nonreactive in the intact molecule and be detected only after reduction and alkylation (Fig. 2F). If one isolates the protein in question, it can be easily shown that the H and L chains are covalently linked. If the patient produces a Bence-Jones protein, either as the sole abnormal protein or in addition to an intact immunoglobulin, one detects a homogeneous precipitin arc with an anti-L-chain serum in the urine and, not infrequently, also in the serum. Here it is generally worthwhile to do the classical heat test in the urine looking specifically for precipitation at 56°–60°C. Since many proteins fail to go back in solution at 100°C, and also because of the frequent coexistence of albumin and other proteins in the urine, the resolubilization is often masked by the concurrent precipitation of the other proteins. If immunological tests are used to search for these L-chain related proteins, it is not necessary to expend a great deal of effort in trying to document this resolubilization.

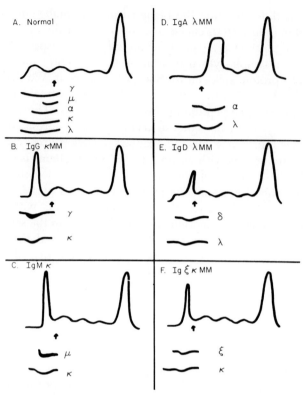

Fig. 1. Electrophoretic (top pattern in each panel) and selected immunoelectrophoretic serum patterns typical of (A) normal serum; (B) IgG κ myeloma; (C) IgM κ macroglobulin; (D) IgA λ myeloma; (E) IgD λ myeloma; (F) IgE κ myeloma. In each figure only the abnormal arcs are indicated; the background normal bands are ignored. In the normal pattern only IgG, IgM, and IgA are shown for simplicity. (From Franklin, 1975.)

An additional word of caution is warranted, since it is generally recognized that the commonly used Albustix dip-stick test often fails to detect Bence-Jones proteins. Hence, in addition to the heat test and quantitation of the 24-hour excretion of protein in the urine, electrophoresis and particularly immunoelectrophoresis are critical in identifying and characterizing Bence-Jones proteins (Fig. 3). Occasionally either because of the presence of the L-chain polymers or because of the marked renal impairment, L chains will accumulate in large amounts in the serum and result in a definite spike, which cannot be distinguished from a myeloma protein without doing immunoelectrophoretic analysis (Fig. 2A). In general, in patients producing both an L-chain and an intact immunoglobulin, the two proteins will have different mobilities and give rise to

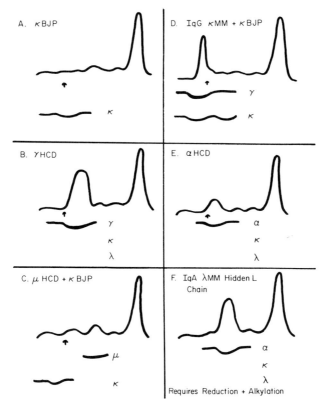

Fig. 2. Electrophoretic (top pattern in each panel) and selected immunoelectro-phoretic serum patterns typical of (A) Bence-Jones proteinemia (BJP); (B) γ heavy-chain disease; (C) μ heavy-chain disease with κ BJP; (D) γG κ myeloma with κ BJP; (E) α heavy-chain disease; (F) IgA myeloma with hidden light chains—this requires reduction and alkylation to demonstrate presence of light chains. (From Franklin, 1975.)

two separate precipitin arcs with anti-L-chain sera (Fig. 2D). When L chains are present, obviously the best place to detect them is in the urine.

Immunoelectrophoresis has been of particular value in recognizing the group of H-chain diseases (Frangione and Franklin, 1973). Three of these are now known—γ, α, and μ H-chain diseases (Figs. 2B, C, and E; 3D). In each type of H-chain disease, there exists in the serum—and in γ and α H-chain diseases, also usually in the urine—a rather broad pre-cipitin band reactive only with an antiserum to the appropriate heavy chains and unreactive with antisera to L chains even after reduction and alkylation. In most patients with μ H-chain disease, free L chains having a mobility differing from the rapidly migrating μ-chain fragments are usually present (Fig. 2C). The diagnosis can be strongly suspected on

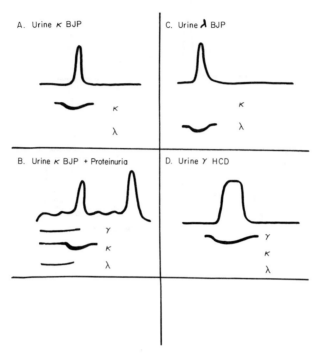

Fig. 3. Electrophoretic (top pattern in each panel) and immunoelectrophoretic pattern of urine; (A) κ Bence-Jones proteinuria (BJP); (B) κ BJP + diffuse proteinuria; (C) λ BJP; (D) γ heavy chain disease. (From Franklin, 1975.)

the basis of these laboratory findings. However, because of the occasional examples of myeloma proteins with hidden L chains, it is best to attempt to isolate the protein and characterize it further as regards molecular weight and other properties. It is worth emphasizing that most patients with μ H-chain disease and several with γ and α H-chain diseases have essentially normal paper or cellulose acetate electrophoretic patterns and can be detected only on immunoelectrophoresis. Hence, the old rule of thumb that one need not do immunoelectrophoresis in the face of a normal electrophoretic pattern is not really valid in these and certain other instances where immunoelectrophoresis provides the only clue to an abnormality. It should be noted here that, even though the γ- and α-chain disease spike is often broad, these are homogeneous components that appear heterogeneous because of differences in carbohydrates or polymer formation.

At this point, it is worth mentioning that not all patients with plasmacellular or lymphocyte neoplasms produce a homogeneous immunoglobulin. Hence in those instances (1–2%) where the clinical and pathological picture is typical in the absence of a spike, the diagnosis should still be made (Franklin, 1974). This occurs either in instances in which the cells have been dedifferentiated so that they no longer make H or L chains or occasionally in patients where there is a block in secretion and where the cells are filled with a monoclonal protein when examined by immunofluorescence. Most of these subjects have depressed immunoglobulins and suffer from hypogammaglobulinemia with a depression of all classes of immunoglobulins. It should be remembered that a depression in the other immunoglobulins—for reasons we do not yet understand—is a common feature also in those patients with large amounts of a monoclonal spike.

Perhaps one should emphasize at this point that a complete workup of patients with homogeneous immunoglobulins should not stop with immunoelectrophoresis. If one wishes to anticipate some of the complications resulting from these proteins, one should look for specific antibody activity—for example, rheumatoid factor and cold agglutinin activity, cryoglobulins, or hyperviscosity syndromes—by the techniques described above.

V. Conclusions

There can be little question that complete immunological workup by the techniques described is necessary in all patients suspected of having a plasma cellular or lymphoid neoplasm or an accidentally discovered monoclonal spike. Not only is precise classification of importance to the patient diagnostically, prognostically, and therapeutically, but in addition it is of great value in classifying these disorders and characterizing the molecular abnormalities associated with these neoplastic states. As techniques have become more standardized and reagents more readily available, their widespread clinical use has resulted in greater awareness, earlier diagnosis, and most important, more effective therapy for these diseases. It would be desirable if immunoglobulin studies could prove equally fruitful in other diseases involving the immune system. Unfortunately, this is true now only of the various deficiency states of humoral immunity. It does not seem likely that the same effectiveness will ever be achieved in the diseases commonly associated with the diffuse increases in all immunoglobulin fractions. However, one should not give up hope of developing even more specific reagents that may be of help. Who would have expected the enormous progress in this area that we have witnessed since the original introduction of electrophoresis by Tiselius in 1937 and of immunoelectrophoresis by Williams and Grabar in 1953?

References

Frangione, B., and Franklin, E. C. (1973). *Semin. Hematol.* **10**, 53.

Franklin, E. C., ed. (1973). *Semin. Hematol.* **10**, 1–177.

Franklin, E. C. (1974). *In* "Harrison's Principles of Internal Medicine" p. 354. McGraw-Hill, New York.

Franklin, E. C. (1975). *In* "Laboratory Diagnosis of Immunologic Disorders" (G. N. Vyas, D. P. Stites, and G. Brecher, eds.), p. 3. Grune & Stratton, New York.

Gally, I., and Edelman, G. M. (1972). *Annu. Rev. Genet.* **6**, 1–46.

Potter, M., and Lieberman, R. J. (1970). *J. Exp. Med.* **132**, 737.

Scheidegger, J. J. (1955). Une micro-méthode de l'immunoélectrophorèse. *Int. Arch. Allergy Appl. Immunol.* **7**, 103.

Solomon, A., and McLaughlin, C. L. (1973). Immunoglobulin structure determined from products of plasma cell neoplasms. *Semin. Hematol.* **10**, 3.

Williams, C. A., and Chase, M. W., eds. (1970). "Methods in Immunology and Immunochemistry," Vol. 3, Chapter 14. Academio Press, New York.

Serum Concentrations of IgG Subclasses[1]

ANDREAS MORELL, FRANTISEK SKVARIL, and SILVIO BARANDUN

Institute for Clinical and Experimental Cancer Research,
Tiefenau Hospital, Berne, Switzerland

I. Introduction

Molecules of the immunoglobulin class IgG include 70–80% of our humoral antibodies. Their wide antibody spectrum is a corollary of the enormous heterogeneity of the antigen binding sites and is structurally confined to the variable region of the IgG molecules. Apart from this

[1] This work was supported by the Swiss National Foundation for Scientific Research.

heterogeneity, which is responsible for their main biological activity, IgG molecules also exhibit some—although much less—heterogeneity in their constant part. In 1960, Dray found that with antisera to chromatographically purified IgG raised in rhesus monkeys, normal IgG can be subdivided immunoelectrophoretically into a number of antigenically distinct components. In the following years, his observations were confirmed and extended by several groups of investigators, who in 1966, under the patronage of a WHO committee, compared their data and agreed on a common nomenclature. Today, four subclasses of IgG are recognized: IgG1, IgG2, IgG3, and IgG4 (World Health Organization, 1966). Molecules of these subclasses differ in the primary structure of the carboxyterminal three-quarters of their heavy polypeptide chains, in number and arrangement of the inter-heavy chain disulfide bridges, and in the localization of the disulfide bridges linking the heavy to the light polypeptide chains. There is evidence that subclass-related structural traits are located in all three homology regions of the IgG heavy chains (Natvig and Kunkel, 1973). In sera of normal individuals, all four IgG subclasses can be demonstrated. IgG myeloma proteins in sera of patients with multiple myeloma and related diseases, however, are the products of one single cell clone and are therefore restricted to only one of the four subclasses.

There is evidence that the antibodies to certain groups of antigens can be limited to one or some of the IgG subclasses: antibodies to carbohydrates, dextran or levan, for instance, were found to be exclusively IgG2 molecules. Antibodies to antigens on cell membranes are predominantly IgG1 and IgG3. Furthermore, antibodies to the blood-clotting factor VIII were identified as IgG4. Antiplatelet antibodies in autoimmune thrombocytopenic purpura appear to be restricted to IgG3. The same has been found for IgG cryoglobulins that react with the Fc portion of IgG molecules like antibodies. In many instances, however, antibodies against a given antigen are distributed among all four subclasses in a way that parallels their serum concentrations.

During the last 10 years, a number of observations have shown that, in addition to their antibody properties, IgG molecules possess biological activities that are controlled by their constant portion, the Fc fragment. These activities may be common to all four of the IgG subclasses, or restricted to some, as indicated in Table I (Natvig and Kunkel, 1973; Spiegelberg, 1974).

We know that IgG is the only immunoglobulin class transmitted from the mother to the fetus. It seems that all four subclasses are transported across the placenta. Complement activation by the classical pathway,

TABLE I

BIOLOGICAL ACTIVITIES OF IgG SUBCLASSES

Activity	IgG1	IgG2	IgG3	IgG4
Placental transfer	+	+	+	+
Complement activation by Clq binding	+	(+)	+	−
Binding to phagocytic cells	+	−	+	−
Skin sensitizing activity for PCA[a]	+	−	+	+
Reaction with staphylococcal protein A	+	+	−	+

[a] Passive cutaneous anaphylaxis.

on the other hand, is accomplished more readily by IgG3 and IgG1 than by IgG2 whereas IgG4 does not activate at all. These differences, however, are not seen in the alternative pathway. A considerable amount of work clearly shows that only IgG1 and IgG3 molecules are cytophilic for phagocytic cells like monocytes, macrophages, and neutrophils. These two subclasses are thus the only ones that can induce phagocytosis of opsonized antigenic particles. IgG2 molecules do not fix to heterologous skin and are unable to elicit the phenomena of passive cutaneous anaphylaxis and reverse passive cutaneous anaphylaxis. IgG3 molecules do not react with staphylococcal protein A, a reaction the biological significance of which is still poorly understood. Finally, IgG subclasses differ in their metabolic behavior: IgG3 is more rapidly catabolized than the other three subclasses. Its biological half-life is 7 days compared to about 21 days for IgG1, IgG2, and IgG4.

In view of these peculiarities associated with the variable or with the constant region of the molecules, it was assumed that the determination of the serum concentrations of the four IgG subclasses could offer some insight into the regulatory mechanisms that control subclass serum levels and could bring some new information on their biological significance. Since the subclasses differ antigenically, the use of immunological methods for this work was obvious. This requires the preparation of specific antisera, an endeavor that has proved to be frustrating. Particularly the preparation of antisera to IgG1 and IgG2 is difficult and time-consuming. Therefore, for reasons of economy, a radioimmunoassay for the four IgG subclasses has been developed in our laboratory. In addition to its higher sensitivity, this method allows the scanning of large numbers of sera with minimal quantities of antisera (Morell et al., 1975).

This article reviews the results of IgG subclass quantitation obtained by this method in our laboratory. Determinations were made in sera from normal individuals of different ages and in sera from patients with a variety of diseases. Also included and discussed are the results of other groups using similar or different techniques.

II. Quantitative Determination of IgG Subclasses

As already mentioned, a radioimmunoassay was used for the quantitation of IgG subclasses in sera. The globulin fraction of subclass specific antisera was precipitated by sodium sulfate and insolubilized by coupling to bromoacetyl cellulose. Immunoadsorbents prepared this way form fine white suspensions and can readily be removed from aqueous solutions by centrifugation.

IgG myeloma proteins of all four subclasses were isolated from the sera of myeloma patients by preparative electrophoresis followed by gel filtration. Immunochemically pure subclass proteins were labeled with radioactive iodine. The binding of these radiolabeled antigens to the antibody preparations can be inhibited by unlabeled antigens of the same specificity. Within a certain dilution range the degree of binding inhibition is quantitatively proportional to the concentrations of the unlabeled antigens. Systems for the four subclasses were standardized with dilutions of isolated myeloma proteins of known concentrations. Sigmoid binding inhibition curves were obtained, and the concentrations in sera were measured by comparing their binding inhibition with the linear portion of these standardization curves. The limit of sensitivity in systems for all IgG subclasses was approximately 1 μg/ml.

In a first series of experiments, IgG subclass levels were determined in the WHO references standard serum pool 67/97, which was kindly supplied by the WHO References Centre in Lausanne. The values are presented in Table II.

For all following determinations in individual sera, the standard binding inhibition curves were established by dilutions of this WHO reference serum pool.

TABLE II

IgG SUBCLASS CONCENTRATIONS IN THE WHO REFERENCE
SERUM POOL 67/97

IgG1	IgG2	IgG3	IgG4
5.1 mg/ml	2.5 mg/ml	0.55 mg/ml	0.35 mg/ml

III. IgG Subclass Concentrations in Sera of Normal Individuals

A. FETAL AND MATERNAL SERA

IgG is the only immunoglobulin class that is transferred across the placenta, and there is evidence that this is due to an active transport mechanism, which in humans develops between about week 20 and week 30 of gestation. Prior to 20 weeks of gestation, only small amounts of IgG are detectable in sera of fetuses. After week 30, total IgG concentrations in the mother and in the fetus are similar. At the physiological end of gestation, IgG levels in umbilical cord sera tend to be even higher than in paired maternal samples.

It is known that the fetus is able to synthesize IgG and other immunoglobulin molecules. But under normal conditions, the amount of IgG of fetal origin is minute and may account for only about 1% of the IgG that is transferred from the maternal circulation.

Quantitative determinations of the four IgG subclasses in 115 pairs of maternal and fetal sera gave evidence that all four subclasses pass the placenta. In early fetal sera from week 13 to week 16 of gestation, serum levels for all subclasses are low. Later, fetal subclass concentrations increase, and at about week 33 they are not much different from the maternal values. This is illustrated in Fig. 1, which shows the ratios of the four subclass values in the fetal and maternal samples at different weeks of gestation.

At the end of gestation, IgG1 concentrations seem to be somewhat higher in fetal than in maternal sera. This has repeatedly been shown. Still a matter of debate are the IgG2 serum levels. It was reported that IgG2 concentrations are significantly lower in cord than in maternal sera and that the placenta might act as a selective barrier for this subclass. This hypothesis, however, could not be confirmed by various other studies, including the data mentioned above. Typing for genetic markers of IgG2 molecules in fact provided additional evidence that IgG2 concentrations in maternal and fetal sera at the end of gestation are similar. There is general agreement that IgG3 and IgG4 levels are identical in maternal and cord sera.

B. DEVELOPMENT IN INFANTS AND CHILDREN

During the first 3 months of life, IgG levels decrease to less than half of the values found in cord blood and then slowly rise again. This

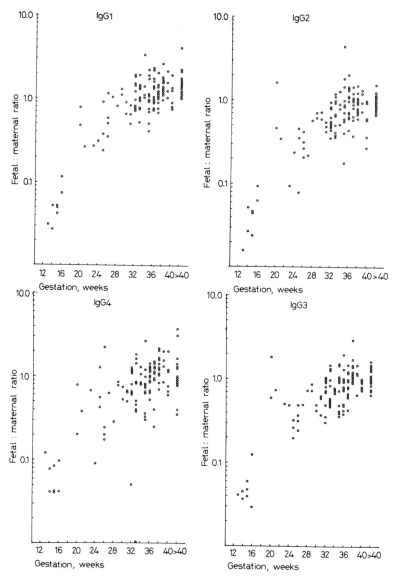

Fig. 1. Ratios of fetal and maternal serum subclass concentrations. The points represent fetal values divided by maternal values of corresponding pairs of sera.

characteristic "trough" is the result of various biological processes, such as catabolism of the maternal supply, expansion of intra- and extra-vascular body compartments, and commencing autonomous synthesis. At the end of the second year of life, concentrations are reached that are

still lower, but comparable to adult values. The following-up of the IgG
subclasses during this time is of special interest since, it is known that
the subclasses differ in their biological behavior.

So far, there is only one study dealing with IgG subclass levels in a
larger number of sera from children of this age group. The data summarized here represent the mean values of 95 children. Figure 2 shows
that during the first months of life serum concentrations of all four subclasses steeply decrease. The decrease of IgG3, however, is more pronounced than that of the other three subclasses, and lowest IgG3 serum
concentrations are already found at the age of 1 month, at a time when
the levels of all the other subclasses continue to drop. This corroborates
the observation made in adults that IgG3 is catabolized faster than the
other subclasses. Afterward, infants synthesize enough IgG3 to stabilize
and then to increase the serum concentration. The IgG1 level decreases
steeply during the first month and then more slowly until it reaches its
lowest value at the age of 3 months. This slowing down of the IgG1
decline may indicate a rapidly increasing IgG1 synthesis after the first

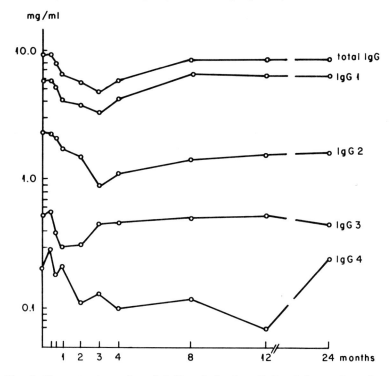

Fig. 2. Concentrations of total IgG and the four IgG subclasses throughout the
first two years of life.

month. In contrast, IgG2 levels more or less uniformly decline to their nadir at 3 months of age. Appreciable IgG2 synthesis, therefore, does not seem to occur before the third month. IgG4 levels decrease during the first 4 months and remain low throughout the first year.

Thus, in response to antigenic stimuli, pronounced antibody production of the IgG class sets in at the age of about 1 month by predominant synthesis of the subclasses IgG3 and IgG1. After the third month, the balance for IgG1 and IgG2 becomes positive. At the age of 2 years, IgG1 and IgG3 levels are not far from adult values, whereas IgG2 and IgG4 at that time are equilibrated around one-half of the serum concentrations observed in adult life.

C. Subclass Serum Concentrations in Adults

1. Young Male Adults (20 Years Old)

Quantitative determinations were made in the sera of 108 young male adults. The mean values, standard deviations, and ranges for the four subclasses are listed in Table III. For IgG4, only the mean and range are given.

Of the sum of the four subclasses, 60.9% was IgG1, 29.6% IgG2, 5.3% IgG3, and 4.2% IgG4. The distribution of the serum concentrations for IgG1, IgG2, and IgG3 were approximately symmetric. The distribution pattern for the IgG4 levels, however, showed some peculiarities: It was clearly asymmetric, and the range of the IgG4 values, from 0.03 to 2.9 mg/ml, was much wider than that for the other three subclasses. This has been found also in studies of other laboratories. Similar values were reported by a number of investigators. The concentrations of IgG1 and

TABLE III

SERUM CONCENTRATIONS OF IgG AND IgG SUBCLASSES IN A POPULATION OF 108 YOUNG MALE ADULTS

Parameter	IgG1	IgG2	IgG3	IgG4	Total IgG (sum)
Mean values ± 1 SD (mg/ml)	6.63 ± 1.70	3.22 ± 1.08	0.58 ± 0.30	0.46	10.89
Ranges (mg/ml)	3.50–11.50	1.30–6.80	0.10–2.10	0.03–2.90	—
Percentage of the sum of the four subclasses	60.9	29.6	5.3	4.2	100

particularly of IgG3, listed in Table III, however, are somewhat lower than those found by others. It is not yet clear whether these differences are inherent to the population and caused by genetic and environmental factors or whether they are simply due to technical diversities.

2. IgG Subclass Serum Concentrations Later in Life

Finally, subclass levels were analyzed in a number of sera from healthy blood donors of various ages. The values are given in Table IV, classified according to age groups. It has to be mentioned here that both men and women are included and that no significant sex-related differences in subclass levels were observed.

The most striking finding in these values is a continuous increase of the IgG3 serum concentrations with age, most pronounced in the sera of individuals more than 80 years old. Nothing is known about the biological significance of this phenomenon. It is probably the result of an increased synthetic rate, which might be due to an age-dependent change in the humoral immune response. Another possibility is a relative decline of the catabolic rate of this subclass. Turnover studies with radiolabeled IgG3 in old individuals, however, have provided no evidence for this latter hypothesis.

TABLE IV

IgG Subclass Concentrations in Sera of Individuals of Different Age Groups[a]

Age (years)	Number of cases	IgG1	IgG2	IgG3	IgG4	Total IgG (sum)
20–30	28	7.35 ± 2.17 (61.6)	3.54 ± 1.30 (29.7)	0.69 ± 0.31 (5.8)	0.35 ± 0.19 (2.9)	11.93
30–40	30	8.21 ± 2.75 (66.7)	3.04 ± 1.01 (24.7)	0.81 ± 0.25 (6.6)	0.25 ± 0.17 (2.0)	12.31
40–50	24	6.48 ± 2.00 (54.8)	4.08 ± 1.35 (34.5)	0.82 ± 0.43 (6.9)	0.45 ± 0.30 (3.8)	11.83
50–60	34	6.83 ± 1.33 (60.3)	3.28 ± 0.88 (29.0)	0.89 ± 0.30 (7.9)	0.32 ± 0.24 (2.8)	11.32
80 and older	49	7.76 ± 1.83 (56.0)	3.99 ± 1.38 (28.8)	1.46 ± 0.63 (10.5)	0.64 ± 0.60 (4.6)	13.85

[a] Mean values ± 1 standard deviation. Percentages of the sum of the four subclasses are given in parentheses.

D. CORRELATIONS BETWEEN SUBCLASS SERUM CONCENTRATIONS AND GENETIC MARKERS OF IgG

IgG molecules are known to carry genetically determined structural variations, the so-called Gm factors (Grubb, 1970), that are located in the constant region of the γ heavy chains. More than 20 different Gm factors have been identified. Most of them are found in association with only one of the four subclasses. These allotypic specificities of the IgG molecules are coded for by structural genes and are inherited as co-dominant Mendelian traits. It appears that molecules of each subclass exist in two genetic variations (Natvig and Kunkel, 1973). Since certain Gm factors are transmitted together, one has to assume that the structural genes for IgG subclasses are closely linked. The serum of normal individuals contains subclass-specific Gm factors constituting a Gm phenotype that makes possible the prediction of a probable genotype. Study of the inheritance of the Gm factors establishes the genotype, and an individual can be described as being homozygous or heterozygous for the various factors.

Some of these Gm factors are listed in Table V. It shows that Gm(a) and Gm(f) are the two genetic variations of IgG1; Gm(g) and Gm(b), of IgG3 molecules. For IgG2 molecules, only one Gm factor has been characterized so far. Thus, IgG2 molecules are either positive or negative for Gm(n).

During the last few years, correlations between Gm phenotypes and IgG subclass serum concentrations were established. This is documented best for IgG3: serum levels of this subclass in homozygous individuals with the phenotype Gm(f+b+) are two times as high as in individuals homozygous for the genes coding for the phenotype Gm(a+g+). In heterozygotes with the phenotype Gm (a+f+g+b+), the IgG3 levels were found to be intermediate. In our experience, however, they tend to

TABLE V

SOME GM FACTORS ON IgG1, IgG2, AND IgG3 MOLECULES

Gm factors	IgG subclasses
Gm(a)	IgG1
Gm(f)	IgG1
Gm(g)	IgG3
Gm(b)	IgG3
Gm(n)	IgG2

TABLE VI

SOME CORRELATIONS BETWEEN IgG SUBCLASS SERUM
CONCENTRATIONS AND GM MARKERS

Gm phenotype	Number of sera	IgG3 (mg/ml)	IgG2 (mg/ml)	IgG4 (mg/ml)
Gm(a+g+)	12	0.27	—	—
Gm(a+f+g+b+)	49	0.59	—	—
Gm(f+b+)	39	0.64	—	—
Gm(n+)	66	—	3.40	0.56
Gm(n−)	34	—	2.93	0.27

be rather high. A similar relationship has been described between the IgG1 serum concentrations and these Gm phenotypes.

IgG2 serum concentrations in general are higher in individuals who carry the IgG2 marker Gm(n) than in those who are Gm(n−); family studies with homozygous and heterozygous members, however, have failed to demonstrate a clear-cut influence of this marker on the IgG2 serum level.

Finally, an interesting observation is the relationship of Gm(n), the IgG2 marker, to the IgG4 levels: serum concentrations of IgG4 are highest in sera of individuals homozygous for this factor having the genotype Gm^{n+}/Gm^{n+}. In heterozygous Gm^{n+}/Gm^{n-} individuals, IgG4 levels are intermediate; and in the Gm^{n-}/Gm^{n-} individuals who lack this Gm factor, they are lowest. Some examples for such correlations are given in Table VI. Taken all together, these genetic data provide evidence that serum concentrations of IgG subclasses are to some extent under a genetic control.

IV. Subclass Levels in Sera of Patients with Increased Concentrations of Total IgG

Basically, high serum immunoglobulin concentrations can be found in two situations. (1) They may be the product of a single plasma cell clone, and are thus by all criteria homogeneous, monoclonal immunoglobulins. Clinically, such "plasmacellular dyscrasias" may be silent, the monoclonal immunoglobulin being the only symptom. Often, however, monoclonal immunoglobulins or myeloma proteins are associated with classical multiple myeloma or with related diseases. It is not yet known to what extent such single plasma cell clones result from antigenic stimuli, but it is conceivable that they represent an immune response to which homeostatic control by the organism was lost. (2) On the other hand, a high increase of the immunoglobulin serum concentrations may be caused by a variety of chronic diseases. One has to assume that high IgG levels in these cases result from the humoral immune response to long-lasting intensive stimulation with antigens of microbial or other "foreign" origin and/or with antigenically active material of the patient's own body. In such situations, large numbers of different plasma cell clones are created, producing the corresponding heterogeneous immunoglobulins of polyclonal origin.

A. Monoclonal IgG Immunoglobulins and Background IgG

In sera of myeloma patients with high levels of monoclonal immuno-globulins, the concentration of normal, heterogeneous immunoglobulins, also called background immunoglobulins, is usually decreased. This reduction is due partly to a diminished synthesis as shown by the reduced number of normal immunoglobulin-producing cells in the bone marrow. It is intensified in IgG myeloma patients by a concentration–catabolism relationship: at elevated serum concentrations of one IgG subclass, the catabolism of all four subclasses is increased.

Sixty-two IgG myeloma sera were studied with regard to the concentrations of the monoclonal immunoglobulin and the normal background IgG composed of the three subclasses not represented by the myeloma protein (Morell and Skvaril, 1973). Concentrations of the monoclonal IgG were estimated from the relative density of the M gradient after electrophoresis on cellulose acetate strips. Subclass concentrations in background IgG were determined by radioimmunoassay. In all these cases, urinary loss of plasma proteins was excluded.

Background IgG was clearly below the age-matched control levels in most of these IgG myeloma sera regardless of the subclass to which the myeloma protein belonged. In general, the levels of all three subclasses of the background IgG were reduced in a balanced way. No tendency for preservation of one particular subclass could be noticed.

Between the concentrations of the myeloma proteins and background IgG an inverse relationship was observed: In most sera with high mono-clonal IgG peaks, background IgG was reduced to 50% or less of the corresponding normal values, whereas in sera with only moderate or small monoclonal gradients, background IgG was closer to normal values. This relationship, however, was not valid for all sera. On the one hand, a few myeloma sera with both high levels of monoclonal and background

IgG could be seen; on the other hand, there was a group of sera where low levels of myeloma proteins were combined with remarkably diminished background IgG. In this group, IgG3 myeloma sera clearly prevailed. One would assume that such IgG3 myeloma patients are more inclined to develop antibody-deficiency syndromes and are more susceptible to infections than other myeloma patients. So far, clinical studies have failed to demonstrate this.

B. HIGH IgG SERUM CONCENTRATIONS OF POLYCLONAL ORIGIN

Subclass compositions were analyzed in sera from patients with polyclonal increase of IgG and other immunoglobulin classes. These patients suffered either from portal cirrhosis of the liver or from rheumatoid arthritis. The second group was subdivided into seronegative cases, who had no rheumatoid factor, and into seropositive cases, who were positive for this test. The results of the quantitative determinations are summarized in Table VII. On the average, the percentage distribution of the IgG subclasses corresponds to the normal values. Thus, generally, all four subclasses seem to participate in such a polyclonal IgG increase due to massive antigenic stimulation.

Similar results were obtained in dysproteinemic sera from patients suffering from other chronic inflammatory diseases or from malignant tumors. In all these cases the percentage distribution of the four IgG subclasses apparently does not significantly differ from normal values.

Another situation, however, was encountered in some sera from patients with kala azar (Table VIII) kindly supplied by Dr. Abbadhi in Algiers. In 7 out of 9 sera that were analyzed, the IgG increase was due predominantly to disproportionately high IgG1. At the same time, IgG2 and

TABLE VII

IgG SUBCLASS DISTRIBUTION IN POLYCLONAL HYPERGAMMAGLOBULINEMIA[a]

Diagnosis	Number of cases	IgG (mg/ml)	IgG1 (%)	IgG2 (%)	IgG3 (%)	IgG4 (%)
Cirrhosis of the liver	8	34.1 ± 10.6	66 ± 9	25 ± 9	6 ± 3	3 ± 3
Seronegative rheumatoid arthritis	7	26.2 ± 8.7	62 ± 8	29 ± 8	7 ± 3	2 ± 1
Seropositive rheumatoid arthritis	7	23.2 ± 4.9	61 ± 7	28 ± 6	6 ± 2	5 ± 5

[a] Mean values ± 1 SD.

TABLE VIII

IgG Subclass Distribution in 7 Hypergammaglobulinemic
Sera from Algerian Patients with Kala Azar

Name	IgG (mg/ml)	IgG1 (%)	IgG2 (%)	IgG3 (%)	IgG4 (%)
Me	23.6	87	8	4	1
Ma	21.3	92	5	3	<1
Ka	32.8	93	4	3	<1
Ay	16.4	82	12	6	<1
Az	36.8	88	6	6	<1
Ao	17.4	82	9	9	<1
Ti	20.8	87	8	5	<1
Pooled normal Algerian serum	13.3	66	25	7	2

IgG4 were markedly diminished whereas IgG3 was close to the normal values.

It is not yet known whether in such sera the IgG1 fraction contains corresponding amounts of antibodies to *Leishmania donovani*. These results, however, should stimulate similar investigations in patients with this and with other protozoal infections.

V. IgG Subclasses in Primary Immunodeficiency Diseases

In primary immunodeficiency diseases, pattern and degree of the immunoglobulin disorders are known to be extremely variable; all or only some of the immunoglobulin classes may be affected. The electrophoretic heterogeneity can be drastically restricted, and disturbances of the normal ratio of κ and λ immunoglobulin light chains are often noticed. Furthermore, several authors have found imbalances of the serum concentrations and even selective absences of one or more IgG subclasses. One of the most interesting observations was made by Yount and coworkers (1970). They saw that in certain cases with "primary immunoglobulin deficiencies of variable onset and expression," the IgG3 serum concentration often was considerably less decreased than the concentrations of the other subclasses. In such sera, IgG3 comprised up to 64% of the total IgG. Typing for Gm genetic markers showed that in most instances of IgG3 preponderance it was the Gm(b) phenotype that was selectively retained whereas IgG3 of the Gm(g) type was markedly depressed. Several studies on IgG subclass levels and Gm phenotypes in sera of patients and their relatives showed that in some instances immunodeficiencies may be genetically transmitted as a result of either a structural or a regulator gene defect.

Our own study included sera from 45 patients with various primary immunodeficiencies. Most of them had low IgG, IgA, and IgM levels. IgG subclass determinations revealed pronounced imbalances of one or more subclasses in 25 of these sera regardless of the clinical type of the disorder. These imbalances are shown in Table IX.

In the remaining 20 sera, all four IgG subclasses were decreased in a parallel way, and their percentage distribution was normal. By far the most common imbalance was a disproportionate decrease of IgG4. In three sera, this subclass was below the limit of the sensitivity of the assay system, i.e., less than 1 μg/ml. A selective absence of one of the other three subclasses was not observed. This does not agree with other reports where selective absences of IgG1, IgG2, or IgG3 were occasionally seen. Relatively high IgG3 levels were present in 5 sera of this study, but in none of them this subclass amounted to more than 25% of the total IgG. Sera of some of the patients and their relatives were also analyzed for Gm markers. The results, however, were uninformative.

Taken all together, no clear pattern emerged from this or from similar work that would allow a correlation between IgG subclass concentrations and the clinical type of the immunodeficiency.

TABLE IX

IgG SUBCLASS IMBALANCES[a] IN SERA OF
IMMUNODEFICIENT PATIENTS

Subclass	Percent of total IgG	Number of patients
IgG1	>90	0
	<40	3
IgG2	>50	3
	<10	1
IgG3	>15	5
	< 1	1
IgG4	>15	2
	< 1	22

[a] An imbalance was defined as a difference of more than two standard deviations from the normal percentage distribution.

VI. IgG Subclasses after Bone Marrow Transplantation in Severe Combined Immunodeficiency

It was possible to follow the concentrations of the IgG subclasses in sera from patients with severe combined immunodeficiencies who underwent successful or partially successful immunological reconstitution of both humoral and cellular immunity by bone marrow transplantation. Quantitative determinations were made at various times after transplantation and showed transient increases of one or more immunoglobulin classes and IgG subclasses. The behavior of the IgG subclass levels in three of these patients is demonstrated and described in Figs. 3–5.

In Fig. 3, subclass levels are followed in patient J. M. He received HLA and MLC matched bone marrow at the age of 5 months (Ràdl et al., 1972). Twenty days after transplantation, a vigorous increase of both IgG1 and IgG3 was observed in his serum. The total IgG concentration of this initial peak was 20 mg/ml. In electrophoresis, it had the

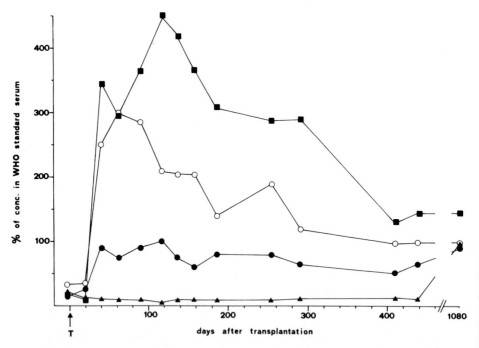

Fig. 3. Patient J. M. IgG subclass concentrations in serum samples taken at different times after bone marrow transplantation. The values are given as percentage of the WHO standard serum concentrations (see Table II). ○, IgG1; ●, IgG2; ■, IgG3; ▲, IgG4.

characteristics of an M gradient. λ light chains were predominant in both subclasses. Gradually, concentrations of these two subclasses declined to approximately normal values. IgG2 rose to a normal value and stayed in this range. IgG4 was low throughout the first year. A significant increase of this subclass was visible only after more than one year. Three years after transplantation, the boy's IgG was normal with regard to the light-chain ratio, subclass concentrations, and electrophoretic mobility.

Figure 4 shows the subclass levels in patient G. C. He received HLA and MLC identical bone marrow at the same age (Vossen *et al.*, 1973). At 40–80 days after transplantation, a high IgG1 peak developed in the serum. Its electrophoretic mobility was restricted to a narrow band. In this IgG1 gradient, both light-chain types were equally represented. Soon the IgG1 concentration sharply declined to about 10 mg/ml, and then stayed in this range. During the observation period, IgG3 increased to subnormal values. IgG2 slowly increased to a normal level whereas a significant increase of IgG4 could not be seen.

K. J. in Fig. 5 was transplanted at the age of 6 months with bone

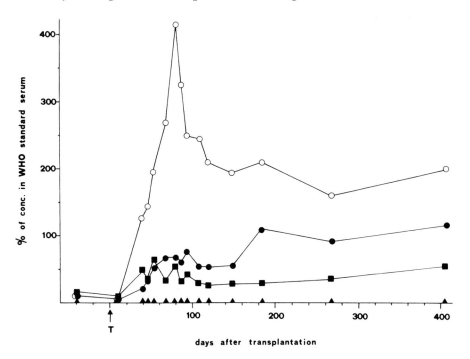

Fig. 4. Patient G. C. Follow-up of the IgG subclass serum concentrations after bone marrow transplantation. The values are given as percentage of the WHO standard serum concentrations (see Table II). ○, IgG1; ●, IgG2; ■, IgG3; ▲, IgG4.

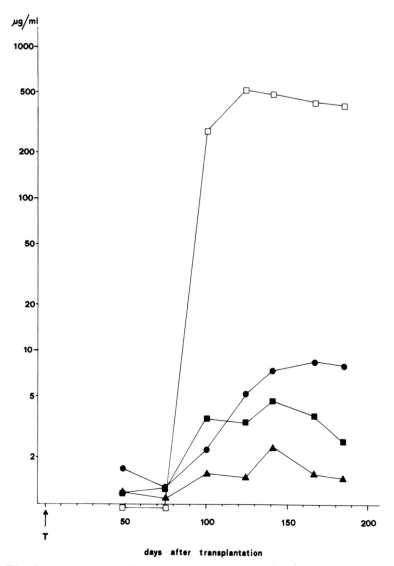

Fig. 5. Patient K. J. Follow-up of the IgG subclass serum concentrations after bone marrow transplantation. □, IgG1; ●, IgG2; ■, IgG3; ▲, IgG4.

marrow from a relative who was MLC identical but differed from the patient in one HLA locus (Koch *et al.,* 1973). This treatment was re-peated 3 and 5 months later. Only after the third transplantation could a modest "take" be observed. IgG1 of type κ steeply increased from about

1 μg to 0.5 mg/ml. The other subclasses concomitantly rose to a few micrograms per milliliter only.

Some common features can be detected in these three cases and in others that have been reported in the literature: After a variable latent period, serum IgG values rapidly increase. The doubling time can be less than 10 days, and values exceeding by far the normal levels may be reached. These immunoglobulins often seem to be of limited heterogeneity concerning subclass distribution, light-chain type, and electrophoretic mobility and thus may appear as oligoclonal or even monoclonal IgG peaks resembling M components. In one case, report by Yount and associates (1974), this initial increase was polyclonal: all four IgG subclasses and both light-chain types were represented, and the IgG had a normal electrophoretic mobility. But also in their patient, the IgG1 and IgG3 levels showed an extremely rapid increase overshooting the normal values. IgG2 levels in their cases and in two of ours rose at the same time, but somewhat more sluggishly and only to subnormal or normal values. A significant IgG4 increase could be observed in one of our patients, and only more than one year after transplantation. This sequence of events has some similarities to the normal development of the IgG subclass levels in infants, as shown in Fig. 2.

Acknowledgments

We thank the following publishers for permission to reproduce material used in this contribution: Mosby, St. Louis, for use of Fig. 2 from *J. Pediatr.* **80**, 960–964, 1972; S. Karger AG, Basel, for use of Tables III, IV, and VI, from Morell *et al.* (1975). "IgG Subclasses of Human Immunoglobulins. Immunochemical, Genetic, Biological, and Clinical Aspects"; and The National Foundation—March of Dimes, for use of Table IX, from Bergsma, D. (ed.) 1975. "Immunodeficiency in Man and Animals, Birth Defects: Orig. Art. Ser.," **11**, No. 1, 108–111. Sinauer Assoc., Sunderland, Massachusetts.

References

Dray, S. (1960). Three γ-globulins in normal human serum revealed by monkey precipitins. *Science* **132**, 1313–1314.

Grubb, R. (1970). *In* "The Genetic Markers of Human Immunoglobulins" (A. Kleinzeller, G. F. Springer, and H. G. Wittman, eds.), pp. 25–36. Springer-Verlag, Berlin and New York.

Koch, C., Henriksen, K., Juhl, F., Wiik, A., Faber, V., Andersen, V., Dupont, B., Hansen, G. S., Svejgaard, A., Jensen, K., and Muller-Berat, N. (1973). Bone marrow transplantation from a HL-A non-identical but MLC-identical donor. *Lancet* **1**, 1146–1149.

Morell, A., and Skvaril, F. (1973). Correlations between the serum concentrations of IgG myeloma proteins and background IgG. *Protides Biol. Fluids, Proc. Colloq.* **20**, 245–249.

Morell, A., Skvaril, F., and Barandun, S. (1975). "IgG Subclasses of Human Immunoglobulins. Immunochemical, Genetic, Biological, and Clinical Aspects" (A. Morell, ed.). S. Karger, Basel.

Natvig, J. B., and Kunkel, H. G. (1973). Human immunoglobulins: Classes, subclasses, genetic variants, and idiotypes. *Advan. Immunol.* **16**, 1–59.

Ràdl, J., Dooren, L. J., Eijsvoogel, V. P., van Went, J. J., and Hijmans, W. (1972). An immunological study during post-transplantation follow-up of a case of severe combined immunodeficiency. *Clin. Exp. Immunol.* **10**, 367–382.

Spiegelberg, H. (1974). Biological activities of immunoglobulins of different classes and subclasses. *Advan. Immunol.* **19**, 259–294.

Vossen, J. M., de Koning, J., van Bekkum, D. W., Dicke, K. A., Eijsvoogel, V. P., Hijmans, W., van Loghem, E., Ràdl, J., van Rood, J. J., van der Waay, D., and Dooren, L. J. (1973). Successful treatment of an infant with severe combined immunodeficiency by transplantation of bone marrow cells from an uncle. *Clin. Exp. Immunol.* **13**, 9–20.

World Health Organization (1966). Notation for human immunoglobulin subclasses. *Bull. W.H.O.* **35**, 953.

Yount, W. J., Hong, R., Seligman, M., Good, R. A., and Kunkel, H. G. (1970). Imbalances of gamma globulin subgroups and gene defects in patients with primary hypogammaglobulinemia. *J. Clin. Invest.* **49**, 1957–1966.

Yount, W. J., Utsinger, P. D., Gatti, R. A., and Good, R. A. (1974). Immunoglobulin classes, IgG subclasses, Gm genetic markers, and C1q following bone marrow transplantation in X-linked combined immunodeficiency. *J. Pediat.* **84**, 193–199.

Imbalances of the κ/λ Ratio of Human Immunoglobulins[1]

SILVIO BARANDUN, FRANTISEK SKVARIL, and ANDREAS MORELL

Institute for Clinical and Experimental Cancer Research,
Tiefenau Hospital, Berne, Switzerland

I. Introduction

Normal human immunoglobulins are a heterogeneous mixture of molecules all of which share the same basic structure of two identical heavy and two identical light polypeptide chains. Structural differences of the non-antigen-binding, constant part of these chains are responsible for the isotypic variations of the immunoglobulins: Five main variants of the heavy and two of the light chains are known. The immunoglobulins can thus be classified in five heavy-chain classes and two light-chain types. There is ample evidence that the five heavy-chain classes differ widely in

[1] This work was supported by the Swiss National Foundation for Scientific Research.

their biological behavior. On the other hand, nothing is known so far about the non-antigen-binding biological properties of the two light-chain types.

Only in recent years attention has been paid to the quantitative relation of κ- and λ-type immunoglobulins in normal sera. The light-chain distribution within the various immunoglobulin classes and subclasses has not yet been investigated in detail. Data derived from the relative frequencies of κ- and λ-type monoclonal immunoglobulins may not be fully representative for normal conditions. Physiological variations of the κ/λ ratio were recently observed during the development of the immunoglobulin-producing tissue in infancy and, to a lesser extent, in aged individuals. In dysproteinemias, particularly in polyclonal hypergammaglobulinemia an imbalance of the κ/λ ratio is unusual.

Disproportionate synthesis of the two light-chain types occurs predominantly in disturbancies of the lymphoreticular system: κ/λ imbalance is characteristic for monoclonal proliferations of immunglobulin-producing cells as it is observed in multiple myeloma, macroglobulinemia and other paraproteinemias. The preponderance of one light-chain type is due to the appearance of an immunoglobulin homogeneous with regard to its heavy and light chains (M protein). Monoclonal proliferation in general seems to hit κ- or λ-producing cells at random. In special conditions, however, there may be a preferential selection for cells of one light-chain type: monoclonal IgM-gradients in idiopathic cold agglutinin disease, for instance, are almost exclusively of the κ-type (Harboe, 1971).

During the last few years, perturbations of the physiological κ/λ ratio have repeatedly been described in humoral immune deficiencies (Yount et al., 1970). In such instances, the light-chain imbalance may be the expression of a developmental or maturation failure of κ- or λ-producing cell lines. The κ/λ imbalance is usually superimposed on an altered heavy-chain synthesis affecting all or only some of the immunoglobulin classes. In most of these sera, the κ/λ ratio is only slightly disturbed. Exceptionally, however, the imbalance can be very pronounced. Such cases are of considerable theoretical interest since they might offer a clue for the biological significance of the light-chain types.

Theoretically, a κ/λ imbalance could possibly also be due to an increased catabolism of immunoglobulin molecules of one light-chain type. But to the best of our knowledge, no such cases have been described so far.

The present review is based on investigations on the κ/λ ratio of serum immunoglobulins in normal individuals and in patients who had abnormal proliferation or developmental failure of the immunoglobulin-producing cells. A method was applied allowing for analysis of the κ/λ ratio of immunoglobulins. Thus a monoclonal increase or a selective diminution of one particular light-chain type could be detected.

II. Methods for Detection of Human Immunoglobulin Light-Chain Imbalances

Screening of large numbers of sera for light-chain imbalances was carried out by double immunodiffusion tests in agar. An immunoreagent consisting of a mixture of antisera to both light-chain types was used (Skvaril and Barandun, 1973).

When anti-κ and anti-λ sera are mixed in an appropriate ratio and this mixture is allowed to react in double immunodiffusion with a dilute normal serum, two parallel precipitin lines appear. The test conditions were found to be most suitable with a mixture of anti-κ antibodies at 1 mg/ml and anti-λ antibodies at 1.7 mg/ml. The sera to be tested were diluted 1:6. Under these conditions λ immunoglobulins precipitate in a line closer to the peripheral antigen well and κ immunoglobulins form a line closer to the antiserum reservoir. In normal adult sera, the distance between these two precipitin lines is constant. In sera with κ-immunoglobulin predominance, the distance between the lines is increased. With a light-chain imbalance in favor of λ immunoglobulins, the lines are closer to each other. In sera with extreme λ-immunoglobulin predominance, the λ line is superimposed upon, or can even cross the κ line. This method is called κ/λ double-line (κ/λ DL) method.

In further experiments, the sensitivity of the method for detecting an imbalance in the κ/λ immunoglobulin ratio was established: Isolated IgG, IgA, and IgM myeloma proteins of both light-chain types were added in various amounts to normal serum and tested in the κ/λ DL method. Both divergence and convergence of the two precipitin lines were seen when κ or λ monoclonal proteins were added to normal human serum. However, the sensitivity of the test system was not equal for all immunoglobulin classes: a clear shifting of the precipitin lines was detectable when 1 mg of monoclonal IgG was added to 1 ml of normal serum. This amount represents about 10% of the total serum IgG. To produce a comparable effect, the addition of 3 mg of monoclonal IgA (i.e., about 100%) or 3 mg of IgM (about 300%) were necessary.

Sera with monoclonal immunoglobulins are characterized by a markedly disturbed κ/λ ratio. When such sera are reacted in immunodiffusion with the κ/λ DL antiserum, the monoclonal protein influences the position of the precipitin line of the corresponding light-chain type by shifting it into the antigen excess zone. Immunoglobulins of the other light-chain type, i.e., nonmyeloma or "background" immunoglobulins are visualized in the other line (Fig. 1).

The κ/λ DL method has been used to screen sera of normal and hypogammaglobulinemic individuals as well as of newborns and old individuals. With respect to the low or high immunoglobulin concentration in some of these sera, several dilutions were used in immunodiffusion. Generally, κ/λ immunoglobulin imbalances observed in some of these sera were only mild. In rare exceptions, however, a pronounced alteration of the κ/λ ratio simulating a monoclonal immunoglobulin was seen. Two such cases are reported (Fig. 2).

In addition to the κ/λ DL method, quantitative determinations of the κ/λ ratio were carried out by means of two methods. Radial immunodiffusion (Mancini et al., 1965) was performed in anti-κ and anti-λ plates. In a few experiments quantitative precipitation of the patients' sera with κ and λ specific antisera was measured nephelometrically according to Schultze and Schwick (1959). In both methods, isolated monoclonal IgG proteins were used as standards. The results were identical.

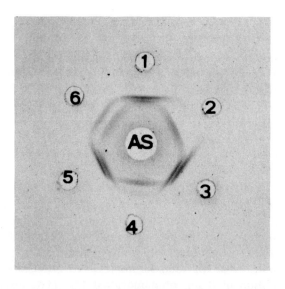

Fig. 1. Double immunodiffusion of normal human serum and of sera with monoclonal immunoglobulins in a 1:6 dilution reacted with the κ/λ double-line (κ/λ DL) antiserum. Peripheral wells: Normal human serum (1, 3, 5); serum from a myeloma patient with IgG1 κ (2), IgG2 λ (4), and IgA1 κ (6) proteins. Center well: AS = κ/λ DL antiserum. A distinct divergence of the precipitin lines is seen at the wells containing monoclonal κ immunoglobulins (2, 6). A crossing of the lines is observed at the well containing a monoclonal λ immunoglobulin (4).

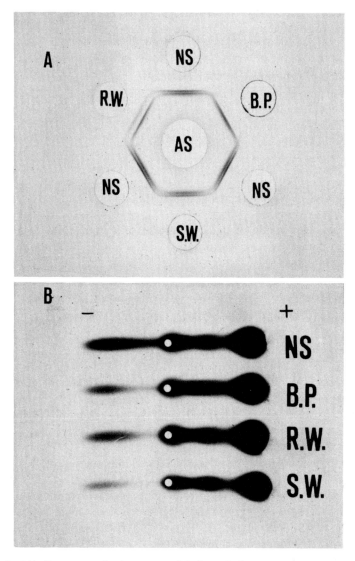

Fig. 2. (A) Detection of κ/λ immunoglobulin imbalances in three patients with immunodeficiency syndrome. NS, normal human serum, diluted 1:6; B. P., serum from the patient with κ-chain deficiency (see text); R. W., serum from the patient with λ-chain deficiency (see text); S. W., serum from a hypogammaglobulinemic patient without κ/λ disturbance. All sera were analyzed in a 1:4 dilution. Note the crossing of the precipitin lines at the well containing serum B. P. and the divergence of the precipitin lines at the well containing serum R. W. (B) Agar gel electrophoresis of a normal human serum (NS) and of sera from the patients B. P., R. W., and S. W. Sera from the patients show a reduced, but electrophoretically heterogeneous, γ-globulin fraction.

The κ/λ DL method is easy to perform and therefore suitable for screening a large number of sera. It allows the detection of pronounced κ/λ imbalances of all immunoglobulin classes. Slight imbalances, however, are detectable in IgG only, since IgG molecules are present in much higher concentration and are more easily precipitable by light-chain antisera than IgA and IgM. In addition, the low diffusion rate of IgM immunoglobulins and of IgA polymers must be taken into account. Therefore, for the determination of the κ/λ ratio in IgA and IgM, these proteins have to be isolated from the serum.

III. Analyses of Normal and Pathological Sera

Analyses were made of the κ/λ ratio in sera from normal individuals and from patients with a perturbation of the immunoglobulin-producing cell system.

A. NORMAL SERA

Preliminary studies performed with the κ/λ DL method in normal individuals have shown that the κ/λ ratio in the serum is subject to slight variations during life. In most sera of newborns and mothers, the κ/λ ratio was identical, as anticipated. In about 10% of paired cord and maternal sera, a slight imbalance in favor of the λ type can be observed. This type of imbalance becomes more marked in infants during the first months of life; between the fourth and the twelfth month, a shifting of the κ/λ ratio in favor of the λ type is the rule. It also could be shown that the pattern changes with increasing age.

More precise data were obtained in a quantitative study of the κ/λ ratio in normal individuals of different age (Skvaril et al., 1975). A marked difference exists between values obtained in children and in young individuals as well as between the latter group and a more heterogeneous population of blood donors (Table I). The distribution of the κ/λ ratio in these three groups was approximately symmetric and close to a normal distribution (Skvaril et al., 1975). On the other hand, a very broad distribution in aged individuals was observed.

B. PARAPROTEINEMIAS

The determination of the κ/λ ratio in the serum represents one of the most reliable laboratory methods for the recognition of a homogeneous immunoglobulin characteristic for a monoclonal proliferation of immuno-

TABLE I

RATIO OF κ/λ IMMUNOGLOBULINS IN SERA FROM NORMAL INDIVIDUALS

Subject	Number of subjects	κ/λ ratios		
		Mean values ±1 standard deviation	Range	Significance of differences from young adult values
Children (4–24 months)	111	1.25 ± 0.20	0.8–1.8	$P < 0.001$
Young adults (20 years)	139	1.68 ± 0.26	1.2–2.7	—
Blood donors (20–60 years)	197	1.91 ± 0.32	1.2–2.8	$P < 0.001$
Aged individuals (over 95 years)	45	1.62 ± 0.33	1.2–2.9	NS[a]

[a] Not significant.

globulin-producing cells. In such cases, the light-chain imbalance is usually pronounced. It is, except in isolated light-chain disease (Bence-Jones paraproteinemia), combined with a corresponding monoclonal increase of one particular immunoglobulin class or subclass. During the last years, approximately 2000 sera with a monoclonal immunoglobulin were analyzed in our laboratory both with conventional techniques and with the κ/λ method. The results agreed without exception. An advantage of the κ/λ DL method is that an M gradient is recognized and typed at the same time. In addition, an eventual Bence-Jones protein can also be seen. In our hands, this method is more sensitive and easier to interpret than immunoelectrophoresis, especially in cases with rudimentary M gradients accompanied by high background immunoglobulin concentrations.

C. HYPOGAMMAGLOBULINEMIAS

In primary hypogammaglobulinemias of early and late manifestation, another type of light-chain imbalance can be found: in some cases, a shifting of the κ/λ ratio in favor of the λ chains was observed, in others the balance was changed in favor of the κ chains. In about 60% the ratio was in the normal range. In three patients, total agammaglobulinemia did not allow an estimation. A superposition of the two precipitin lines in the κ/λ DL test (κ-chain deficiency) and a marked divergence (λ-chain deficiency) were observed in two hypogammaglobulinemic children—one 2 years old and the other 6 years old. Neither suffered from recurrent bacterial infections. Both, however, had gastrointestinal disorders: the younger child suffered from a protein-losing gastroenteropathy of unknown origin; the older one from a familial celiac disease-like syndrome.

When studied quantitatively, the κ/λ ratio in hypogammaglobulinemic patients showed a broad and asymmetric distribution (Skvaril *et al.*, 1975). Extreme alterations of κ- or λ-type immunoglobulin synthesis are rare: one case of "κ-chain deficiency" has recently been published by Bernier *et al.* (1972), another by Maertzdorf *et al.* (1972). Two other patients, one with an extreme κ-chain defect, the second with a λ-chain deficiency, have been observed by us (Barandun *et al.*, 1976). Some relevant data from these two patients are presented in the following sections.

1. κ-Chain Deficiency

Patient P. B. was born in 1942 and had a normal development in infancy and childhood up to the age of 14 years. At this time, his current disease started with severe chronic diarrhea complicated by frequent acute exacerbations, gastric pain, and occasional vomiting. Other symptoms of an increased susceptibility of infections, in particular bacterial infections of the respiratory tract, were never found. The patient received several blood transfusions while undergoing minor surgical interventions. In 1970, severe pernicious anemia (Hb 4.7 gm/100 ml) was detected with profoundly disturbed megaloblastic maturation of all three cell lines in the bone marrow. The patient's gastric juice was totally anacid even after maximal stimulation. The production of intrinsic factor was markedly depressed (192 IF units in the first 60 minutes after stimulation with a normal range of 2000–20,000 units). Autoantibodies to parietal cells or intrinsic factor could not be found. The first-stage Schilling test showed a 2.5% urinary excretion of orally administered ^{58}Co-labeled vitamin B_{12} in a 48-hour urine. The test was corrected to normal (20.4%) by the simultaneous oral administration of hog intrinsic factor. Symptoms of malabsorption, e.g., steatorrhea were not present. The D-xylose and glucose resorption were within normal limits.

Accidentally, a humoral immune deficiency was detected at this time with a clearly decreased IgG concentration (375 mg/100 ml) and a severe IgA- (28 mg/100 ml) and IgM- (21 mg/100 ml) deficiency. The κ/λ ratio of the immunoglobulin light chains was markedly altered: more than 98% of the serum immunoglobulins were of the λ light-chain type (κ/λ ratio ± 0.01). A similiar shift of the κ/λ ratio could also be demonstrated in isolated immunoglobulins of the classes IgG and IgM and in the secretory IgA. In electro- and in immunoelectrophoresis, no signs of a monoclonal disturbance were found. No free light chains could be detected in the serum or urine. In a disc electrophoresis of light chains isolated from the patient's serum IgG, a heterogeneous pattern similar to that of isolated light chains from normal IgG was observed (Fig. 3).

The number of the patient's peripheral immunoglobulin-bearing B lymphocytes was normal and so was their percentage distribution regarding the main immunoglobulin classes IgG (7%), IgA (1%), IgM (10%), as well as the κ-positive (8%) and λ-positive (7%) cells. In the bone marrow and in the intestinal mucosa there was a distinct diminution of immunoglobulin-secreting cells, but the percentage distribution of these cells in the bone marrow was normal except for a minor reduc-

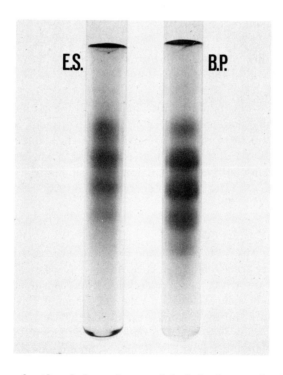

Fig. 3. Polyacrylamide gel electrophoresis of the light chains isolated from reduced and alkylated IgG at alkaline pH in the presence of urea. B. P., light chains from the IgG of the patient with κ-chain deficiency; E. S., light chains from the IgG of a normal individual with the same Inv-phenotype as patient B. P. The same pattern can be observed with both light-chain preparations.

tion of IgA-positive cells (positive cells for IgG 61%, IgA 34%, IgM 5%). Of these immunoglobulin-producing cells, however, 98% were λ positive and only 2% were κ positive. Estimations of the κ- and λ-immunoglobulin-producing cells in the mucosa of the small bowel showed the same type of light-chain imbalance. Antibody production after natural exposition and repeated vaccinations with a variety of vaccines was in the low normal range (various viral antigens, Te, Per) or was totally absent (TAB, Di).

Skin test showed normal or even increased delayed-type reactions. The number of T lymphocytes determined by rosette formation with sheep erythrocytes was normal (55% lymphocytes with more than three adherent erythrocytes). When the patient's lymphocytes were isolated on a Ficoll gradient and stimulated with various mitogens, soluble antigens, and allogenetic cells (MLC), the response was normal.

The analysis for autoantibodies to various immunoglobulin allotypes and to heavy- and light-chain determinants was negative. In turnover studies with isolated and radiolabeled monoclonal IgG1 type-κ and IgG1 type-λ proteins it could be demonstrated that the survival of immunoglobulin molecules of both light-chain types in the patient's organism was equal and within the normal range ($t/2$ of IgG1/κ = 21 days, $t/2$ of IgG1/λ = 24 days).

Under substitution therapy with vitamin B_{12}, the patient's pernicious anemia was fully compensated. Intermittent treatment with Bactrim® (Hoffmann-La Roche) prevented relapse of diarrhea. The patient is now able to carry on a full-time job and is showing no increased susceptibility to infections, although the immunological findings including the imbalance of the κ/λ ratio have not changed since 1970.

2. λ-Chain Deficiency

Patient R. W. was born in 1941 and has suffered from frequent febrile upper respiratory tract infections since infancy. A classical antibody deficiency syndrome with recurrent otitis media, purulent pansinusitis, bronchitis with bronchopneumonic relapses, frequent furunculosis, etc., developed already during his first year of life. There were no gastrointestinal troubles, however, and the patient never suffered from diarrhea or other gut-related disturbances. Humoral immunodeficiency was detected in 1972 when a severe bilateral pneumonia required hospitalization: All serum immunoglobulins were diminished (IgG, 390 mg/100 ml, IgA, less than 10 mg/100 ml, IgM, 40 mg/100 ml). The κ/λ ratio was markedly shifted in favor of the κ-immunoglobulins with a κ/λ ratio of 6.0: 85% of the serum immunoglobulins had κ and only 15% had λ light chains. When IgG and IgM were isolated from the patient's serum, the same κ/λ imbalance was detected. Similar results were found in the patient's secretions. As in patient P. B., no evidence for the presence of a monoclonal immunoglobulin could be found. The hematological investigation showed a moderate anemia (Hb 11 gm/100 ml, hematocrit 35%). Precursors of all three cell lines in the bone marrow demonstrated unequivocal megaloblastic changes. Serum vitamin B_{12} was 44 pg/ml, serum folic acid was 66 ng/ml. After maximal stimulation, total anacidity and markedly diminished production of intrinsic factor (144 U/hour stimulation) was noticed. The Schilling test revealed a 3.7% urinary excretion in 48 hours without intrinsic factor and 18.1% when hog intrinsic factor was given per os. No symptoms of malabsorption were observed, and no antibodies to parietal cells or to intrinsic factor could be demonstrated.

In the patient's peripheral blood, the number of the immunoglobulin-bearing B lymphocytes was reduced during infections, but normal during infection-free intervals. Their percentage distribution, in repeated examinations, with regard to membrane-associated immunoglobulin heavy chains and light chains was in the normal range. In the bone marrow and in lymphoreticular tissues, cells with intracellular, cytoplasmic immunoglobulins were diminished and showed an unusual percentage distribution: The relative frequency of IgG (67%) and particularly of IgM (32%) was higher than normal, whereas the number of IgA-positive plasma cells (1%) was severely decreased. Of the immunoglobulin-secreting cells 88% were positive for κ light chains, 12% for λ chains. A similar distribution pattern for κ and λ cells was found in immunofluorescence studies of the mucosa of the small bowel. Here, IgA-positive cells were more frequent than in the bone marrow.

The production of humoral antibodies after spontaneous exposition or after repeated vaccination with various antigens was equivocal. In part, it was normal (Polio I, II, III, Di, Per). With some antigens, however, no or only weak antibody response could be elicited (TAB-O and H-antigens, Te) even after repeated vaccinations.

The patient's cell-mediated immune system was normal as shown by delayed-type skin reactions to a battery of standard antigens. With sheep erythrocytes 65% of the patient's peripheral lymphocytes formed rosettes. Stimulation of the lymphocytes with mitogens, soluble antigens, and allogenetic cells (MLC) was found to be normal.

No antibodies against immunoglobulin could be detected.

Since 1972, the patient has been under regular substitution therapy with γ-globulin and vitamin B_{12}. Antibiotics were given during exacerbation of the chronic infections of his upper respiratory tract. The patient is now in good condition and able to assume a full-time job, but he still has chronic bronchitis and sinusitis. The immunological findings, particularly the κ/λ imbalance, has not changed during the last two years.

IV. Conclusions

The κ/λ light-chain ratio in normal serum is subject to some variations during life: between the fourth and the twelfth month and again in old age, a shift in favor of λ chains is more frequent than in middle age. No correlation between the κ/λ light-chain ratio and the concentrations of the various immunoglobulin classes and subclasses in the serum could be detected. It therefore appears that the synthesis of the two light-chain types is under separate control.

A disproportionate synthesis of κ and λ immunoglobulins characterizes a monoclonal proliferation of Ig-producing cells as observed in multiple myeloma, macroglobulinemia, and other paraproteinemias. Differences in the clinical course between κ or λ paraproteinemias are not known.

Light-chain imbalances of variable degree can be observed in humoral immunodeficiencies. So far, only a few observations of a pronounced disturbance of the κ/λ ratio have been reported. Therefore, a clear picture of the immunobiological and clinical peculiarites of selective light-chain defects has not yet emerged. Immunofluorescence studies of peripheral B lymphocytes and of Ig-producing cells in the bone marrow and other lymphoreticular tissues permit us to assume that at least in our cases a selective light-chain defect is the consequence of a developmental or maturation failure in the B-cell system. A differentiation arrest between the Ig-bearing B lymphocytes and the mature Ig-secreting cells is proposed. The capability of patients with κ- or λ-chain deficiency to respond to antigenic stimuli by producing corresponding antibodies varied: Some antigens triggered a normal or subnormal immune response, others did not. A regular response pattern could not be recognized. Cellular immunity, on the other hand, seemed to be intact. The clinical course was not uniform. A typical antibody deficiency syndrome with repeated bacterial infections was dominant in patient N. C. reported by Bernier *et al.* (1972) (κ/λ ratio 0.66) and in our patient R. W. (κ/λ ratio 6.0). Our other case, B. P. (κ/λ ratio 0.01), however, showed no signs of increased susceptibility to infections, except for his chronic diarrhea.

A remarkable and exceptional finding in all three patients was a more or less severe megaloblastic alteration of the bone marrow. Simultaneously, histopathological and functional disturbances of the gastrointestinal tract were present. In our patient B. P., a severe pernicious anemia was detected at the age of 28 years, but chronic diarrhea had existed since childhood. In the second case, R. W., only a moderate anemia was found in spite of typical findings in the bone marrow. In Bernier's patient who was 3.75 years old, only slight bone marrow alterations were observed, and their interpretation is difficult. In our two cases, a severe atrophy of the gastric mucosa, a total anacidity, and a markedly diminished or even absent intrinsic factor secretion were found. There was no malabsorption, and the serum concentration of folic acid was high. All these findings are compatible with the diagnosis of a primary pernicious anemia. This diagnosis, however, is justified only if the atrophy of the gastric mucosa was not the consequence of the humoral immune defect responsible for the other histopathological changes, e.g., the inflammatory infiltrations and the follicular hyperplasia.

In contrast to the classical primary pernicious anemia, the cases presented show some peculiarities, namely, the young age of the patients, the humoral immune defect, and the lack of antibodies to parietal cells and intrinsic factor. On the basis of the sparse information available so far, it cannot be decided whether there is a causal relationship between the hematological finding and the gastrointestinal disturbancies, on the one hand, and the immune deficiency, particularly the κ/λ light chain imbalance, on the other. Nevertheless, the probability seems remote that the simultaneous occurrence of two such rare disorders as juvenile pernicious anemia and selective light-chain deficiency is merely coincidental. Thus, it is possible that a sufficient supply of vitamin B_{12} is essential for both the proliferation and the differentiation of immunologically active cells, as it is for other rapidly dividing cell systems.

References

Barandun, S., Morell, A., Skvaril, F. and Oberdorfer, A. (1976). *Blood* **47**, 79.

Bernier, G. M., Gunderman, J. R., and Ruymann, F. B. (1972). *Blood* **40**, 795.

Harboe, M. (1971). *Vox Sang.* **20**, 289.

Mancini, G., Carbonara, A. G., and Heremans, J. F. (1965). *Immunochemistry* **2**, 235.

Maertzdorf, W., Stoop, J. W., Mul, N. A. J., Zegers, B. J. M., and Ballieux, RE. (1972). *Eur. J. Clin. Invest.* **2**, 294.

Schultze, H. E., and Schwick, G. (1959). *Clin. Chim. Acta* **4**, 15.

Skvaril, F., and Barandun, S. (1973). *J. Immunol. Methods* **3**, 127.

Skvaril, F., Barandun, S., Morell, A., Kuffer, F., and Probst (1975). *In* "Protides of Biological Fluids, 23th Colloquium." (H. Peeters, ed.). Pergamon Press, Oxford and New York (in press).

Yount, W. J., Hong, R., Seligmann, M., Good, R. A., and Kunkel, H. G. (1970). *J. Clin. Invest.* **49**, 1957.

Metabolism of Immunoglobulins

THOMAS A. WALDMANN *and* WARREN STROBER

Metabolism Branch, National Cancer Institute, NIH, Bethesda, Maryland

I. Introduction

Over 40 years ago Glenny and Hopkins (1923) and Freund and Whitney (1928) demonstrated that passively infused antibody disappeared from the plasma of the recipient owing to the combined effects of distribution to extravascular sites and protein breakdown. These pioneering studies presaged the work of Borsook and Keighley (1935) and Schoenheimer (1942), who showed with the use of isotopes that body proteins do not serve the organism for life but are continually being degraded and replaced by newly synthesized molecules.

In recent years the work of Glenny and Freund has been greatly extended by using proteins with radioiodine labels instead of antibody labels and by using purified, chemically homogeneous classes of immunoglobulins instead of crude, undefined protein fractions. Studies utilizing such radiolabeled immunoglobulins have led to a general understanding of the normal metabolism of the various classes of immunoglobulin molecules. In broadest outline the immunoglobulins are synthesized in cells of the lymphocyte and plasma cell series and, for the most part, are then delivered into the plasma compartment. Immunoglobulin molecules circulate in the plasma compartment as well as in one or more extravascular protein compartments which exchange with the plasma compartment. Immunoglobulin catabolism occurs in close connection with the plasma compartment and the degradative process is largely complete, i.e., does not result in the circulation of partial degradation products. In the normal individual in the steady state, the rates of synthesis and catabolism of immunoglobulin molecules are equal and, hence, the immunoglobulin concentration in the various body compartments remains stable. Finally, it is important to note that although the immunoglobulins are made up of molecules with individual antibody specificity, interactions between antibodies and antigens with subsequent immune elimination makes only a negligible contribution to the overall metabolism of the immunoglobulin molecules; the latter is controlled, for the most part, by bodily processes that act on most of the circulating serum proteins.

The techniques for the study of immunoglobulin metabolism have been of value in elucidating the physiological factors controlling the rates of immunoglobulin synthesis, catabolism, and transport (Waldmann and Strober, 1969). These techniques have also been of value in studying the pathogenesis of the abnormalities of immunoglobulin levels seen in disease. Frequently new abnormalities in recognized diseases have first been revealed through the use of immunoglobulin metabolic studies. For example, antibodies to IgA in patients with isolated IgA deficiency or ataxia-telangiectasia were first recognized following the demonstration of exceedingly short IgA survivals in such patients (Strober et al., 1968). A number of new classes of diseases have been elucidated through the use of immunoglobulin turnover studies. For example, the class of diseases associated with protein loss into the gastrointestinal tract and the group of diseases associated with abnormalities of endogenous catabolism of one or more classes of immunoglobulin molecules were discovered through the use of protein turnover studies. In addition, immunoglobulin turnover studies have been of value in the differential diagnosis of immunodeficiency states with similar clinical features. For example, one may use turnover studies to differentiate patients with severe combined immunodeficiency disease associated with decreased rates of synthesis of immunoglobulins and lymphocytes from patients with intestinal lymphangiectasia wherein a comparable pattern of hypogammaglobulinemia and lymphocytopenia is due to excessive loss of these elements into the gastrointestinal tract. Finally, immunoglobulin turnover studies have provided the information necessary for the rational use of γ-globulin or its subunits as therapeutic agents.

II. Methods Used in Immunoglobulin Turnover Studies

A. GENERAL PRINCIPLES

The aim of metabolic studies of immunoglobulins (or other circulating proteins) is to obtain reliable estimates of pool sizes as well as synthetic and catabolic rates of these proteins. In special studies, data on additional aspects of metabolism such as the site of synthesis and catabolism, the rates and pathways of transport of the molecules, and the precursor–product relationships between immunoglobulins and their subunits can be obtained. Labeled molecules used in immunoglobulin turnover studies have included actively produced or passively infused antibody, infused immunoglobulins without radioactive labels, or immunoglobulins labeled biosynthetically *in vivo* with labeled amino acids or *in vitro* with radioisotopes of iodine. Of these labeled molecules, immunoglobulins labeled with isotopes of iodine have proved to be the most versatile and widely used for the study of immunoglobulin metabolism; this follows from the fact that radioiodine labels are not reutilized for protein synthesis (if thyroidal uptake of iodine is inhibited by the administration of unlabeled iodine) and, in addition, radioiodine is quantitatively and rapidly excreted in the urine after protein breakdown. Thus the amount of label retained in the body is a good estimate of the amount of injected protein not yet degraded. Finally, radioiodine labels are easy to follow and radioiodinated proteins can be rapidly prepared.

In order to prepare radioiodinated proteins that are metabolically identical to native molecules, great care must be taken in the isolation, radiolabeling, and storage of proteins. The techniques for protein isolation that are generally satisfactory for metabolic studies include ion exchange chromatography, electrophoresis, gel filtration, and ammonium sulfate precipitation. The techniques for protein isolation that may be unsatisfactory include cold alcohol fractionation, procedures involving release of protein from antigen–antibody precipitates, and procedures involving lyophilization or heating to 60°C for prolonged periods of time (which would be used to inactivate hepatitis virus).

After purification the protein may be radioiodinated without damage by a number of techniques. In all techniques at least two reactions occur. There is a preliminary oxidation of free sulfhydryl groups and then incorporation of iodine into the tyrosine ring. The most widely used procedure is the iodine monochloride technique of McFarlane (1958). Other valid techniques involve electrolytic iodination of proteins or the use of lactoperoxidase as the oxidizing agent. Techniques using strong oxidizing agents, such as chloramine-T, have, in general, been found to be unsatisfactory for metabolic studies by most investigators, but may be useful in some cases if great care is taken to use very low concentrations of oxidizing agent and high concentrations of the protein. Whatever method is employed the iodination should be minimal, with the result that less than 1 atom of iodine per molecule of protein is incorporated into the final product.

B. Specific Procedures for Immunoglobulin Turnover Studies

In the performance of radioiodinated protein turnover studies, the test subject is placed under stable conditions of intake and activity in order to maintain a steady state. To this end also the patient must be free of acute illness and not subject to major physiological perturbations.

The purified radioiodinated immunoglobulin is administered intravenously. Samples of blood are then withdrawn (at a second venipuncture site) every few minutes for 30 minutes and daily for 10–14 days. These samples are counted in a gamma counter, and the rate of decline of radioactivity from the serum is thereby determined. Complete urine collections are also usually made to determine the rate of excretion of the iodide label released as a result of radiolabeled protein degradation; the daily excretion values may be subtracted cumulatively from the injected dose (determined from the activity and volume of the injected solution containing radiolabeled immunoglobulin) to obtain a decline of radiolabeled protein in the whole body. This latter decline can also be obtained directly by counting the test subject initially and daily thereafter in a whole-body counter.

Over the past 20 years a number of mathematical techniques have evolved to convert the raw tracer data into physiologically meaningful estimates of plasma immunoglobulin, pool sizes, fractional catabolic and, in the steady state, synthetic rates. The exact techniques used and the assumptions inherent in the various methods of analysis of iodinated protein turnover have been reviewed previously (Waldmann and Strober, 1969), and only a single method using serum data alone will be considered here.

Serum data alone can be analyzed to determine the metabolic parameters of immunoglobulin metabolism as follows: the decline (die-away) of plasma radioactivity is plotted as a function of time on semilogarithmic paper as indicated in Fig. 1. This plasma radioactivity curve is

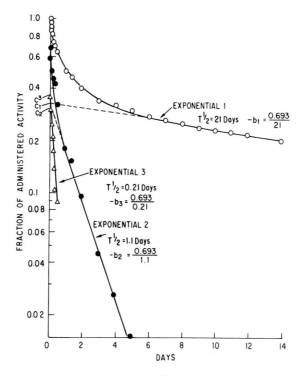

Fig. 1. Graphic analysis of the plasma ^{125}I-labeled IgG curve. The open circles represent actual measurements. The other points are graphically determined by "curve peeling." The original curve was plotted on semilogarithmic paper, and its straight linear terminal portion was extrapolated to the ordinate to obtain the intercept c_1. The slope of this line is $-b_1$. By subtracting the extrapolated line from the original curve, a new curve is obtained from which the slope and intercept value c_2 and $-b_2$ are obtained in the same manner as with the original curve. A third "peeling" yields c_3 and $-b_3$. Thus, the original curve may be described by three exponentials with slopes $-b_1$, $-b_2$ and $-b_3$ and corresponding intercepts c_1, c_2, and c_3. These values for slopes and intercepts are used to determine the metabolic parameters for the protein as indicated in the text.

resolved by graphic analysis into 2 or 3 exponential functions, each with an ordinate intercept c_i and slope $-b_i$. The metabolic parameters are determined using these slopes and intercepts in the following formulas:

Plasma volume (PV)

$$= \frac{\text{Activity of radiolabeled immunoglobulin injected iv}}{\begin{array}{c}\text{Activity per ml of plasma at zero time (extrapolated from samples}\\ \text{taken at intervals during the first few minutes of study)}\end{array}} \quad (1)$$

Plasma pool of immunoglobulin
$$= \text{PV} \times \text{serum concentration of immunoglobulin protein under study} \quad (2)$$

Fraction of the total body pool present in the intravascular space

$$= \left(\sum_{i=1}^{n} c_i/b_i \right)^2 \bigg/ \sum_{i=1}^{n} c_i/(b_i)^2 \quad (3)$$

Fractional catabolic rate (FCR) (fraction of the intravascular pool
of protein catabolized per day) $= 1/[(c_1/b_1) + (c_2/b_2) \cdots (c_i/b_i)] \quad (4)$

$$\text{Absolute catabolic rate} = \text{FCR} \times \text{plasma pool} \quad (5)$$

If a patient is in the steady state the absolute catabolic rate is equal to the synthetic rate for the protein.

III. Metabolism of Immunoglobulins in Normal Individuals

Each of the major classes of immunoglobulin molecules has a unique pathway and rate of synthesis and catabolism and in many cases specific transport pathways as well. The results of studies of the metabolism of the five major classes of immunoglobulins in normal human subjects are summarized in Table I. There is a wide range in the serum concentration of the immunoglobulin classes from approximately 100 ng/ml for IgE to over 12 mg (12×10^6 ng/ml) for IgG. These differences in serum concentrations reflect differences in the rates of synthesis and the rates of catabolism of the different classes of molecules. The synthetic rate of IgG is 33 mg/kg per day, which is quite similar to that of IgA, but about 5 times that of IgM, 100 times that of IgD, and about 10,000 times that of IgE. There are also significant differences in the survivals of the different immunoglobulin molecules expressed either as a survival half-time, where there is a range in survival from 2.4 days with IgE to 23 days with IgG, or expressed as the fraction of the intravascular pool of these proteins catabolized per day. The fraction of the intravascular pool catabolized

TABLE I
SURVIVAL OF IMMUNOGLOBULINS IN NORMAL MAN[a]

Immuno- globulin class	Serum concen- tration (mg/ml)	Percent intra- vascular	Total circulating pool (mg/kg)	$T_{1/2}$ (days)	FCR[b]	Synthetic rate[c] (mg/kg/day)
IgG	12.1	45	494	23	0.067	33
IgM	0.93	76	37	5.1	0.18	6.9
IgA	2.5	42	95	5.8	0.25	24
IgD	0.023	75	1.1	2.8	0.37	0.4
IgE	0.000076	51	0.003	2.4	0.71	0.002

[a] All proteins were prepared by DEAE-cellulose chromatography and gel filtration and were iodinated by the iodine monochloride method.

[b] Fractional catabolic rate: fraction of intravenous pool per day.

[c] Synthetic rates recorded refer to molecules delivered into the circulating pool. Immunoglobulins synthesized beneath mucosal surfaces and delivered directly into external secretions are not included in these synthetic rate estimates.

per day ranges from 6.7% for IgG to 71% for IgE. In addition to the differences in the fractional catabolic rates among the major classes of immunoglobulins, there are differences in this parameter of metabolism among the subclasses of these proteins as well. For example. IgG1, IgG2, and IgG4 have similar fractional catabolic rates with approximately 7% of the intravascular pool of these proteins degraded per day whereas, IgG3 has a much higher fractional catabolic rate with 17% of the intra-vascular pool catabolized daily (Spiegelberg et al., 1968; Morell et al., 1970). Thus, it is clear that the differences in catabolic rates as well as differences in synthetic rates play a profound role in determining the serum concentrations of the various classes and subclasses of immunoglobulins.

By studying the metabolism of naturally occurring immunoglobulin subunits and those experimentally produced it has been shown that the differences in metabolic behavior between different immunoglobulin classes are determined in large measure by differences in the Fc fragment of the molecule (Spiegelberg and Weigle, 1965; Wochner et al., 1967). It is clear that immunoglobulin fragments that will be useful for therapy in man will have to retain at least that part of the Fc fragment that controls the survival of the protein, inasmuch as treatment of proteins that result in the production of fragments such as the Fab piece may be capable of antibody–antigen interaction but have biological survivals that are too short to be of use in vivo.

IV. Problems in Interpretation of the Data

The most common problem in performing iodinated immunoglobulin metabolic studies results from the use of labeled preparations that are damaged and hence do not have the metabolic characteristics of the native molecules. As indicated above, such damaged preparations may occur secondary to a variety of factors including the use of harsh separation techniques for the isolation of the protein, denaturization resulting from prolonged storage or excessive oxidation or overiodination of the protein during radiolabeling. Such damaged proteins lead to spuriously short estimates of the half-times of survival, high estimates of the fractional catabolic rate, high estimates of the fraction of the body protein that is in the extravascular space, and ultimately high estimates for the plasma volume and total circulating pool of the protein under study. A number of approaches are possible to detect damaged proteins. First, one may define the fraction of the circulating label excreted daily as radioactivity in the urine throughout the study period. Normally, a constant fraction of the circulating label is cleared into the urine daily. However, when damaged proteins are utilized the damaged molecules are catabolized rapidly, and a very high fraction of the circulating radioactive label is excreted during the first 1 to 3 days of study as compared to the fraction excreted subsequently. If this occurs, one can be certain that one is dealing with damaged radiolabeled protein. An additional approach to the detection of damaged preparations is to perform the turnover study in control individuals with the same preparation that is used to study the patients with disorders of immunoglobulin concentration. The parameters of protein metabolism obtained in the normal individuals should be comparable to those indicated in Table I for the different immunoglobulin classes. This approach is not applicable when new classes or subclasses of proteins are to be studied wherein the normal metabolic pattern has not yet been defined. In these cases an effort should be made to obtain independent estimates of the metabolic parameters by methods that do not involve *in vitro* radiolabeling procedures. Such estimates may be obtained by determining the rate of decline of the serum concentration of immunoglobulins under study after the passive infusion of immunoglobulin molecules or whole serum containing immunoglobulin molecules to patients who do not have these proteins, that is, patients who have hypogammaglobulinemia. Alternatively, one may obtain estimates of the survival of the immunoglobulin class by following the time course of specific activity in that particular class after administration of precursor-labeled amino acids.

V. Disorders of Immunoglobulin Metabolism

Abnormalities of the serum immunoglobulin concentration (hypo- and hypergammaglobulinemia) may occur secondary to a variety of pathophysiological mechanisms (Table II). These different mechanisms affect

TABLE II

DISORDERS OF IMMUNOGLOBULIN METABOLISM IN DISEASE

I. Hypogammaglobulinemia associated with endogenous hypercatabolism of serum proteins
   A. Hypercatabolism affecting all immunoglobulin classes as well as other serum proteins
      1. Familial hypercatabolic hypoproteinemia
      2. Wiskott–Aldrich syndrome
      3. Hypermetabolic states
   B. Hypercatabolism affecting a single immunoglobulin class
      1. Myotonic dystrophy—hypercatabolism of IgG
      2. Connective tissue disorders—hypercatabolism of IgG
      3. Isolated IgA deficiency and ataxia-telangiectasia with IgA deficiency-hypercatabolism of IgA may occur when anti-IgA antibodies are produced by the patient
II. Hypogammaglobulinemia associated with excessive loss of immunoglobulins
   A. Nephrotic syndrome
   B. Protein-losing gastroenteropathy
III. Hypogammaglobulinemia associated with decreased immunoglobulin synthesis
   A. Deficiency of all immunoglobulin classes
      1. Severe combined immunodeficiency
      2. X-linked agammaglobulinemia
      3. Common variable immunodeficiency
      4. Hypogammaglobulinemia with thymoma
   B. Selective immunoglobulin deficiencies
      1. Isolated IgA deficiency
      2. Ataxia-telangiectasia—deficient IgA and IgE synthesis
      3. Other dysgammaglobulinemias with variable immunoglobulin levels
IV. Hypergammaglobulinemia associated with increased immunoglobulin synthesis
   A. Diffuse increase in synthesis of immunoglobulins
      1. Cirrhosis of liver
      2. Connective tissue disease
      3. Infectious diseases
   B. Increased synthesis of a single class of monoclonal immunoglobulin
      1. Multiple myeloma
      2. Macroglobulinemia of Waldenström
      3. Benign monoclonal gammopathy
V. Hypergammaglobulinemia (of immunoglobulin fragments) with prolonged immunoglobulin fragment survival
      Uremia and nephron loss with decreased endogenous catabolic rates of light chains and other low-molecular-weight serum proteins

serum concentrations through a more primary effect on one or more metabolic parameters, the rate of synthesis, the rate of catabolism, or the
pattern of distribution of the immunoglobulins. One class of hypogammaglobulinemia is due to decreased survival of many immunoglobulin classes
as well as other serum proteins. This is observed in patients with abnormalities of endogenous immunoglobulin catabolism or in patients with
excessive loss of immunoglobulins into the urinary, respiratory, or gastrointestinal tracts. A second class of hypogammaglobulinemia is due to
hypercatabolism affecting a single immunoglobulin class. This may be
observed in patients with complex cryogels, myotonic dystrophy, or
rheumatoid arthritis. A third class of hypogammaglobulinemia is due to
decreased synthesis of one or more classes of immunoglobulin molecules.
This occurs as a primary disease of the lymphoid system or as a secondary
effect on the lymphoid system associated with primary disease in another
system. Finally, hypogammaglobulinemia of modest proportions has also
been reported secondary to those pathophysiological mechanisms that
result in the dilution of a normal pool of immunoglobulins in an abnormally large plasma volume. It should be noted that in many patients
hypogammaglobulinemia may be caused by a combination of disorders
that lead to effects on both catabolic and synthetic processes; in such
patients minor effects on each parameter may summate and thereby lead
to a major degree of serum immunoglobulin depression.

Increased serum concentrations of immunoglobulins or immunoglobulin
fragments (hypergammaglobulinemia) have been noted in association
with disease mechanisms that affect metabolism in one of two ways. In
the first, there is either a diffuse increase in synthesis of immunoglobulins
or an increase in synthesis of a single class of immunoglobulin molecules.
In the second, synthetic rates are normal but the rate of catabolism of the
immunoglobulins is decreased.

A. Hypogammaglobulinemia Associated with Decreased Immunoglobulin Survival

Decreased immunoglobulin survival has been shown through metabolic
turnover studies to be a major cause of hypogammaglobulinemia. By the
use of iodinated immunoglobulin molecules in metabolic turnover studies,
patients with hypogammaglobulinemia (in this category) can be shown
to have a reduction in immunoglobulin pool sizes, normal rates of immunoglobulin synthesis, and markedly reduced survival half-times and
increased fractional catabolic rates for the major immunoglobulin classes.
Decreased immunoglobulin survival may result from a disorder or endogenous catabolism or from a disorder leading to loss of immunoglobulin
into the urinary or gastrointestinal tract. Iodinated protein turnover

studies will not distinguish between these two classes of disorders because in both cases there is an increase in the rate at which labeled protein leaves the circulating pool and the whole body. Excessive loss of immunoglobulin into the urinary tract may usually be detected by determination of the urinary immunoglobulin concentration. This is usually done as a quantitation of unlabeled urinary immunoglobulin excretion but may also be done in connection with an iodinated turnover study in which the fraction of the circulating pool of immunoglobulin lost into the urine may be determined. This calculation assumes no catabolic breakdown within the kidney, an assumption that may hold for all intact immunoglobulin molecules but not for immunoglobulin fragments (see below).

As noted, excessive loss of immunoglobulin into the gastrointestinal tract cannot be detected with iodinated protein turnovers alone. In patients with this kind of disorder there is rapid reabsorption of the radioiodide label following catabolism of the labeled protein in the intestinal lumen, and, in addition, there is active secretion of radioiodide into the intestinal lumen in the salivary, gastric, and certain small intestinal secretions. Thus, the analysis of the data obtained from the serum and urinary radioactivity curves shows that a short survival as opposed to decreased synthesis is the cause of the hypogammaglobulinemia, but does not differentiate endogenous hypercatabolism from gastrointestinal loss. In order to determine whether a short immunoglobulin survival is due to excessive loss into the gastrointestinal tract, one must use macromolecules with labels that are lost into the gastrointestinal tract only when bound to intact protein and, once in the gastrointestinal tract, are not reabsorbed in the bound or unbound form. Macromolecules that fulfill these requirements and, therefore, that can be used to diagnose and quantitate gastrointestinal protein loss include intravenously administered ^{131}I-labeled polyvinylpyrrolidone, ^{51}Cr-labeled serum proteins, ^{59}Fe-labeled dextran, and ^{95}Nb-labeled albumin. Of these, the most widely used for the diagnosis of gastrointestinal protein loss are the ^{51}Cr-labeled serum proteins including ^{51}Cr-labeled albumin or serum proteins labeled *in vivo* by intravenous administration of ^{51}CrCl$_3$ (Waldmann *et al.*, 1969).

To use ^{51}Cr-labeled albumin in a simple screening test, approximately 25 μCi of this radiolabeled macromolecule are administered intravenously. The stools over the subsequent 4 days are collected in 24-hour lots in half-gallon paint cans. The stools are brought to constant volume with water, homogenized in a paint shaker, and counted along with a can containing a known fraction of the injected dose (the stool "standard") in a bulk gamma ray scintillation counter. The results obtained are usually expressed as the percentage of the injected dose of radioactivity that is excreted in the stools in the 4 days following the intravenous administration of the isotope. Normal individuals or those with a short immunoglobulin survival due to disorders limited to endogenous hypercatabolism excrete from 0.1 to 0.7% of the administered dose in the stool during this period, whereas patients with excessive gastrointestinal protein loss excrete from 2 to 40% of the administered dose.

Although the 4-day ^{51}Cr-albumin excretion study is a simple test of value in making the diagnosis of excessive gastrointestinal protein loss, it does not provide data that can be easily related to other parameters of protein metabolism determined with the radioiodinated immunoglobulins. In this regard, a more meaningful study of enteric protein loss is obtained if one determines the clearance of ^{51}Cr-labeled serum protein into the gastrointestinal tract; in other words, one determines the fraction of the plasma pool or the milliliters of the plasma pool of protein cleared into the gastrointestinal tract per day. For such a determination, stools are collected in daily lots for a 12-day period and are processed and counted as described above. In addition, serum samples are obtained, both 10 minutes after injection and daily thereafter; these serum samples are then counted along with a known fraction of the injected dose (the serum "standard"). The serum and stool standards are used to correct for the differences in counting efficiency due to differences in geometry when counting serum as opposed to stool samples. The milliliters of plasma cleared into the gastrointestinal tract daily are then determined as follows:

$$\text{Ml of plasma cleared of protein/day} = \frac{\text{Counts in the stool in the 24-hour collection period}}{\text{Counts/ml of serum 1 day before collection}}$$

This value assumes a transit time of 1 day between excretion of labeled protein into the gastrointestinal tract and its appearance in the stool. The value for milliliters of plasma cleared of protein per day over the period from the third to twelfth days of study are determined, and the mean value is obtained; this is the clearance value. To calculate the fraction of the circulating protein pool cleared into the gastrointestinal tract per day, the milliliters of plasma cleared per day are divided by the plasma volume. Normal individuals or those with disorders of endogenous immunoglobulin hypercatabolism clear the protein from 5 to 40 ml of plasma into the gastrointestinal tract per day. This is equal to 0.2 to 1.6% of intravascular pool of protein per day. In contrast, patients with excessive gastrointestinal protein loss clear into the gastrointestinal tract 50–1800 ml of plasma per day, or about 2–60% of the intravascular pool of protein per day.

1. Hypogammaglobulinemia Associated with Protein Loss into the Gastrointestinal Tract

The loss of proteins into the gastrointestinal tract occurs in a wide variety of diseases (the protein-losing enteropathies) (Waldmann, 1966). In each case it is a process affecting all serum proteins, meaning that patients with protein-losing enteropathy will have not only hypoalbuminemia but hypogammaglobulinemia as well. Moreover, in protein-losing enteropathy proteins appear to be lost in bulk fashion; i.e., the loss affects each class equally as though whole serum were being lost. The evidence for this is that in protein-losing enteropathy the increase in fractional catabolic rate above the normal mean value is approximately the same for all classes of immunoglobulins. In stating this we do not imply that a given magnitude of protein-losing enteropathy has an equal effect on the serum level of all immunoglobulin classes. On the contrary, although the increase in fractional loss into the gastrointestinal tract for the various classes is generally the same the effect of this on the serum concentration for the various classes is different. For example, the IgG level was depressed from the normal level of 11.8 mg/ml to a geometric mean serum concentration of 4.4 mg/ml in a group of patients with intestinal lymphangiectasia and protein-losing enteropathy, whereas the IgE level was virtually normal in these patients (Waldmann et al., 1972a). This difference can be understood by analyzing the normal rates of metabolism of these immunoglobulin classes: normal individuals catabolize 6% of the intravascular pool of IgG whereas the rate of IgE catabolism is much higher with 71% of the intravascular pool degraded per day. A bulk process, such as gastrointestinal protein loss in which a certain fraction of the intravascular pool of proteins is lost daily in excess of the normal loss rate, would have a much more profound effect on the serum concentration of a protein that normally has a low fractional catabolic rate than one with a high fractional catabolic rate. If the plasma volume and rates of synthesis and endogenous catabolism of an immunoglobulin remain constant, the ratio of the serum immunoglobulin concentration of a patient with bulk loss of proteins to that of normals can be predicted from the following formula:

$$\frac{\text{Patient immunoglobulin level}}{\text{(fraction of normal level)}} = \frac{\text{Normal fractional catabolic rate}}{\text{Normal fractional catabolic rate} + \text{fractional rate of bulk loss}}$$

Thus, if a patient had a bulk loss of 15% of intravascular pool of immunoglobulins per day, one would expect to have an IgG level of 28% of normal (i.e., $6/6 + 15$). By the same method of analysis the mean IgE level would be predicted to be over 80% of normal in the same patient. In actual fact, there is no reduction in IgE levels whatsoever observed in these patients: This may be explained in part by the observation that patients with protein-losing enteropathy have an approximate 15% reduction in their total plasma protein volume resulting from their hypoproteinemia.

Protein-losing enteropathy has been found in association with over 90 diseases, and direct studies of the gastrointestinal tract, such as gastro-intestinal X-ray examinations and peroral intestinal biopsies, must be performed in those patients with documented excessive gastrointestinal tract protein loss in order to identify the specific disease process in-volved. In reviewing the various causes of protein-losing enteropathy, it is clear that in many cases one of several disease mechanisms can be demonstrated whereas in other cases no disease mechanism can be identi-fied. One cause of protein-losing enteropathy is a disorder of lymphatics leading to leakage of lymph into the gastrointestinal lumen. Intestinal lymphangiectasia, cardiac diseases, and Whipple's disease exhibit this kind of loss mechanism. A second cause is that of gastrointestinal inflam-mation leading to leakage of protein-rich inflammatory exudate. Finally, the local release of vasoactive amines with consequent change in the mucosal permeability may be a third mechanism of protein-losing enter-opathy; allergic gastroenteropathy, and perhaps gluten-sensitive enter-opathy, are candidates for this disease mechanism. These various disease mechanisms explain some but not all of the causes of protein-losing enter-opathy, and in many instances the cause of this physiological derange-ment is undefined. Whatever the mechanism of protein-losing enteropathy involved, it is clear that in many instances hypoalbuminemia and hypo-gammaglobulinemia may be the presenting problem, and gastrointestinal symptoms may be quite minimal or nonexistent. In such instances the techniques for demonstrating abnormalities of immunoglobulin metab-olism and for demonstrating excessive gastrointestinal protein loss may be the only way of identifying the intestinal tract as the site of disease.

The prototype of the lymphatic disorders is intestinal lymphangiectasia, a generalized disorder of lymphatic channels characterized by extreme hypoalbuminemia, hypogammaglobulinemia, edema, and, in certain cases, chylous effusions (Waldmann et al., 1961; Strober et al., 1967). The hallmark morphological lesion of this disease is dilated lymphatic channels in the small bowel. It can result from abnormalities in the development of central and peripheral lymphatics, or alternatively it can result from a disease process with secondary blockage of lymphatics as in protein-losing enteropathy associated with cardiac disease or protein-losing en-teropathy associated with lymphoma. The protein-losing enteropathy with hypogammaglobulinemia and short immunoglobulin survival of intestinal lymphangiectasia is associated with a striking lymphocytopenia. This is due to the gastrointestinal loss of lymphocyte-rich lymph, and it may be said that the patients with intestinal lymphangiectasia have a functional equivalent of a thoracic duct fistula. In intestinal lymphangiectasia one observes a preferential depletion of the cells involved in *in vitro* lymphocyte cell-mediated immune functions and impaired *in vitro* transformation to nonspecific mitogens, specific antigens, and allogeneic cells when compared with equal numbers of mononuclear cells from normal individuals. On a clinical level this is associated with depressed, delayed hypersensitivity responses and inability to reject skin grafts from unrelated donors.

It is clear that patients with protein-losing enteropathy secondary to disorders of intestinal lymphatics may present with clinical features that are quite similar to those of patients with combined immunodeficiency. Both groups of patients may have hypoalbuminemia, hypogammaglobulinemia, diarrhea, extreme lymphocytopenia, abnormalities of *in vitro* lymphocyte transformation, and skin anergy. The use of immunoglobulin metabolic studies and tests using ^{51}Cr-labeled albumin may be of value in differentiating these disorders; the patient with combined immunodeficiency will be found to have profoundly decreased synthesis of immunoglobulin molecules as their abnormality whereas those with intestinal lymphangiectasia have a reduction in immunoglobulin survival and have excessive excretion of ^{51}Cr-labeled albumin into the gastrointestinal tract. The distinction between these two diseases may be critical, since the mode of therapy of these disorders is quite different. The immunodeficiency of patients with combined immunodeficiency has been completely reversed following transplantation of bone marrow from a compatible donor (Good, 1971) whereas the immunodeficiency of patients with protein and lymphocyte loss into the gastrointestinal tract due to cardiac disorders have been completely reversed by surgical correction of the cardiac defects and have been ameliorated in patients with intestinal lymphangiectasia by the use of a diet wherein middle-chain triglycerides are substituted for long-chain triglycerides.

2. Hypogammaglobulinemia Associated with Protein Loss into the Urinary Tract

Urinary protein loss of intact immunoglobulin molecules resulting in hypogammaglobulinemia is usually associated with a disorder of the glomerulus characterized by increased permeability to serum proteins. In such cases the sieving function of the glomerulus is only partially lost, and the predominant proteins that escape into the urine are those of intermediate molecular weight (MW 50,000–200,000) whereas very large molecules continue to be retained. Albumin is by far the predominant protein in the urine of such patients, but in addition there is massive proteinuria involving other proteins of slightly larger size, such as IgG and IgA. In contrast, the very large IgM molecules are retained by the glomerulus and do not appear in high concentrations in the urine. This evidence of selective loss of proteins through the glomerular filter contrasts with the nonselective bulk loss of immunoglobulins described above for patients with protein-losing enteropathy.

When patients with urinary loss are studied by means of metabolic turnover techniques, the total circulating and total body pools of immunoglobulins of intermediate molecular weight are found to be reduced. These pool size abnormalities cannot be explained by deficient protein synthesis since the absolute synthetic rate of IgG is above the normal range in almost all the patients studied. On the contrary, the explanation for the reduced pool abnormality is found in the survival side of the metabolic process. Serum survivals of IgG are decreased, and the fractional disappearance rates of these proteins are elevated.

The major factor in the increased disappearance rates of these proteins is a marked increase in the rate of their loss as intact protein into the urine. However, an additional factor accounting for the increased fractional disappearance rate in about 80% of the patients with glomerular disease is an increased endogenous fractional catabolic rate for IgG. In the majority of patients this is due to the passage of molecules through the diseased glomerulus and into the tubular lumen where they are taken up by and catabolized in tubular cells. In addition to this tubular catabolism, in a minority of cases another cause of the increased fractional catabolic rate in the patients with glomerular disease is occult protein-losing enteropathy of obscure origin. In summary, the predominant factor in the hypogammaglobulinemia of the nephrotic syndrome is loss of intact protein into the urine with increased tubular uptake and catabolism of these proteins playing a minor supplementary role.

3. Hypogammaglobulinemia Associated with Endogenous Hypercatabolism Affecting Several Serum Proteins

Another group of disorders that have the pattern of hypogammaglobulinemia and a short survival of several serum proteins are the disorders of endogenous serum protein catabolism in which more than one immunoglobulin class is affected. The first example we shall describe is familial hypercatabolic hypoproteinemia (Waldmann et al., 1968). This latter term has been applied to the condition observed in two siblings, the product of a first-cousin marriage, who had bone abnormalities including bilateral bowing of the radii bones, abnormal glucose metabolism, and low albumin and IgG levels. One of the patients also had necrobiosis, lipoidica diabeticorum, thrombocytopenia, and increased incidence of infections. The patients had a marked reduction of serum IgG and albumin concentrations associated with slightly reduced IgM concentrations and a normal or slightly elevated IgA and IgE concentrations. The patients had total circulating IgG pools that were less than 15% of normal. The rate of IgG synthesis was essentially normal, but the fractional catabolic rate was markedly increased. The fractional catabolic rate for IgG was 35% of the intravenous pool per day, 5 times the normal mean of 6.7% per day. The survivals of albumin and IgA were also significantly reduced in these patients. These patients did not have proteinuria and, in addition, protein loss into the gastrointestinal tract was excluded by normal ^{51}Cr-labeled albumin excretion rates. Other causes of generalized protein hypercatabolism (as discussed below) were investigated but were not present. It was concluded that the hypogammaglobulinemia could not be explained on the basis of a mechanism heretofore described, and these patients can be said to have a new disease, the chief feature of which appears to be endogenous hypercatabolism affecting several serum proteins.

A second disorder with a generalized hypercatabolism of several classes of immunoglobulin molecules as well as albumin is observed in patients with the Wiskott–Aldrich syndrome (Blaese *et al.*, 1971). Metabolic turnover studies with purified immunoglobulins have shown that the synthetic rate of all classes of immunoglobulins studied were elevated in these patients. On the other hand, the fractional catabolic rate of all immunoglobulins and albumin was increased. These high fractional catabolic rates were obscured by the elevated synthetic rates resulting in normal or elevated serum concentrations of all the major immunoglobulins with the exception of IgM. There was a slight increase of loss of serum proteins into the gastrointestinal tract in these patients; however, the predominant disorder in immunoglobulin metabolism was accelerated catabolism. This was quite possibly related to increased activity of the reticuloendothelial system, but this is by no means proved.

4. Hypogammaglobulinemia Associated with Endogenous Hypercatabolism Affecting a Single Class of Immunoglobulin Molecules

Another pattern of disordered immunoglobulin metabolism is characterized by hypercatabolism affecting a single immunoglobulin class. The first representative of this pattern to be characterized was the disorder myotonic dystrophy (Wochner *et al.*, 1966), a hereditary muscle abnormality with dominant transmittance and associated with frontal baldness, testicular atrophy, and endocrinopathy. Patients with this disorder had normal albumin, IgM, IgA, IgD, and IgE concentrations associated with normal metabolic parameters for these proteins. In contrast, the serum IgG concentration and circulating IgG pool size was distinctly reduced and the survival of ^{125}I-labeled normal IgG or IgG purified from patients with myotonic dystrophy was markedly shortened. IgG survival half-times averaged 11.4 days in the patients compared to 22.9 days in the controls and a mean of 14% of the circulating IgG was catabolized per day in the patients compared to 6.8% per day in the controls. Thus, the reduced IgG concentration of patients with myotonic dystrophy appears to be due solely to a disorder of endogenous hypercatabolism involving the IgG immunoglobulin class specifically.

Hypogammaglobulinemia associated with a short IgG immunoglobulin survival also has been demonstrated in a variety of patients with connective tissue disorders. Rheumatoid arthritis and systemic lupus erythematosus (SLE) are instances where one finds decreased survival of IgG (Wochner, 1970). In these cases one may also find decreased survival of IgM associated with normal or increased synthetic rates for the immunoglobulins. One might expect abnormal protein–protein interactions to account for the short survival, but studies to define such interactions as the cause of hypercatabolism have not been fruitful and the cause of the altered protein survival in these connective tissue diseases remains unexplained.

Another clinically significant condition in which a short survival of a single protein is observed is in patients with isolated IgA deficiency or IgA deficiency associated with ataxia-telangiectasia. In the study of the metabolism of all classes of immunoglobulins in such patients it was found that the primary defect leading to IgA deficiency was decreased IgA synthesis (Strober *et al.*, 1968). In addition, however, several patients had a markedly decreased survival of injected radiolabeled IgA proteins associated with fractional catabolic rates 4–20 times normal. Using a variety of techniques it was shown that this shortened IgA survival was due to the presence of circulating anti-IgA antibodies in such patients. Subsequently it was found that anti-IgA antibodies are common in many patients with IgA deficiency (Vyas *et al.*, 1968) and an exceedingly short survival of IgA is present in all patients with isolated IgA deficiency who have antibodies directed against this immunoglobulin class. Patients with such antibodies against IgA may have severe anaphylactoid reactions when blood products containing even very small amounts of IgA are administered, suggesting that, in general, the transfusion of plasma must be given with care to patients who lack one or another serum component.

B. HYPOGAMMAGLOBULINEMIA ASSOCIATED WITH DECREASED IMMUNOGLOBULIN SYNTHESIS

1. Hypogammaglobulinemia Associated with Decreased Synthesis of All Immunoglobulin Classes

Combined immunodeficiency, X-linked agammaglobulinemia, and common variable immunodeficiency constitute a complex of diseases with different defects in the pathways of cellular differentiation, cellular interaction, and cellular biosynthesis that are required for the normal immune response (Good, 1971). These defects include failure of the development of stem cell precursors of immunocompetent cells, failure of differentiation of stem cells into B cells, and failure of terminal differentiation of B cells into plasma cells that produce immunoglobulins. In addition, we have recently observed that a subset of the patients with common variable hypogammaglobulinemia have an abnormality of regulatory T cells which act to suppress B-cell maturation and antibody production (Waldmann *et al.*, 1974).

Although the primary defects are different, these various immunodeficiencies have a common pattern of immunoglobulin metabolism. In all patients of this group one finds a marked reduction in the circulating and total body pool sizes of all immunoglobulin classes associated with a profound defect in the synthesis of each of the immunoglobulin classes. In all patients the survival and fractional catabolic rates of IgM, IgA, IgD, and IgE are normal whereas the fractional catabolic rate of IgG is reduced and the survival is prolonged. This reduced fractional catabolic rate for IgG is in accord with the physiological concentration–catabolism effect which is specific to IgG metabolism. By concentration–catabolism effect we refer to the fact that the fractional catabolic rate for IgG molecules varies directly with the serum concentration of IgG in both man and rodents; thus, as the concentration of IgG rises as a result of endogenous IgG production or as a result of IgG infusion, the fractional catabolic rate increases (Fahey and Robinson, 1963; Waldmann and Strober, 1969). In man the fraction of the intervascular pool of IgG catabolized daily rises as the serum concentration rises from 2% in patients with extreme hypogammaglobulinemia to a limit of 16–18% in patients with very elevated serum IgG concentrations. Evidence is available to suggest that this concentration–catabolism effect could be explained by postulating the presence of a saturable carrier-mediated protection system for IgG molecules that is similar to the mechanism involved in transplacental transport of IgG molecules from maternal circulation to the fetal circulation or the transport of IgG molecules across the gut of the newborn rodent (Waldmann and Jones, 1973; Brambell *et al.*, 1964). In the case of IgG catabolism this carrier-mediated protection system could operate as IgG molecules are transported across vascular barriers as they move from one body compartment to another.

It should be noted that patients with hypogammaglobulinemia primarily due to decreased immunoglobulin synthesis may develop gastrointestinal disorders associated with excessive protein loss into the gastrointestinal tract. In this case the primary defect in γ-globulin synthesis may coexist with decreased immunoglobulin survival secondary to loss of proteins into the gastrointestinal tract. Thus, the latter abnormality should be suspected as an associated feature in patients with defective synthesis of immunoglobulin when the survival of IgG molecules is shorter than would be predicted on the basis of the IgG serum concentration. When the gastrointestinal disorder is identified and successfully treated, the survival of the proteins will return to normal, but the underlying defect in immunoglobulin synthesis will persist.

2. Hypogammaglobulinemia Associated with Decreased Synthesis of Some, but Not All, Immunoglobulin Classes

Defects of immunoglobulin synthesis may not affect all classes of immunoglobulin molecules but be restricted to one or two classes of proteins. Here the primary defect is the failure of development of certain classes of B cells or, more frequently, the failure of terminal differentiation of Ig-bearing B cells of certain classes into immunoglobulin-secreting plasma cells. In such patients the survival of the deficient classes of immunoglobulins is usually normal, but as noted it may be markedly shortened when the patients produce antibodies to the deficient class. The most common form of selective immunoglobulin deficiency is the absence of IgA with normal levels of IgG and IgM. In addition, IgA deficiency may be frequently accompanied by a similar deficiency of IgE synthesis. This immune abnormality may occur either as an isolated defect or in association with the features of ataxia-telangiectasia.

A second form of selective immunoglobulin deficiency is characterized by reduction in the serum concentration of IgG and IgA and an increased concentration of IgM. This disorder of serum immunoglobulin concentration is due to abnormalities of synthesis of the different classes of immunoglobulin molecules, not to disorders of catabolism. The mechanism in this group is obscure and may involve a maturation arrest of lymphoid cells.

C. HYPERGAMMAGLOBULINEMIA ASSOCIATED WITH INCREASED IMMUNOGLOBULIN SYNTHESIS

An increased serum concentration of immunoglobulins or their sub-units may occur secondary to a variety of pathophysiological mechanisms with different patterns of immunoglobulin metabolism. Such hyper-gammaglobulinemia may be due to a diffuse increase in the synthesis of all classes of immunoglobulin molecules as in patients with cirrhosis of the liver, connective tissue diseases, or the chronic infectious diseases. Such patients have an increase in the pool sizes of all classes of immuno-globulin molecules due to increased synthesis. The survival of IgA and IgM is frequently normal in these patients. The survival of IgG is usually reduced, in part due to the IgG concentration-catabolism effect and in part due to hypermetabolism associated with these disorders and, in patients with the connective tissue diseases, due to additional factors that have not been fully defined.

A second pattern of immunoglobulin metabolism resulting in hyper-gammaglobulinemia is the increased rate of synthesis of a single class of immunoglobulins seen in patients with paraproteinemias: multiple myeloma, benign monoclonal gammopathy, or macroglobulinemia of Waldenström. In patients with such disorders there is a defect leading to the increased production of immunoglobulins restricted in electro-phoretic mobility usually containing one class of heavy chain and one class of light chains. In the majority of patients with paraproteinemia there are also reduced pool sizes and synthetic rates of normal poly-clonal immunoglobulins.

D. HYPERGAMMAGLOBULINEMIA (OF IMMUNOGLOBULIN FRAGMENTS) ASSOCIATED WITH PROLONGED IMMUNOGLOBULIN FRAGMENT SURVIVAL

Increased concentration of immunoglobulin fragments may also occur owing to decreased catabolism in patients with certain forms of renal diseases.

Metabolic studies using representative small proteins or immuno-globulin fragments such as λ light-chain dimers (MW 44,000) and representative proteins of intermediate size, IgG (MW 160,000) have provided insights into the role of the kidney in the metabolism of immunoglobulin molecules and their fragments as well as an understanding of the disorders of the metabolism of these proteins in renal disease (Waldmann *et al.*, 1972b). Low-molecular-weight proteins, such as light chains, readily pass through glomerular filter and are largely taken up and catabolized by tubular cells. For this class of molecular fragments, the kidney is the primary organ of catabolism. Proteins of intermediate and high molecular weight are generally retained by the glomerular filter and therefore do not normally have a significant exposure to tubular catabolic sites. For this class of proteins the kidney is not normally a primary organ of catabolism. In patients with uremia and loss of entire nephrons the serum concentration of light chains is markedly increased. This cannot be explained by an increased rates of synthesis of light chains, which is normal in these patients, but can be accounted for by prolonged serum light-chain survival associated with comparable reductions in the fractional catabolic rate for these proteins. Presumably the reduced fractional catabolic rate and prolonged survival of light chains results from the loss of functional renal tissue and entire nephrons. Thus, the light chains were not filtered through the glomerulus and not exposed to their normal catabolic site, the renal tubule, resulting in the decreased metabolism of these molecules and their accumulation in the circulation. In patients with proximal tubular diseases, as seen in individuals with cystinosis or the adult Fanconi syndrome, the serum concentrations, pool sizes, synthetic rates, and survival of IgG and light chains are normal. Similarly the glomerular permeability for light chain is normal in the patients with tubular disorders. These normal metabolic parameters in patients with tubular disease occurred in association with vastly increased quantities of low-molecular-weight proteins, such as light chain in the urine and vastly increased fractional proteinuric rates for these proteins. It appears that this high rate of excretion of light chains in the patients with tubular disease is due to the failure of the proximal tubule of the kidney to take up and catabolize these small proteins, which are normally filtered through the glomerulus. However, since the normal route of light-chain disposal tubular catabolism, is counterbalanced by urinary excretion of the intact protein, the overall rate of metabolism remains unchanged and no protein accumulates in the circulation.

VI. Summary

Techniques for the study of immunoglobulin metabolism using purified radioiodinated serum proteins have been developed to define the factors controlling the rates of immunoglobulin synthesis, catabolism, and transport. These techniques have been of value in studying the pathogenesis of abnormalities of immunoglobulin levels seen in various immunodeficiency diseases and have even resulted in the discovery of new forms of immunodeficiency disease. These techniques have also been of value in differential diagnosis of immunodeficiency states and in addition provide the information necessary for the rational use of γ-globulin or its subunits as therapeutic tools.

Disorders of immunoglobulin pool size and concentration occur secondary to a variety of pathophysiological mechanisms that are associated with a variety of different patterns of immunoglobulin metabolism. At one end of the metabolic processes are the disorders characterized by decreased immunoglobulin synthesis. This may involve decreased synthesis of all classes of immunoglobulins or it may involve decreased synthesis of selective classes of immunoglobulins. At the other end of the metabolic process are disorders characterized by a short survival of immunoglobulin. This short immunoglobulin survival may be caused by excessive loss of immunoglobulins into the urinary or gastrointestinal tracts. Alternatively, hypogammaglobulinemia may be due to a disorder of endogenous catabolic pathways that affect a single immunoglobulin class or all immunoglobulin classes.

Hypergammaglobulinemia also may occur owing to a variety of pathophysiological mechanisms that are associated with different patterns of immunoglobulin metabolism. Hypergammaglobulinemia may be caused by a diffuse increase in synthesis of immunoglobulins or increased synthesis of a single class of monoclonal immunoglobulin. Alternatively in patients with renal disease there may be an increased level of immunoglobulin fragments such as light chains in the serum secondary to decreased catabolism of these immunoglobulin subunits.

References

Blaese, R. M., Strober, W., Levy, A. L., and Waldmann, T. A. (1971). Hypercatabolism of IgG, IgA, IgM and albumin in the Wiskott Aldrich syndrome. *J. Clin. Invest.* **50**, 2331–2338.

Borsook, H., and Keighley, G. L. (1935). The "continuing" metabolism of nitrogen in animals. *Proc. Roy. Soc., Ser. B* **118**, 448–521.

Brambell, F. W. R., Hemmings, W. A., and Morris, I. G. (1964). A theoretical model of γ-globulin catabolism. *Nature (London)* **203**, 1352–1355.

Fahey, J. L., and Robinson, A. G. (1963). Factors controlling serum γ-globulin concentration. *J. Exp. Med.* **118**, 845–868.

Freund, J., and Whitney, C. E. (1928). The distribution of antibodies in the serum and organs of rabbits. II. The effect of perfusion upon the antibody content of serum and organs. *J. Immunol.* **15**, 369–380.

Glenny, A. T., and Hopkins, B. E. (1923). Duration of passive immunity. Part III. *J. Hyg.* **22**, 12–36.

Good, R. A. (1971). Immunodeficiency in developmental perspective. *Harvey Lect.* **67**, 1–107.

McFarlane, A. S. (1958). Effective trace-labelling of proteins with iodine. *Nature* (*London*) **182**, 53.

Morell, A., Terry, W. D., and Waldmann, T. A. (1970). Metabolic properties of IgG subclasses in man. *J. Clin. Invest.* **49**, 673–680.

Schoenheimer, R. (1942). "The Dynamic State of Body Constituents." Harvard Univ. Press, Cambridge, Massachusetts.

Spiegelberg, H. L., and Weigle, W. O. (1965). Studies on the catabolism of γG subunits and chains. *J. Immunol.* **95**, 1034–1048.

Spiegelberg, H. L., Fishkin, B. G., and Grey, H. M. (1968). Catabolism of human γG-immunoglobulins of different heavy chain subclasses. I. Catabolism of γG-myeloma proteins in man. *J. Clin. Invest.* **47**, 2323–2330.

Strober, W., Wochner, R. D., Carbone, P. P., and Waldmann, T. A. (1967). Intestinal lymphangiectasia: A protein-losing enteropathy with hypogammaglobulinemia, lymphocytopenia and impaired homograft rejection. *J. Clin. Invest.* **46**, 1643–1656.

Strober, W., Wochner, R. D., Barlow, M. H., McFarlin, D. E., and Waldmann, T. A. (1968). Immunoglobulin metabolism in ataxia telangiectasia. *J. Clin. Invest.* **47**, 1905–1915.

Vyas, G. N., Perkins, H. A., and Fudenberg, H. H. (1968). Anaphylactic reactions associated with anti-IgA. *Lancet* **2**, 312–315.

Waldmann, T. A. (1966). Protein-losing enteropathy. *Gastroenterology* **50**, 422–443.

Waldmann, T. A., and Jones, E. A. (1973). The role of cell-surface receptors in the transport and catabolism of immunoglobulins. *In* "Protein Turnover," Ciba Found. Symp. No. 9 [New Ser.], pp. 5–23. Associated Scientific Publishers, Amsterdam.

Waldmann, T. A., and Strober, W. (1969). Metabolism of immunoglobulins. *Progr. Allergy* **13**, 1–110.

Waldmann, T. A., Steinfeld, J. L., Dutcher, T. F., Davidson, J. D., and Gordon, R. S., Jr. (1961). The role of the gastrointestinal system in "idiopathic hypoproteinemia." *Gastroenterology* **41**, 197–208.

Waldmann, T. A., Miller, E. J., and Terry, W. D. (1968). Hypercatabolism of IgG and albumin: A new familiar disorder. *Clin. Res.* **16**, 45.

Waldmann, T. A., Wochner, R. D., and Strober, W. (1969). The role of the gastrointestinal tract in plasma protein metabolism. *Amer. J. Med.* **46**, 275–285.

Waldmann, T. A., Polmar, S. H., Balestra, S. T., Jost, M. C., Bruce, R. M., and Terry, W. D. (1972a). Immunoglobulin E in immunologic deficiency disease. II. Serum IgE concentration of patients with acquired hypogammaglobulinemia, thymoma and hypogammaglobulinemia, myotonic dystrophy, intestinal lymphangiectasia and Wiskott-Aldrich syndrome. *J. Immunol.* **109**, 304–310.

Waldmann, T. A., Strober, W., and Mogielnicki, R. P. (1972b). The renal handling of low molecular weight proteins. II. Disorders of serum protein catabolism in patients with tubular proteinuria, nephrosis, or uremia. *J. Clin. Invest.* **51**, 2162–2174.

Waldmann, T. A., Broder, S., Durm, M., Blackman, M., Blaese, R. M., and Strober, W. (1974). The role of suppressor T cells in the pathogenesis of common variable hypogammaglobulinemia. *Lancet* **2**, 609–613.

Wochner, R. D. (1970). Hypercatabolism of normal IgG an unexplained immunoglobulin abnormality in connective tissue diseases. *J. Clin. Invest.* **49**, 454–464.

Wochner, R. D., Drews, G., Strober, W., and Waldmann, T. A. (1966). Accelerated breakdown of immunoglobulin G (IgG) in myotonic dystrophy: A hereditary error of immunoglobulin catabolism. *J. Clin. Invest.* **45**, 321–329.

Wochner, R. D., Strober, W., and Waldmann, T. A. (1967). The role of the kidney in the catabolism of Bence Jones proteins and immunoglobulin fragments. *J. Exp. Med.* **126**, 207–221.

Cell-Mediated Immunity: *In Vivo* Testing[1]

CARL M. PINSKY

Memorial Sloan-Kettering Cancer Center, New York, New York

I. Introduction

In this chapter, we present methods that have been useful in assessing cell-mediated immunity (CMI) *in vivo*. These techniques involve the elicitation of cutaneous hypersensitivity reactions. We test the efferent arm of the immune response by injecting a series of bacterial, fungal, and viral antigens intradermally and measuring the delayed (usually 48 hours) reactions. In addition, we test the patient's capability for *de novo* immune response by applying 2,4-dinitrochlorobenzene (DNCB) on the skin and challenging him with graded doses of the chemical 2–3 weeks later.

It had been known since the work of Landsteiner and Chase in the 1940s, that both intradermal and contact delayed cutaneous hypersensitivity reactions are mediated by immunologically committed cells. They showed that contact sensitivity to DNCB (and other halogenated nitrobenzenes), as well as tuberculin sensitivity, could be transferred to nonimmunized guinea pigs by cells (but not sera) from immunized animals.

[1] Aided by grants from National Cancer Institute (CA05826) and American Cancer Society (CIA275).

The clinical importance of cell-mediated immune reactions is beyond the scope of this discussion. Suffice it to say that CMI is responsible for resistance against protozoa, viruses, fungi, and many bacteria, and may be responsible for resistance against progressive neoplasia. In addition, the rejection of allografts and xenografts, as well as the pathogenesis of many "autoimmune" diseases depends, in large part, on the existence of cellular (delayed-type) hypersensitivity.

From the turn of the twentieth century, it has been known that individuals who were exposed to the tubercle bacillus developed delayed cutaneous hypersensitivity reactions following the intradermal injection of tuberculin. In fact, until the last several decades virtually all adults were reactive to tuberculin. In areas where tuberculosis is endemic or where BCG (Bacillus Calmette-Guérin) is widely used, this situation persists today.

On the other hand, patients with Hodgkin's disease or with sarcoidosis were usually nonreactive to tuberculin. This anergy, coupled with the fact that tuberculosis often developed in such patients, suggested to early workers that these diseases were unusual forms of tuberculosis. Evidence to the contrary arose from reports, employing a "battery" of skin test antigens, which demonstrated that the anergy was not confined to tuberculin but extended to all skin test antigens that were used. Such patients usually fail to become sensitized to DNCB, as well. Yet they are capable of mounting antibody responses after appropriate immunization. By contrast, patients with agammaglobulinemia, who do not make antibodies well and resist many bacterial infections poorly, but are able to resist fungal, viral, and other bacterial infections quite well, can develop delayed cutaneous hypersensitivity on intradermal challenge and usually respond normally to sensitization with DNFB or DNCB. These observations suggested to Good, and others, that the immune system was composed of two major sections—one responsible for antibody-mediated reactions and the other for cell-mediated reactions (Ehrlich, Metchnikoff, Chase, and others, had speculated along these lines years earlier).

These pioneering studies (and many others that are referred to in the review articles cited under References) clearly establish the necessity of testing cellular immunity as part of immunological studies. While *in vitro* methods are rapidly becoming available (e.g., Cunningham-Rundles *et al.*, this volume), *in vivo* tests employing skin test "batteries" are indispensable for this purpose. Not only are the results one experts in normal populations well known, but also, only with *in vivo* techniques can one avoid many of the artifacts inherent *in vitro*. Of course, skin testing has some disadvantages, and these will be pointed out.

II. Skin Test Battery

In order to ensure that suspected defects in CMI are real, not just apparent owing to inadequate test procedures, clinical investigators have combined several tests. This is particularly important when using antigens which the patient is presumed to have encountered previously. If a patient is unresponsive to any single antigen (even if its distribution is widespread), one cannot conclude that the system is defective; the individual may not have had prior exposure. One way to obviate this difficulty is to combine tests with several antigens, proving with appropriate control groups (concurrent or historical) that all normal individuals (or virtually all) do respond to at least one of the antigens in the group. If the patient under investigation fails to respond at all, then the presumption of immunodeficiency is supported.

How many, and which, antigens to use has not been conclusively determined. We, and most other investigators, have found that challenging with four antigens, from commonly encountered bacterial, viral, and fungal organisms, induces at least one clear reaction in close to 100% of apparently healthy individuals. We use: Dermatophytin "0"® (1:100), an extract from *Candida albicans*, distributed by Hollister-Stier, Co.; mumps skin test antigen, Eli Lilly and Co.; tuberculin purified protein derivative (PPD)-intermediate strength (5TU), Connaught Laboratories; and streptokinase/streptodornase (Varidase®, Lederle Division of American Cyanamid Company), diluted so that the final concentration is streptokinase 4 units/0.1 ml and streptodornase $\geq$1 unit/0.1 ml). Careful intradermal injection of exactly 0.1 ml of each antigen is performed usually on the forearm (but we have occasionally used the thigh). All tests are read at 48 hours. When possible, the reactions are also examined at 6 and 24 hours. If logistics prevent seeing the patients subsequently, they are instructed to inform us of new reactions or intensification of existing reactions that occur later. At the time of each reading, the diameter (in round reactions) or the two maximum diameters at right angles (in oval reactions) of both erythema and induration are recorded. By convention, induration $\geq$5 mm at 48 hours is considered positive, but the actual readings should be recorded.

Another way to avoid the difficulty of not knowing about a patient's prior exposure to antigens in the test battery is to expose him to a new antigen at the time of testing. This technique has the additional advantage of testing the entire immunological arc from exposure to response, not just the efferent arm. Once immunization and challenge has been accomplished, however, subsequent rechallenges with the same antigen test only the efferent arm of the immune response.

The antigen we use to test a patient's ability to develop CMI *de novo* is DNCB. Solutions of DNCB in acetone are prepared, as follows. Stock Solution: 2 gm/100 ml = 2 mg/0.1 ml; appropriate dilution in acetone to achieve solutions with 25, 50, 100, and 200 μg/0.1 ml. Sensitization requires 2 mg (or 0.1 ml of stock solution). The usual test dose is 100 μg, but the other strengths may be used to grade the response.

We usually administer the sensitizing dose on the inner upper arm, with testing carried out on the ipsilateral forearm. The skin is first cleansed with acetone. With the tester wearing gloves, the DNCB is applied to each site, confined within a plastic ring, 2 cm in inside diameter. The doses used on the first day are 25 μg, 100 μg, and 2 mg. If one starts with the lowest concentration and works up, the same ring can be used throughout. The solution is allowed to evaporate, and the site is covered by a 1-inch bandage for 48 hours, care being taken to keep the areas dry. After 48 hours an intense erythematous reaction is expected at the 2-mg site. If this does not occur, a defect in the inflammatory system is probably present and failure to mount reactions at the lower test doses, later, cannot be taken as evidence of deficient CMI. On the other hand, induration at the 100-μg site is evidence for preexisting immunity to DNCB. In such cases, DNCB testing is unable to measure *de novo* immunity.

After 9 or 10 days, some patients who previously had no reaction at the 100-μg site of DNCB, develop a reaction without further challenge. This is taken as evidence of *de novo* immunity, and no further testing is necessary. In occasional patients, such reactions appear even later. Applying 25 μg and 100 μg on the day of sensitization serves two purposes. First, it detects patients with preexisting immunity to DNCB; and, second, it prevents the application of a full test dose to a patient who has developed a high degree of sensitivity.

If no reaction is seen at the test sites by 14–21 days, challenge doses of 25 μg and 100 μg are applied (other doses may be used, as well). A test at any site is considered positive if there is induration (with or without erythema) $\geq$5 mm in diameter at 48 hours.

Several groups of investigators have described modifications of the DNCB technique described above. In general, these are designed to avoid equivocal reactions. Since equivocal reactions are encountered rarely, in our experience, and since the newer techniques have not yet been adequately standardized in normal populations, we continue to use the technique described.

III. Results

Individuals with normal CMI are expected to react to at least one of the intradermal skin tests and to develop contact hypersensitivity to 100 μg of DNCB. Actually, when apparently normal individuals are studied, up to 5% of them are nonreactive. To our knowledge there has not been a study in which such individuals are followed periodically. One wonders whether they would be prone to frequent infections and the subsequent development of neoplasia. Chase, who developed two strains of guinea pigs, one with high and the other with low frequencies of contact hypersensitivity reactions, did not observe neoplasia in either strain, but prolonged observation was not carried out in the latter.

Of the two techniques, intradermal tests for preexisting immunity seem to have more inherent technical difficulties than *de novo* tests for contact sensitization. In the first place, no battery can be developed which ensures that the patient being tested has had adequate prior exposure to antigen. Immunity wanes with time, and even a history of exposure does not imply present immunity. Also, the initial exposure may have been weak in the first place.

Another disadvantage of intradermal testing is that the presence of antibodies to the test antigen may interfere with delayed reactions in various ways. Local, fixed antibodies of the reaginic type, lead to anaphylactic, wheal-and-flare reactions after the injection of the appropriate antigen. While these reactions disappear long before one attempts to measure a delayed reaction, and hence do not make reading the test more difficult, the inflammation and dilation of small blood vessels that accompanies such reactions may permit the antigen to be carried away before the delayed reaction can be mounted. This, in effect, obviates one major advantage in intradermal injection, namely, establishing an antigenic depot.

The presence of circulating antibodies can result in a reaction intermediate between the immediate type and the delayed type, called an Arthus reaction. It usually appears at 4–6 hours after administration of antigen and may last 24–36 hours. Therefore, it may be fading at just the time that a delayed reaction will be appearing. So that, in addition to allowing for early antigen loss, the Arthus reaction may make it more difficult to read a subsequent delayed-type response. The gross appearance of Arthus and delayed hypersensitivity reactions are both characterized by erythema and thickening of the skin. But Arthus reactions are more edematous than indurated. This distinction may not be easy to make, and often one decides on the basis of time relationships, not of gross appearance. Histologically, Arthus reactions contain more acute inflammatory and fewer mononuclear cells than delayed hypersensitivity reactions, but vasculitis is present in both and biopsy is usually unwarranted just to make this decision.

Finally, aside from making subsequent interpretation of the gross reaction difficult and leading to antigen loss, antibody-mediated reactions may interfere in one other way. Antigen–antibody complexes can "block" the full expression of lymphocyte-mediated reactions to the same antigen. While this observation is best shown with *in vitro* techniques, there is no doubt that the phenomenon operates *in vivo* as well.

Both contact and intradermal tests are difficult to interpret occasionally for another reason. Some reactions do not have clear-cut edges, and judging where the induration ends is difficult. This is particularly true when erythema extends beyond the indurated border.

Systemic hypersensitivity reactions (anaphylaxis, tuberculin "shock," etc.) also are theoretically more likely after intradermal injection than after application of an antigen to the skin, since intravenous administration is virtually impossible in the latter instance. It is not too cautious to suggest that the tester should have appropriate medications and staff available to manage anaphylaxis when antigens are injected.

Extensive local necrotizing reactions are possible if full doses of antigen are administered to sensitive individuals. A carefully obtained history is not always adequate, but will probably help to avoid most problems. Most patients know whether they have had tuberculosis or reactive tuberculin tests, mumps, frequent streptococcal infections, or thrush.

On the other hand, prior exposure to DNCB (or DNFB) is almost never remembered by the patient. While preexisting immunity was seen in only 1 or 2% of our patients, most did not know of any prior exposure. Their histories suggest that DNCB may be present in some dyes (used by pottery-makers or photographers) and in some refrigeration solutions. At any rate, hydrocortisone 1% cream applied several times a day, liberally, clears up local reactions within a few days.

When immunizing a patient with DNCB, one should be aware that challenge doses at 2–3 weeks may result in negative tests, but that rechallenge later may yield a normal response. We have frequently seen this type of response in patients with cancer. The investigator must be aware of this possibility to avoid incorrectly ascribing changes in skin tests to changes in disease activity or to the administration of an immunopotentiating agent. "Conversions" in skin test reactivity due to such an agent can be considered convincing only if a group of untreated anergic patients has a conversion rate lower than the treated group. On occasion, a similar delayed reaction is seen after intradermal injection of antigen. These delayed-positive responses may be the *in vivo* counterpart of the observation that lymphocytes which seem hyporeactive to antigen or mitogen at a given time, *in vitro*, respond quite well after longer incubation.

IV. Differential Diagnosis

Several patterns are possible when both intradermal tests for preexisting immunity and contact tests for *de novo* immunity are being used. When normal reactions are elicited in both types of tests, the presumption is made that the patient has a normal cellular immune system. When reactions are seen in neither type, there is strong presumption of a cellular immune defect. When there are reactions of preexisting immunity but failure to become immune to *de novo* challenge, various possibilities exist: (1) the defect has been acquired more recently than the time of exposure to the intradermal antigen(s); (2) the defect is in the recognition arm, only; (3) the defect is partial, and a stronger antigenic stimulus than DNCB might result in cell-mediated reaction, etc. When DNCB sensitization is successful, but no reactions of preexisting immunity are seen, again there are various possibilities: (1) intradermal injection was not accomplished; (2) one or more of the antigens may have been "blocked" by an Arthus reaction; (3) the patient may never have had adequate exposure to any of the antigens used; (4) exposure to one or more of the antigens may have been too long ago for immunity to persist, etc.

CMI is known to be defective in patients with lymphoma, sarcoidosis, many advanced cancers, and congenital or acquired immunodeficiency diseases; several other conditions may also be associated with measurable deficiencies—e.g., old age, advanced infections (particularly those associated with granulomata, such as tuberculosis and lepromatous leprosy), uremia. Also, some self-limited viral infections, such as measles, and vaccination may be associated with temporary cutaneous anergy. Irradiation therapy, thoracic duct lymphocyte drainage, and administration of corticosteroids and/or cancer chemotherapeutic agents are associated with immunosuppression. For the most part, discontinuance of such therapy is followed by immunological recovery, although this may take years (e.g., in the case of irradiation therapy). It has also been shown that, on occasion, successful treatment of malignancy is accompanied by recovery of CMI. In most cases, those patients who show immunological recovery are those who do (or are doing) well.

At this Center, we have concentrated on the study of skin-test re-activity in a group of patients with carcinoma, melanoma, and sarcoma. While patients with Hodgkin's disease, other lymphomas, and sarcoidosis have been well studied (see references), patients with the conditions we studied have largely been ignored in the past. It was generally assumed that patients with "solid" tumors are immunologically normal until the cancer becomes widely metastatic. This is not the case. While defective DNCB responses are seen earlier in some cancers than in others (e.g., DNCB reactivity is less frequent in patients with localized epidermoid carcinoma of the head and neck region than in patients with disseminated melanoma or sarcoma), in no instance, when prognosis of patients with the same disease and stage of disease is correlated with DNCB result, do patients who are DNCB-negative fare better than those who are DNCB-positive. The correlation is not complete, however, and patients with cutaneous anergy are found at all stages of cancer.

In summary, the use of skin tests for delayed hypersensitivity continues to be of value in the assessment of CMI in patients. Until *in vitro* techniques are developed that reflect all the factors affecting immunity in a patient, skin tests will be indispensable.

References

General

Aisenberg, A. C. (1966). *Cancer Res.* **26**, 1152–1160.
Benacerraf, B., and Green, I. (1969). *Annu. Rev. Med.* **20**, 141–154.
Chase, M. W. (1959a). *Toxicol. Appl. Pharmacol., Suppl.* **3**, 45–57.
Chase, M. W. (1959b). *In* "Cellular and Humoral Aspects of the Hypersensitive States" (H. S. Lawrence, ed.), pp. 251–279. Harper (Hoeber), New York.
Chase, M. W. (1966a). *Harvey Lect.* **61**, 169–203.
Chase, M. W. (1966b). *Cancer Res.* **26**, 1097–1120.
Chase, M. W., and Macher, E. (1971) *Advan. Biol. Skin* **11**, 63–93.
Eisen, H. N. (1959). *In* "Cellular and Humoral Aspects of the Hypersensitive States" (H. S. Lawrence, ed.), pp. 89–119. Harper (Hoeber), New York.
Friou, G. J. (1952). *Yale J. Biol. Med.* **24**, 533–539.
Good, R. A., Bridges, R. A., and Zak, S. J. (1959). *In* "Mechanisms of Hypersensitivity" (J. H. Shaffer, G. A. LoGrippo, and M. W. Chase, eds.), pp. 467–477. Little, Brown, Boston, Massachusetts.
Miller, S. D., and Jones, H. E. (1973). *Amer. Rev. Resp. Dis.* **107**, 530–538.
Park, B. H., and Good, R. A. (1974). "Principles of Modern Immunobiology." Lea & Febiger, Philadelphia, Pennsylvania.
Pepys, J. (1968). *In* "Clinical Aspects of Immunology" (P. G. H. Gell and R. R. A. Coombs, eds.), pp. 189–221. Davis, Philadelphia, Pennsylvania.
Schier, W. W. (1954). *N. Engl. J. Med.* **250**, 353–361.

Sokal, J. E. (1966). *Cancer Res.* **26**, 1161–1164.
Southam, C. M. (1968). *Cancer Res.* **28**, 1433–1440.
Uhr, J. W. (1966). *J. Neurophysiol.* **46**, 359–419.
Waksman, B. H. (1960). *Cell. Aspects Immunity, Ciba Found. Symp., 1959* pp. 280–323.
Waksman, B. H. (1971). *In* "Immunological Diseases" (M. Samter, ed.), Vol. I, pp. 220–252. Little, Brown, Boston, Massachusetts.

DNCB Testing

Brown, R. S., Haynes, H. A., and Foley, T. H. (1967). *Ann. Intern. Med.* **67**, 291–302.
Eilber, F. R., and Morton, D. L. (1970). *Cancer* **25**, 362–367.
Kligman, A. M., and Epstein, W. L. (1959). *In* "Mechanisms of Hypersensitivity" (J. H. Shaffer, G. A. LoGrippo, and M. W. Chase, eds.), pp. 713–722. Little, Brown, Boston, Massachusetts.
Pinsky, C. M., El Domeiri, A., Caron, A. S., *et al.* (1974). *Recent Results Cancer Res.* **47**, 37–41.

Cellular Immunity: Antibody-Dependent Cytotoxicity (K-Cell Activity)

PETER PERLMANN

Department of Immunology, Wenner-Gren Institute, University of Stockholm, Stockholm, Sweden

I. Introduction

Cell-mediated reactions are of major importance for tissue damage in connection with transplant or tumor rejection, autoimmune disease or delayed hypersensitivity. Tissue destruction is the end result of a long chain of specific and nonspecific reactions, difficult to analyze in the living animal. Therefore, many *in vitro* models have been designed in order to establish the cytotoxic potential of lymphocytes and macrophages, implicated as major effector cells in tissue-damaging immune responses.

When "immune" lymphocytes are incubated *in vitro* with target cells of relevant antigenicity, the latter are killed in an immunologically specific reaction. Thymus-derived lymphocytes (cytotoxic T-lymphocytes, CTL) act as effector cells in many of these reactions. CTL do not require IgG antibodies as specific recognition factors for target cell antigens. However, IgG antibodies also induce cell-mediated target cell destruction, but in this case different types of effector cells are involved.

Many cell types do have receptors for IgG (Fc receptors) and are capable of killing antibody-coated target cells *in vitro*. Good evidence exists that apparently *nonphagocytic, nonadherent lymphocytic cells* exhibit this activity. These killer cells are often called *K cells*, and this term will be used throughout this chapter. It should be noted that it is a strictly operational term, primarily chosen to help us to distinguish IgG-dependent killing of target cells (*K-cell activity*) from the antibody-independent CTL-mediated cytotoxicity mentioned above. Moreover, while lymphocytic K cells as defined above are distinct from mononuclear phagocytes, these latter cells are also known to have the potential of antibody-dependent nonphagocytic lysis of certain target cells. Thus, although in this chapter we will concentrate on a discussion of K-cell activity exhibited by lymphocytic effector cells, it should be realized that the antibody-dependent mononuclear effector cells found in many experimental systems are not always well defined entities.

We shall first discuss the results of model studies in which effector cells from normal donors and various target cells have been utilized to elucidate the mechanisms of the cytotoxic reaction and the nature of K-type effector cells. Thereafter we will discuss K-cell activity displayed by cells and antibodies from immune animals or patients and the possible biological relevance of these reactions.

II. Model Studies with Effector Cells from Nonimmune Donors

A. TARGET CELLS

While freshly explanted cells from normal tissue or tumors have the advantage of well preserved antigenicity as compared to cells which are kept in tissue culture, they are frequently too fragile to withstand the conditions of incubation required for the cytotoxicity experiments. Moreover, they may be coated with immunoglobulin and hence give rise to either false-positive or false-negative reactions. Cells that have been kept in tissue culture for a longer time, particularly cells from established tissue culture cell lines, are more stable under *in vitro* conditions. However, such cells may have lost some of their original antigens or may have acquired new ones owing to viral transformations, mycoplasm infection, etc. They may therefore be less suitable when the immunological specificity of the reaction is the issue under investigation.

Red blood cells from certain species are also used as target cells. Some red blood cells, e.g., those from chicken or sheep, are highly susceptible to antibody-dependent cell-mediated lysis. Others, such as human erythrocytes, are hardly lysed at all by K cells, but are easily destroyed by monocytic effector cells. It should be noted that antibody-coated erythrocytes are in general much more susceptible to both phagocytosis and extracellular lysis by monocytes or macrophages than are similarly treated tissue culture cells, which sometimes are not at all affected by these latter cell types (Fig. 1). The reasons are not clear, but it is likely that this has to do with both cell size and the greater capacity of nucleated cells to repair small surface lesions. Erythrocytes are also excellent tools for the study of immune systems comprising hap-

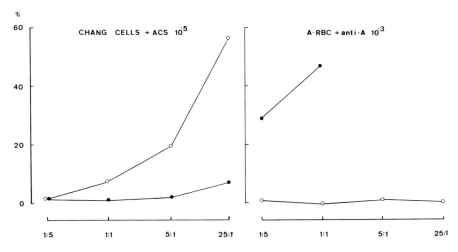

Fig. 1. Tissue culture cells (Chang cells) from suspension cultures or human erythrocytes (blood group A) were labeled with [^{51}Cr]chromate and incubated for 30 minutes at 37°C with rabbit anti-Chang cell serum (ACS) or human immune anti-A (IgG antibodies), respectively. After washing, 5×10^4 target cells were incubated with purified human blood lymphocytes (O———O) or purified monocytes (●———●) from the same donor, at the effector cell: target cell ratios indicated on the abscissa. Time of incubation, 16 hours. The ordinate shows percentage of ^{51}Cr release as a measure of lysis. [From G. Holm. For further details, see Huber and Holm (1975).]

tens or antigens which can be chemically or physically attached to the red cell surface. In contrast, erythrocytes are unsuitable for the study of antigens of the major histocompatibility locus since such antigens are phenotypically poorly or not all expressed on erythrocytes. In these instances, lymphoid cells have recently been widely used as target cells. Some authors have found it useful to use lymphoblastoid target cells obtained by treating lymphocytes with the mitogen phytohemagglutinin (PHA), a treatment that seems to make the cells more susceptible to lysis with retained antigenicity.

B. Assay Systems

An important factor determining the choice of target cells is the assay system. In essence, there are two principally different procedures which are most commonly used. (1) Effector cells and antibodies are mixed with target cells in suspension; or (2) they are added to target cells growing as colonies or monolayers on plastic or glass surfaces.

In the first procedure, a moderate excess of effector cells over target cells is usually sufficient to give a strong reaction within hours. In most cases, lysis of the target cells is recorded by measuring the release of isotopic markers from target cells labeled before the onset of the experiments. The most widely used marker is ^{51}Cr, added as sodium chromate. The chromate is enzymically reduced within the cells and is not reutilized. Most of the isotope is released in noncovalent association with macromolecular substances, which are set free only from target cells that are irreversibly lysed. The radioactivity of the cell-free medium therefore represents a good index of actual target cell death. Minor and more rapidly occurring changes in target cell surface permeability are recorded by measuring uptake or release of radioactive ions or low molecular metabolites, but high backgrounds and rapid changes in control mixtures may make evaluation of the results difficult. Radioactive precursor substances built into DNA, e.g., ^{14}C- or ^{3}H-labeled thymidine or ^{125}I-labeled deoxyuridine are useful markers since background release from living cells is usually insignificant. However, incorporation requires proliferating target cells, and release may be considerably slower than that of ^{51}Cr. Unless special precautions are taken, some of these metabolites will also be reutilized in the cytotoxic test.

The second procedure requires target cells adapted to grow as colonies or monolayers. Effector cells have to be added in considerable excess over the target cells, and incubation time is usually prolonged over several days. In the colony inhibition assay, the number of outgrowing target cell colonies from single-cell cultures in the experimental samples is compared with that found in the controls. In the microcytotoxicity test, mostly performed in microtitration plates, the number of surviving target cells is counted. Alternatively, isotopic metabolites, such as thymidine, proline, or ^{125}I-labeled deoxyuridine are also used. Cytotoxicity is in all modifications assessed in relative terms by comparing target cells surviving in samples incubated with antiserum + effector cells with those containing normal serum + effector cells. It is, however, also necessary to have controls containing target cells + serum without effector cells, and cell survival in the different controls may sometimes vary considerably.

From this brief description it should be clear that these two experimental procedures differ in several aspects. While isotope release from suspended target cells is a direct measure of cytolysis, the microcytotoxicity test with target cell monolayers reflects the net result of both cytolysis and cytostasis. Moreover, the long incubation times needed in the latter assays may give rise to *in vitro* sensitization, activation, or maturation of effector cells. At the same time, proliferation of part of the target cells may be promoted by various nonspecific feeder effects. Cytostasis and feeder effects can be prevented by inhibiting target cell growth with mitomycin C or X-irradiation. Use of ^{125}I-labeled deoxyuridine as the isotopic marker also prevents target cell proliferation. Nevertheless, even under such conditions, the mechanisms leading to target cell destruction in the two types of assay may frequently be different. Release of the cells from the monolayer appears to be a prerequisite of lysis in the microcytotoxicity test. This implies that different effector cell types may predominate in the different assay systems even when the same antigen–antibody system is involved and the same antiserum is the inducing agent. Monolayer cells seem frequently to be more susceptible to the action of several antibody-dependent effector cells (including macrophages) than tissue culture or tumor cells grown in suspension.

A recent plaque assay combines features of the two types of methods. In this assay, target erythrocytes are attached to cover slips, e.g., by means of poly-L-lysine, to form dense layers. Addition of properly diluted antiserum to the erythrocytes and incubation with lymphocytes leads to locally restricted lysis of erythrocytes in the vicinity of antibody-dependent effector cells. These clear areas (plaques) are of varying size and irregular shape, quite distinct from the plaques seen in the Jerne assay. Usually one lymphocyte can be seen to be associated with each plaque. Counting of plaques formed under standardized conditions makes it possible to estimate the minimal numbers of K-cells present in

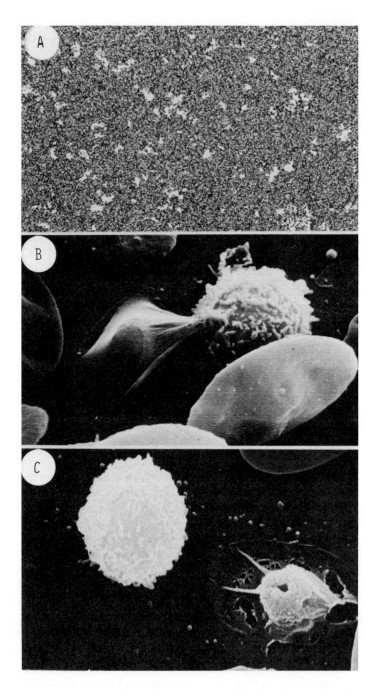

a lymphocyte preparation. In addition, morphology, ultrastructure, and surface markers of K-cells can be studied on the level of the individual effector cell by direct observation (Fig. 2).

C. Effector Cells

In order to be able to exhibit K-cell activity, the effector cells must interact with the Fc portion of antibody molecules. Cell types such as polymorphonuclear leukocytes (PMN), monocytes or macrophages, platelets, mast cells, as well as some tumor cells, possess "Fc receptors" and can therefore be regarded as potential killer cells. Hence, when mononuclear spleen cells consisting of 80–90% "lymphocytes" are being used as killer cells, the effector cells may be found among the 10–20% of nonlymphoid cells. They may also be among the cells that have a lymphocytic appearance but nevertheless belong to a nonlymphocytic lineage. Since target cells differ in their susceptibility toward different antibody-dependent effector cells and different assay systems may reveal the killing activity of different cell types, it is impossible to make any general statements as to the nature of "the" antibody-dependent effector cell.

A large number of highly elaborate methods have been devised for characterizing the lymphocyte-like K cells active in the various model systems presently in use. Lymphocytes from peripheral lymphoid organs or from blood are purified by standard procedures, which in most instances include removal of phagocytic and adherent cells and of erythrocytes. Such preparations from human blood should contain $\geq 98\%$ lymphocytic cells and $<0.5\%$ mature monocytes. It should be noted that the proportion of different lymphocyte subpopulations found in the purified samples may differ from what was present in the unpurified material. This requires careful consideration when purified lymphocyte preparations are used to monitor effector-cell activities in different diseases.

In order to establish the nature of antibody-dependent effector cells, the purified lymphocyte preparations are further fractionated. While some fractionation methods make use of physical properties, such as cell

Fig. 2. (A) Light micrograph showing plaque formation in an antibody-sensitized sheep erythrocyte monolayer incubated overnight with purified human blood lymphocytes. The plaques vary in form and size. (B) Tearing of a target chicken erythrocyte within a plaque by an effector K cell. Note the villous appearance of the lymphocyte. Scanning electron micrograph. (C) Characteristic appearance of a lysed target cell within a plaque and a predominantly villous lymphocyte. Scanning electron micrograph. Micrographs taken by P. Biberfeld. [From Perlmann *et al.* (1975).]

size, density, or surface charge, others utilize surface characteristics typical for the various subpopulations. Adherence to glass- or plastic surfaces may be useful although this property varies significantly with the experimental conditions. Other important fractionation procedures make use of structural cell surface markers, such as antigens, lectin receptors, surface-bound immunoglobulin, Fc or complement receptors. Thus, antisera in combination with complement may be used to eliminate subpopulations of lymphocytes. Various cell types may also be fractionated by affinity chromatography or by means of their capacity to form rosettes with erythrocytes. Whatever fractionation procedure is being followed, the various fractions are assessed analytically with regard to certain surface markers and functional characteristics, such as K-cell reactivity.

Both the fractionation procedures presently in use and the analytical assays have inherent errors that pose serious limitations on effector cell characterization. Thus, conclusions as to effector cell characterization are usually based on assessment of the cytolytic potential of cell populations, more or less enriched in or depleted of certain cell types. In other words, contamination of a fraction with small numbers of potent effector cells may grossly distort the picture. Nevertheless, combination of the methods mentioned above with kinetic studies has permitted certain characterizations.

The majority of lymphocytes possessing *T-cell characteristics* such as θ-antigen (mouse) or sheep erythrocyte receptors (man) are devoid of K-cell activity. Thus, most T cells in human blood are not retained on columns which bind lymphocytes with surface immunoglobulin (Table I, column charged with HGG/rabbit F(ab')$_2$-anti-HGG), or lymphocytes with Fc receptors (Table I, column charged with HGG/rabbit IgG anti-HGG). As seen from Table I, it is only the second type of fractionation which abolished K-cell mediated cytotoxicity. Since the majority of the T cells in human blood have no Fc receptors for IgG, this is not surprising. However, this type of experiment does not prove that all T cells are devoid of antibody-dependent cytolytic activity. In fact, from 5 to 15% of the lymphocytes in human blood have recently been shown to have both T-cell markers (e.g., receptors for sheep erythrocytes) and Fc receptors for IgG. That such cells, which are distinct from B cells and thus may be thymus derived, also display K-cell activity has been shown by the plaque assay. It should be noted, however, that these cells are distinct from CTL which are IgG independent and are not known to have Fc receptors.

A large part (but probably not all) of the *mature B cells* present in blood and peripheral lymphoid organs have Fc receptors and may thus possess K-cell potential. As also demonstrated by the experiment of Table I

TABLE I

ANTIBODY-INDUCED LYSIS OF CHICKEN ERYTHROCYTES AFTER COLUMN
FRACTIONATION OF EFFECTOR LYMPHOCYTES[a]

Column[b]	% Residual erythrolysis[c]		Effector cell preparations defined by surface markers before and after column fractionation		
	20 Hours	40 Hours	% SIg[+]- cells[d]	% CRL[e]	% T cells[f]
None	100	100	18	15	53
HGG	83	93	14	16	50
HGG/F(ab')$_2$-anti-HGG	93	100	4	11	57
HGG/anti-HGG	14	17	1	5	62

[a] See Perlmann et al. (1973).

[b] Effector cells were either purified unfractionated human blood lymphocytes, or fractionated by passage through glass bead columns charged with (a) human immunoglobulin (HGG), control columns; (b) HGG + excess of rabbit anti-HGG, F(ab')$_2$ fragments; or (c) HGG + intact rabbit anti-HGG.

[c] Effector cells and ^{51}Cr-labeled chicken erythrocytes, treated with rabbit antiserum, diluted 10^{-5} were incubated at ratio 5:1 as indicated. Lysis expressed as percentage of ^{51}Cr release in unfractionated control.

[d] Cells with positive surface immunofluorescence after staining with rabbit antiserum to F(ab')$_2$ fragments of human IgG.

[e] Lymphocytes forming rosettes with complement-carrying sheep erythrocytes.

[f] Lymphocytes forming rosettes with sheep erythrocytes.

(HGG/rabbit F(ab')$_2$-anti-HGG column), cells with high concentration of surface-bound immunoglobulin have in several instances been reported to be devoid of K-cell activity. However, available data are conflicting, and some reports suggest that such cells also may be cytolytically active. Lack of reactivity of cells with surface immunoglobulin in certain instances does not imply that K cells could not belong to the B-cell family, defined as lymphocytes of the bone marrow-derived plasma cell precursor series. Thus, it is feasible that high concentrations of surface immunoglobulin, characteristic for certain phases of B-cell development, may block Fc-receptor reactivity and thereby inhibit antibody-dependent cytolysis.

Available evidence indicates that the K cells discussed above are nonphagocytic and have lymphocytic morphology on both light- and electron microscopic levels. In human blood they are nonadherent to glass or plastic surfaces in high protein concentration and are heterogeneous in regard to size and surface charge. In mouse spleen, K-cell activity has been found in both adherent and nonadherent fractions. Part of the cytolytically active cells are also equipped with complement receptors (man, rat, mouse). In contrast to the complement receptor specific for C3b on PMN, human blood lymphocytes have distinct complement receptors for both C3b and C3d, and this seems also to be the case with the cytolytic effector cells.

Data obtained by studying individual K cells in the plaque assay confirm and extend these results. Thus the minimum number of cells with K-cell activity for erythrocytic target cells comprises from 4 to 8% of the purified lymphocytes from normal human blood. The actual number is probably $\leq 10\%$. About 50–60% of these cells have complement receptors. Moreover, about 30% have T-cell markers and belong to the subpopulation of lymphocytes equipped with both T-cell markers and Fc receptors.

It is evident that K cells represent a heterogenous family of effector cells which all possess Fc receptors. However, not all lymphocytes with Fc receptors are necessarily cytolytic and their K potential may differ for different types of target cells. Thus, while obviously several different lymphocytic cells are cytolytic for erythrocytes, nucleated target cells (e.g., lymphocytes or tumor cells) may be susceptible to only some of these cell types. Moreover, the data summarized above are almost exclusively based on results obtained with methods measuring target-cell lysis directly. Data available for microcytotoxicity assay systems (target cells growing in monolayers) point in the same direction but are less complete. It is likely that additional cell types, not active in the ^{51}Cr-release assay, exhibit K-cell reactivity under these conditions.

D. ANTIBODY–EFFECTOR CELL INTERACTIONS

Induction of K-cell-mediated lysis of target cells requires antibodies of the IgG class. With a few exceptions, IgM antibodies have been found to be inactive in this respect. When IgG and IgM antibodies occur in mixture, the latter will often inhibit the reaction. Antibodies belonging to the other major immunoglobulin classes and capable of inducing K-cell activity have so far not been found. In man, inhibition studies with myeloma proteins belonging to classes, M, A, D, and E also suggest that these immunoglobulins are inactive.

Antibody-dependent cytolysis requires the presence of an intact Fc fragment on the inducing antibody. Thus, Fab or F(ab')$_2$ fragments of IgG antitarget cell antibody have no capacity to induce K-cell-mediated cytolysis but are efficient inhibitors of the reaction induced by intact antibodies. For human IgG, the reactive site has been reported by some authors to be located in the CH3 homology region of the γ chains and to be different from the complement (C1q) activating site. Others have presented evidence for the importance of the CH2 region and K-cell-inducing capacity may depend on the interaction of these regions within the intact Fc fragment.

Effector cells from a given species may mediate cytolysis by means of IgG antibodies from other species with seemingly equal efficiency. Possible differences in affinity for IgG from different species may exist but have so far not been delineated. However, there may exist differences in inducing capacity of antibodies between and perhaps within the known IgG subclasses. In man, K-cell-mediated target-cell lysis induced by rabbit or human IgG can be inhibited by human myeloma proteins belonging to subclasses IgG1, 2, 3, and probably also 4. However, the inhibitory capacity of individual proteins within these subclasses is variable and highly dependent on their state of aggregation. Nevertheless, this inhibitory pattern seems to distinguish K cells from monocytic effector cells, which are most easily inhibited by IgG belonging to subclass 1 or 3. It should be noted, however, that antibody belonging to human IgG subclass 2 may induce cytolytic reactivity of human K cells as well as monocytes.

For induction of target-cell lysis, antiserum or purified antibodies may be added directly to the effector cell/target cell mixture. With antiserum from hyperimmunized donors, significant reactions are induced at extremely high dilutions (10^{-6} to 10^{-9}), and it has been shown that a few hundred antibody molecules per target cell are sufficient to produce strong reactions. Cytolysis may almost as efficiently be induced by pretreatment of the target cells with the antibody before addition of the effector cells. In contrast, pretreatment of the effector cells with antibody is very inefficient, requiring about 10,000 times more antibody than in the two first-mentioned cases. It can be concluded that the affinity of the Fc receptor on the effector cells for monomeric IgG is low, and this has also been shown by binding experiments. However, when IgG is presented to the effector cells in aggregated form or as antigen–antibody complexes, adsorption to the Fc receptors is much stronger and the adsorbed material cannot be removed by washing. It has been demonstrated that effector cells in certain instances may pick up antibody in complex with antigen from the surface of target cells and utilize these antibodies in a cytotoxic reaction with fresh target cells of relevant antigenicity. Thus, antigen–antibody complexes may confer specific receptor structures to effector cells while monomeric antibody cannot (Table II). However, effector cells sensitized in this way are cytolytically less efficient than effector cells that interact with equal amounts of target cell bound antibody.

TABLE II

TRANSFER OF ANTIBODY FROM TARGET CELLS TO EFFECTOR CELLS[a,b]

Expt. No.	Antibody adsorbed to 2.5×10^6 lymphocytes pretreated with		Cytotoxicity of lymphocytes pretreated with	
	Anti-Crbc + Crbc[c] (ng)	Anti-Crbc (ng)	Anti-Crbc	Anti-Crbc + Crbc
1	20	0.3	2	17
2	39	1.2	12	35
3	20	0.9	—	—
4	16	0.4	7	23
5	14	0.4	3	33

[a] Purified lymphocytes from human blood were first incubated overnight with the ^{125}I-labeled IgG fraction of rabbit antichicken erythrocyte serum (Anti-Crbc) in the presence or in the absence of Crbc. The lymphocytes were then separated from Crbc and thoroughly washed. The amount of rabbit IgG adsorbed to 2.5×10^6 lymphocytes/tube was measured on part of the lymphocytes. The other part was added to fresh ^{51}Cr-labeled Crbc without adding anti-Crbc (2.5×10^6 lymphocytes, 10^5 Crbc.) After incubation for 20 hours, cytotoxicity was determined as a percentage of ^{51}Cr release.

[b] For further details, see Perlmann et al. (1972).

[c] The amount of antibody adsorbed in anti-Crbc/Crbc tubes varied frcm $\approx 2 \times 10^4$ (Expt. 5) to $\approx 6 \times 10^4$ molecules/lymphocyte (Expt. 2).

These properties of the Fc receptor have a number of important implications. Thus, K-cell-mediated lysis of target cells can take place in the presence of high concentrations of monomeric nonantibody IgG. In contrast, it is easily inhibited by aggregated IgG or antigen–antibody complexes present in the test serum. Small soluble complexes have been shown by MacLennan (1972b) to be efficient inhibitors. In the presence of serum, the balance between the concentrations of various inhibitory and inducing factors will be decisive in determining the extent of a cytolytic reaction. K-cell-mediated cytolysis is also highly susceptible to inhibition by antigen–antibody complexes formed on the surface of "third party" cells present in preparation of either effector cells or of target cells. This fact has recently been utilized by Halloran et al. (1974) for designing a sensitive assay (cytotoxicity inhibition assay, CIA) for determination of antibodies against cell surface antigens in general.

E. MECHANISM OF K-CELL-MEDIATED DESTRUCTION OF TARGET CELLS

Most investigations of the mechanisms of K-cell-mediated destruction of target cells have been performed with lytic systems in which effector cells and target cells are incubated in suspension. With antibody added at optimal concentration, effector cell:target cell ratios of 5:1–25:1 are usually sufficient to achieve complete lysis within less than 20 hours. With some susceptible lymphoid target cells, 4–6 hours or even shorter incubation times have been found to suffice for complete lysis. Extent of lysis increases with effector cell concentration, similarly to what has been described for specific T-cell-mediated lysis. The number of target cells lysed also depends on the number of target cells present, incubation volume, and the geometry of the incubation vessel.

With ^{51}Cr as indicator, target cell lysis usually exhibits a lag period. This reflects the fact that this label is associated with macromolecular material that needs surface lesions above a certain size to be released. With low molecular metabolites or ions as indicators, no lag period is seen.

For initiation of lysis, contact between effector cells and target cells is necessary. Immunological specificity of lysis is determined by the inducing immunoglobulin. As in the case of CTL-mediated lysis, very short contacts between effector cells and target cells seem to suffice to initiate lysis, which then will procede to completion even in the absence of living effector cells. However, for initiation the effector cells have to be alive and metabolically active. Contact per se is thus not sufficient to initiate the lytic events. It seems that the interaction between target cell-bound IgG and the Fc receptor of the effector cells is of special importance for the triggering of the reaction. Thus, while interaction between effector cells equipped with complement receptors and target cells bearing activated complement (C3) but no IgG only leads to target cell binding (rosette formation), addition of minute amounts of anti-target cell IgG induces lysis. On the other hand, target cell-bound C3b amplifies the lytic reaction, probably by improving the contact between effector cells and target cells.

Treatment of the effector cells with neuraminidase or low concentrations of trypsin also enhances K-cell reactivity. The effect of trypsin on K-cell reactivity is different from its effect on specific CTL-mediated lysis, which is inhibited. Most likely trypsin acts by making Fc receptors more accessible, thereby making individual effector cells more efficient, and perhaps also by recruiting more cells into the reaction. Cytochalasin B, which inhibits microfilament function and various metabolic pathways, blocks both K-cell- and CTL-mediated lysis, probably by inhibiting effector cell/target cell contact.

The precise structural and biochemical background of the lytic reaction is unknown. Good evidence exists that the lytic effector components of the complement system (C5–C9) do not participate in K-cell-mediated lysis, which can take place in complete absence of serum in the supporting medium. In model systems in which the inducing antibody is added to effector cells from nonimmune donors, some studies with metabolic inhibitors suggest that neither nucleic acid synthesis nor protein synthesis are needed for the cytolytic reaction. However, the results of these studies are conflicting. On the other hand, inhibitors of energy supply (e.g., antimycin A, oligomycin, DFP), acting irreversibly on the effector cells, efficiently block cytolytic K-cell as well as CTL activity. Effector cell activity in both K and CTL systems is controlled by cyclic nucleotide levels in these cells at the time of interaction with the target cells. High levels of cAMP, produced either by β-adrenergic stimulation, by activators of adenyl cyclase, or by inhibitors of phosphodiesterase, decrease or block cytolytic activity in a dose-dependent fashion. In contrast, elevation of cGMP, e.g., by cholinergic stimulation, increases the cytolytic effector cell potential.

It is clear from these data that the interaction between effector cell- and target cell-bound IgG triggers the activation of a lytic machinery which seems to be the same for both K- and T-effector cells. Activation involves modulation of effector cell surface, including microtubular functions. Addition of certain alkaloids known to interact with microtubules also inhibit cytolytic effector cell (Table III). Since microtubules are important for secretion, it has been suggested that cell-mediated target-

TABLE III

EFFECT OF COLCHICINE ON LYMPHOCYTE-MEDIATED CYTOTOXICITY[a,b]

| | % Suppression of | | | | | |
| | Spleen cells from immune donors | | | Spleen cells from nonimmune donors | | |
Drug concentration (M)	10^{-4}	10^{-5}	10^{-6}	10^{-4}	10^{-5}	10^{-6}
Present in incubation mixture	50	32	18	58	26	10
Prior incubation of effector cells	37	25.5	1.7	63	53	47
Prior incubation of target cells[c]	0	—	—	0	—	—

[a] Effector cells were either from Lewis rats, immunized by skin grafts from Brown Norway (BN) rats, or from nonimmunized Lewis rats. In the latter case, cytotoxicity was induced by incorporation of diluted Lewis anti-BN antiserum in the incubation mixtures. Target cells were ^{51}Cr-labeled BN-thymocytes. The numbers in the table show percentage of suppression of the ^{51}Cr release seen in untreated controls.

[b] For complete data and details, see Strom et al. (1973).

[c] The susceptibility to cytolysis of pretreated target cells was unaltered.

cell lysis is based on a secretory process. However, nonspecifically cyto-toxic substances (so called "lymphotoxins") released from activated K cells into the incubation medium have so far not been found. Neither have such substances been found in effector cell lysates. This negative evidence does not exclude a secretory nature of the lytic reaction, since toxic mediators may be released locally in small amounts and may also be short-lived when free in the medium. It is also possible that target-cell lysis is started by structural changes of the effector cell surface and is not a secretory process.

III. K-Cell Activity in Different Immune Systems

A. ANTIBODIES AND EFFECTOR CELLS

Antibodies that induce K-cell reactivity *in vitro* in syngeneic or auto-logous lymphocytes have been found frequently in a large variety of antigen–antibody systems. Since such antibodies are of the predominat-ing IgG class, this is not necessarily of biological significance. However, the sensitivity of the K-cell assay being superior to that of other common antibody assays, determination of the K-cell-inducing potency of im-mune sera offers highly sensitive methods for monitoring immune res-ponses in experimental animals or patients.

Immunization of animals with xenogeneic, allogeneic, or syngeneic (or autologous) material may give rise to generation of killer cells specific for the immunizing antigen. Killer cells specific for tumor-associated antigens have been found in tumor-bearing animals or patients, as have killer cells specific for "normal" tissue antigens in experimental or human autoimmunity. Such effector cells have been shown to be of different types which may occur separately or in mixture. Antigen-specific effector cells may be of the CTL variety. T cells have also been shown to arm macrophages with antigen-specific cytotoxic reactivity by means of a recognition factor claimed not to be immunoglobulin. Macrophages may also acquire specific reactivity by interaction with cytophilic antibodies. In other cases, good evidence exists that the IgG-dependent effector cells belong to the K-cell variety discussed in this chapter.

All attempts to prove that B cells which produce antibodies specific for target-cell antigens by themselves act as killer cells have so far failed. However, cells that release IgG antibodies have been shown to be responsible for the generation of specific K-cell reactivity in immune donors. Thus, mice immunized with protein antigen or hapten possess spleen cells that are specifically cytolytic for chicken erythrocytes coated with these antigens. Although the generation of this effector mechanism is thymus dependent, the effector cells are neither CTL nor antibody-producing cells. *In vitro* cytolysis exhibited by these spleen cells is a cell-cooperation phenomenon dependent on the presence of at least two cell types. Thus, as shown by Schirrmacher and colleagues (1974), antibody-producing cells release antibody which reacts with the target cells, and this recruits effector cells with Fc receptors into the reaction. It is likely that the same mechanism prevails in many other systems where specific K-cell reactivity has been demonstrated *in vitro*. This is particularly true for many of the experiments in which the microcytotoxicity assay has been utilized, since this involves prolonged incubation periods. Even if very few antibody-releasing cells are present, this gives ample time for release of sufficient antibody to cause K-cell-mediated destruction of target cells.

Antigen-specific K cells may be generated *in vitro* by transfer of antigen–antibody complexes from target cells to effector cells and utilization of the adsorbed antibody as recognition factor (see Section II,D). A similar arming of K cells could also occur in animals immunized by tissue grafts or tumors. However, evidence for *in vivo* generation of specific effector cells in this manner is lacking.

B. ANTIGEN RECOGNITION

For elucidation of the biological importance of different cell-mediated effector mechanisms, it is essential to establish whether the antigenic specificities involved in K-cell killing are fundamentally distinct from those involved in CTL-mediated killing. Since IgG constitutes the recognition factor for K-cell reactivity, antigenic determinants known to be recognized by IgG antibodies, will also be involved in K-cell-mediated reactions. The antigen-specific receptor of T-killer cells is unknown but presumably distinct from IgG. It is therefore possible that CTL may recognize target cell surface structures different from those involved in K-cell-mediated killing. However, evidence available for some of the major histocompatibility antigens would seem to suggest that the determinants recognized by CTL are identical with those recognized by humoral alloantibodies. For other systems, including tumor-associated antigens or various cell- or tissue-specific antigens, knowledge of antigenic fine structures is not sufficient for such conclusions.

Generation of CTL to altered alloantigens (H2, HLA) and certain tumor-associated transplantation antigens is known to slow syngeneic restriction. It has therefore been speculated that immunization with xenogeneic antigens would generally lead to the generation of antibody-dependent effector mechanisms. No general statements to this effect can be made at present since both types of effector cells have been found in animals immunized either with allogeneic or with xenogeneic material. The only target cells that do not seem capable of inducing formation of CTL are xenogeneic erythrocytes. However, T cells do not lack the capacity to lyse erythrocytes. The finding would thus fit with the above-mentioned hypothesis in that erythrocytes lack the surface structures which the recognition factors of specific T-killer cells recognize. However, other explanations, such as the kinetics of the immune response, may easily account for this phenomenon.

C. Discrimination between CLT and K Cells by Means of Antibodies, Antigens, or Antigen–Antibody Complexes

There has been much speculation in recent years how various "blocking" and/or "unblocking" factors in blood and tissues of immunized animals or patients affect the course of cell-mediated effector mechanisms. In this section, the *in vitro* effects of various antibodies, antigens, or complexes on CTL or K-cell-mediated destruction of target cells will be discussed (Table IV). Such experiments help us to discriminate between these two effector mechanisms. In addition, they have obvious implications as to how antigen, antibodies or complexes may affect tissue-damaging immune responses *in vivo*.

Treatment of effector cell mixtures containing both T and K cells with antibodies against *T-cell antigens* (e.g., anti-θ in mice) + complement, and subsequent removal of the lysed cells, abolishes CTL-mediated cytotoxicity, with a corresponding relative increase of K-cell reactivity in some cases. However, the same antibodies applied without complement may decrease K-cell reactivity as well. K-cell reactivity is also inhibited by antibodies against H-2 or HLA antigens on the lymphocytes used as effector cells. These antibodies affect CTL dependent cytotoxicity not at all or very little. Inhibition of K-cell activity in all those cases is obtained with intact IgG antibodies, but not with Fab or F(ab')$_2$ fragments. It usually reflects blocking of Fc receptors on the effector cells by antigen–antibody complexes formed on some cells in the preparation. Thus, these inhibitions do not necessarily imply that the antigens reacting with the added antibodies are located on the actual effector cells (see Section II,D).

Antiimmunoglobulin antibodies do not affect CTL-mediated cytotoxic-

TABLE IV

CTL- OR K-CELL DEPENDENT CYTOTOXICITY OF UNFRACTIONATED
EFFECTOR CELL PREPARATIONS FROM IMMUNE DONORS.
In Vitro EFFECTS OF ANTIBODIES, ANTIGENS, OR COMPLEXES[a]

Reagents	CTL	K
IgG antibodies to antigens of effector cell donor		
Anti-θ, anti-T, etc.	I[a]	P or I[c]
Anti-H-2, anti-HLA	O	I
Antiimmunoglobulin (donor type)		
Fab (IgG) fragments	O	I
IgM antibodies	O	I
Antitarget cell antigens		
IgG antibodies	I[d]	P
IgM antibodies	I	I
Target cell antigen		
Soluble, purified (e.g., H-2)	O	I
Membrane fragments, particles	I	I
Aggregated IgG	O	I
Immune complexes		
Third party	O	I
Target-cell surface antigen	I	P or I[e]

[a] For further explanations see text. I, Inhibition; P, potentiation (or induction); O, no effect.

[b] In the presence or in the absence of complement.

[c] In the presence of complement, P; in the absence, O or I.

[d] May be masked by K-cell induction, but F(ab')$_2$ inhibits. May also "unblock" when added in excess to antigen-blocked effector cells.

[e] Dose dependent.

ity. When added as Fab fragments in an immune K-cell system in which effector cells and the inducing antibodies are of the same species origin, cytotoxicity is inhibited. IgM antiimmunoglobulin has the same effect. When antiimmunoglobulin is added as intact IgG or as F(ab')$_2$ fragments, the effects may vary in a dose-dependent fashion. Inhibition or potentiation of K-cell reactivity may be seen, the latter presumably due to cross-linking of effector cells and target cells.

In several well defined systems, both IgG and IgM *alloantibodies to target-cell surface antigens* (e.g., H-2, HLA) have been shown to inhibit CTL cytotoxicity. In contrast, K-cell cytotoxicity is potentiated (or induced) by IgG antitarget cell antibodies and inhibited by IgM. When CTL and K cells are present in a mixture, addition of IgG antitarget antibodies may give variable results, depending on dosage as well as on affinity and specifity of the added antibodies.

The effect of solubilized *antigen* on CTL cytotoxicity varies. For instance, while soluble purified H-2 antigens have been reported to have no effect even when added at high doses, solubilized H-2-active membrane fragments or particles seem to be inhibitory. K-cell cytotoxicity is inhibited by both soluble and particulate antigen, except in certain dose ranges in which antigen may have "unblocking" effects (see below).

Aggregated IgG has not been reported to affect CTL cytotoxicity but inhibits K cells. The same is the case with *immune complexes* comprising third-party antigens (i.e., antigens not involved in the cell-mediated reaction). However, when added complexes contain *antigens involved in the actual cell-mediated reactions,* CTL cytotoxicity is often inhibited. This inhibition is assumed to reflect a blocking of the T-cell receptor for antigen. Addition of excess antibodies to such blocked T-cell systems has been shown to unblock (by antigen neutralization). The effects of target cell-specific complexes on K-cell reactivity vary widely according to the composition of the complexes and the prevailing balance between the different components of the system. Thus, such complexes may potentiate a reaction by recruiting new effector cells into the system, or may inhibit it by Fc-receptor blockade (see Section II,D). Addition of excess antigen may have "unblocking" effects, presumably by formation of complexes with little or no affinity for the Fc receptors of the effector cells.

D. Transplantation Systems (H-2, HLA)

K-cell-inducing alloantibodies directed against major transplantation antigens have been found in many animal species. Mice immunized with H-2 allogeneic normal tissues or tumors develop alloantibodies that induce *in vitro* cytotoxicity in K-type spleen cells syngeneic to those of the immunized recipients. The development of these antibodies has been shown to be thymus dependent, and specifically cytotoxic lymphocytes in such immunized mice are most frequently of CTL type. However, specific effector cells of K-cell type have also been seen. Thus, mice immunized with allogeneic tumor cells have been shown by Forman and Britton to develop both types of effector cells, directed against H-2 antigens, with K-type effector cells appearing early after immunization and CTL activity predominating later when *in vitro* cytotoxicity was maximal. In accordance with this, immune serum which also induced K-cell reactivity in normal spleen cells augmented cytotoxicity of the immune spleen cells present early after immunization, but inhibited that of the cells appearing during the peak phase of the response (see Section III,C). The data are not sufficient to correlate the *in vitro* findings with graft rejection *in vivo*. In general, evidence available for rodents points to the importance of CTL-effector mechanisms for primary rejection of both vascularized organ grafts and allogeneic tumors. Whether or not antibody-dependent K-cell reactivity is important in those instances in which humoral mechanisms have been implicated, e.g., in hyperacute rejections or other special cases is presently not known.

In man, K-cell-inducing antibodies directed against alloantigens within the HLA system have been found in multiply transfused patients, multiparous women, and kidney transplant recipients. In the *in vitro* tests, allogeneic blood lymphocytes, usually activated with PHA, are used as target cells. Nonphagocytic, nonadherent blood lymphocytes from normal donors serve as effector cells. The cytotoxic potential of normal lymphocytes may be adversely affected by antieffector cell antibodies in the test serum (anti-HLA and others). These problems can be partly circumvented by using a panel of effector cells of known HLA type. The assays detect antibodies to the same HLA antigens as the complement-dependent cytotoxicity test in conventional tissue typing, but at a much higher sensitivity level ($\geq 100\times$). Because of this, the K-cell induction assay often reveals occurrence of antibodies which are missed in the conventional typing systems (Table V). It is therefore a powerful tool for the analysis of the major histocompatibility system. Moreover, testing of patients' sera for K-cell-inducing reactivity provides important means for monitoring the immune response in transplant recipients.

Cytotoxic effector cells, specific for donor-type transplantation antigens have been detected in the blood of kidney graft recipients concomitantly

TABLE V

HLA Specificities and Titers of Some Human Alloantisera Tested by Complement-Dependent and K-Cell Dependent Cytotoxicity[a]

| Serum | Complement dependent | | K-cell dependent | |
	Specificity[b]	Titer	Specificity[b]	Titer
BsSH	A7	1:4	A7, W27, W10, W22	1:400
PR2.24	—	0[c]	A14	1:100[c]
PR8.19	A5, W5	1:4[c]	A5, W5	1:100[c]
PR10.15	W18	1:2[b]	W18, A5, W5	1:400[c]
ToBn	—	0[c]	W16	1:10,000[c]

[a] From Trinchieri *et al.* (1973).
[b] Specifications established by population analysis from $p < 0.01$.
[c] Titer against immunizing blood donor.

with K-cell-inducing antibodies. In longitudinal studies of a number of patients, the latter activities, according to Carpenter and colleagues (1974) have been seen to be correlated with irreversible rejection episodes, in contrast to the direct lymphocyte-mediated cytotoxicity, reflecting a CTL reactivity. However, the relative importance of different effector mechanisms in human transplantation cannot as yet be evaluated from the results of available *in vitro* studies.

E. IMMUNE RESPONSES TO TUMOR-ASSOCIATED ANTIGENS

Serum activity that induces cell-mediated cytotoxicity *in vitro* against tumor-associated antigens has been found in tumor-bearing animals or in animals whose tumors have regressed spontaneously. In the case of certain virally induced tumors, infusion of such sera into tumor-bearing mice has been shown to cause tumor regression rather than enhancement, the latter being a well established phenomenon. In the case of certain transplantable rat lymphomas, infusion of tumor-specific rabbit antisera into tumor-bearing rats has been seen by Hersey (1973) to have protective effects, correlated with the appearance of K-cell inducing serum activity in the recipients. Such results do not prove that *in vivo* protection against tumor growth is due to K-cell reactivity, since virus neutralization, various complement-dependent reactions, or several other serum activities may be responsible for this. It should be noted that K-cell-inducing sera often contain antibodies which are also detectable by direct complement-mediated cytotoxicity.

Inoculation of rats or mice with syngeneic tumors gives rise to the appearance of cytotoxic lymphocytes. Occurrence of CTL with specificity for tumor-associated antigens is well established. Tumor-specific T-killer cells have also been produced *in vitro* by cocultivation of syngeneic lymphocytes and tumor cells. Transfer of specific CTL to tumor-bearing syngeneic recipients has in certain instances been shown to have protective effects, but tumor growth enhancement has also been reported. During recent years, effector cells of K-cell type with tumor-associated killing activity have been detected as well. Thus, mice infected with Moloney sarcoma virus develop local tumors at the site of virus injection, frequently regressing spontaneously after a few weeks. Such mice have been seen to develop effector cells that exhibit *in vitro* cytotoxicity for target cells with tumor-associated antigens. When analyzed by the microcytotoxicity assay, both Lamon *et al.* (1973) and Plata *et al.* (1974) found the response to be biphasic, with a first peak early during tumor development and a second peak during and after regression. CTL (spleen and lymph nodes) were seen transiently just before tumor development and after regression. Cytotoxicity due to specific K-type effector cells also showed a prominent but transient peak before tumor development and a second long-lasting peak starting soon after regression. During the phase of maximal tumor growth both effector cell types seemed to be inactive. In contrast, similar studies performed with the ^{51}Cr-release assay show only the first transient CTL reactivity, but with a peak at the time of optimal tumor growth. While several explanations may account for these discrepancies, the results indicate that both antibody-dependent and antibody-independent cell-mediated effector mechanisms operate in tumor-bearing animals. This is also evident from many other studies in which serum from tumor-bearing animals has been found to potentiate as well as to inhibit lymphocyte cytotoxicity *in vitro* in a dose-dependent fashion.

Reactivities similar to those reported for animal tumors have been reported for a variety of human tumors. Evaluation of these data is difficult since the specificity of the human reactions is not sufficiently known in many cases. Nevertheless, study of these reactions is of importance because of their potential diagnostic or prognostic value. Thus, in transitional cell carcinoma of the human urinary bladder, blood lymphocytes of most patients with less advanced tumor growth are cytotoxic *in vitro* for both autologous and allogeneic bladder carcinoma cells, but not for carcinoma cells of other histogenetic origin, or for cells from normal tissue, including urinary bladder epithelium. In contrast, only 50% of the patients with advanced tumors show this activity. After local radiotherapy, lymphocyte cytotoxicity *in vitro* is found during the first year to be inversely related to presence of residual tumor or metastases in these patients. This transient activity disappears later on, but reappears with tumor recurrence. Removal of tumor by surgery results in more rapid loss of cytotoxicity which, however, also reappears in case of tumor recurrence. In almost all cases investigated thus far, cytotoxicity reflects an immunoglobulin-dependent activity with effector cells of K type (Table VI).

Numerous *in vitro* studies have established the presence in the blood of tumor patients of serum factors that block, unblock, or potentiate cell-mediated cytotoxicity *in vitro*. Since blocking serum activities have occasionally been found to be correlated to tumor growth, it has been speculated that similar reactions might be responsible for failures in immune protection against the tumors *in vivo*. However, while specific blocking of the *in vitro* reaction by a patient's serum reflects occurrence of antigen, antibodies, or complexes in the blood (see Section II,C, Table IV), it gives no clues as to the decisive balance of the various components in the

TABLE VI

TUMOR-DIRECTED CYTOTOXICITY OF LYMPHOCYTE FRACTIONS

Target	Lymphocyte fraction	E:T	Surviving target cells/well		Percent reduction
			Patient	Control	
T24	T-cell enriched	250:1	64 ± 1.9	63 ± 2.3	0
		125:1	63 ± 1.9	62 ± 1.3	0
	T-cell depleted	250:1	24 ± 1.9	57 ± 2.7	58
		125:1	33 ± 3.5	70 ± 2.5	53
	Unfractionated	250:1	57 ± 2.0	75 ± 3.2	24
		125:1	56 ± 2.2	71 ± 3.7	21
MEL-1	T-cell enriched	250:1	44 ± 4.0	42 ± 3.6	0
		125:1	40 ± 3.2	40 ± 2.4	0
	T-cell depleted	250:1	36 ± 3.2	24 ± 2.4	0
		125:1	36 ± 2.0	32 ± 3.2	0
	Unfractionated	250:1	28 ± 2.4	28 ± 2.0	0
		125:1	36 ± 6.0	32 ± 2.4	0
HCV/29	T-cell enriched	250:1	54 ± 3.0	56 ± 3.8	4[c]
		125:1	61 ± 2.3	58 ± 2.8	0
	T-cell depleted	250:1	50 ± 3.7	52 ± 3.4	4[c]
		125:1	50 ± 4.6	54 ± 3.0	7[c]
	Unfractionated	250:1	50 ± 4.5	54 ± 3.8	7[c]
		125:1	52 ± 3.3	53 ± 2.6	2[c]

[a] Purified lymphocytes from a patient with transitional cell carcinoma of urinary bladder and from a healthy control were separated into T-cell-enriched and T-cell-depleted fractions by rosette formation with sheep erythrocytes and subsequent centrifugation. Unfractionated effector cells or fractions were added to the wells of microtitration plates containing target cells, at the effector cell:target cell ratios indicated. The number of surviving target cells was counted after 24 hours of incubation. Percent reduction = number of surviving cells in samples with patient's lymphocytes as percentage of that in samples containing control lymphocytes. (Surviving cells incubated in medium only were for T24, 62 ± 3; MEL-1, 44 ± 3; HCV/29, 56 ± 5.) T24, cell line from bladder carcinoma; MEL-1, primary culture from metastatic malignant melanoma, passage 13–16: HCV/29, cell line derived from nonmalignant specimen of bladder epithelium.

[b] For complete data and details, see O'Toole et al. (1973).

[c] Statistically not significant.

vicinity of the growing tumor. Protection against tumor growth evidently depends on a large variety of factors. From the *in vitro* data available, no general conclusions can be drawn as to the relative significance of the many different mechanisms that may be implicated in affecting tumor growth. It is also reasonable to expect that the relative protective importance of different effector mechanisms varies not only for different tumors, but also for different phases of tumor growth. Nevertheless, the fact that specific K-cell reactivity occurs in tumor patients and varies with the clinical course of the disease emphasizes that its possible protective function should not be disregarded.

F. Various Applications

In the previous sections it has repeatedly been pointed out that measuring the specific K-cell activity provides extremely sensitive tools for monitoring both cellular and humoral immune responses. Examples have been given for transplantation immunology and tumor immunology. Similar analyses have been performed in other immune systems, including experimental or animal autoimmunities and viral diseases.

Since K-cell reactivity is very susceptible to inhibition by soluble antigen–antibody complexes, it may also be utilized to establish the occurrence of such complexes in the serum of patients with various disease. Thus, Jewell and MacLennan (1973) have made use of a model system consisting of normal human lymphocytes, Chang liver tissue culture cells, and rabbit anti-Chang cell serum to assay sera of patients with chronic gastrointestinal diseases. The content of inhibitory complexes in these sera was found to vary with the clinical course of the disease.

In other instances, circulating lymphocytes of patients with various diseases are used as effector cells in similar model systems in order to monitor for nature and functional properties or the effects of therapy. This has been described for patients with multiple myeloma, leukemias, and cancer and for patients with various immunodeficiencies.

References

Biberfeld, P., Wåhlin, B., Perlmann, P., and Biberfeld, G. (1975). A plaque technique for assay and characterization of antibody dependent cytotoxic effector (K) cells. *Scand. J. Immunol.* 4, 859–864.

Carpenter, C. B. (1974). Transplantation: Immunogenetics and effector mechanisms. *In* "Biology of Lymphoid Systems" (A. Gottlieb, ed.). CRC Press, Cleveland, Ohio.

Cerottini, J. C., and Brunner, K. T. (1975). Cell-mediated cytotoxicity, allograft rejection, and tumor immunity. *Advan. Immunol.* 18, 67–132.

Forman, J., and Britton, S. (1973). Heterogeneity of the effector cells in the cytotoxic reaction against allogeneic lymphoma cells. *J. Exp. Med.* 137, 309–386.

Halloran, P., Schirrmacher, V., and Festenstein, H. (1974). A new sensitive assay for antibody against cell surface antigens based on inhibition of cell dependent antibody-mediated cytotoxicity. *J. Exp. Med.* 140, 1348–1363.

Hersey, P. (1973). New look at antiserum therapy of leukemia. *Nature (London) New Biol.* 244, 22–24.

Huber, H., and Holm, G. (1975). In "Mononuclear Phagocytes in Immunity, Infection, and Pathology" (R. van Furth, ed.) pp. 291–301. Blackwell, Oxford.

Jewell, D. P., and MacLennan, I. C. M. (1973). Circulating immune complexes in inflammatory bowel disease. Clin. Exp. Immunol. 14, 219–226.

Lamon, E. W., Wigzell, H., Klein, E., Andersson, B., and Skurzak, H. M. (1973). The lymphocyte response to primary Moloney sarcoma virus tumors in BALB/c mice. J. Exp. Med. 137, 1472–1493.

MacLennan, I. C. M. (1972a). Antibody in the induction and inhibition of lymphocyte cytotoxicity. Transplant. Rev. 13, 67–69.

MacLennan, I. C. M. (1972b). Competition for receptors of immunoglobulin on cytotoxic lymphocytes. Clin. Exp. Immunol. 10, 275–283.

Mellstedt, H., and Holm, G. (1973). In vitro studies of lymphocytes from patients with plasma cell myeloma. I. Stimulation by mitogens and cytotoxic activities. Clin. Exp. Immunol. 15, 309–320.

O'Toole, C., Stejskal, V., Perlmann, P., and Karlsson, M. (1974). Lymphoid cells mediating tumor specific cytotoxicity to carcinoma of the urinary bladder. Separation of the effector population using a surface marker. J. Exp. Med. 139, 457–466.

Perlmann, P., and Holm, G. (1969). Cytotoxic effects of lymphoid cells in vitro. Advan. Immunol. 11, 117–193.

Perlmann, P., and Wåhlin, B. (1976). Analysis of antibody dependent lymphocytic effector cells (K-cells) in human blood by a plaque assay. In "Proceedings of the 10th Leucocyte Culture Conference, Amsterdam 1975" (V. P. Eijsvoogel, D. Roos, and W. P. Zeylemaker, ed.). Academic Press, New York (in press).

Perlmann, P., Perlmann, H., and Wigzell, H. (1972). Lymphocyte-mediated cytotoxicity in vitro. Induction and inhibition by humoral antibody and nature of effector cells. Transplant. Rev. 13, 91–114.

Perlmann, P., Wigzell, H., Golstein, P., Lamon, E. W., Larsson, Å., O'Toole, C., Perlmann, H., and Svedmyr, E. A. J. (1974). Cell mediated cytolysis in vitro. Analysis of active lymphocyte subpopulations in different experimental systems. Advan. Biosci. 12, 71–85.

Perlmann, P., Biberfeld, P., Larsson, Å., Perlmann, H., and Wåhlin, B. (1975). Surface markers of antibody-dependent lymphocytic effector cells (K cells) in human blood. In "Membrane Receptors of Lymphocytes" (M. Seligmann, J. C. Preud'Homme, and F. M. Kourilsky, eds.) pp. 161–169. North-Holland, Amsterdam.

Plata, F., Gomard, E., Leclerc, C., and Levy, J. P. (1974). Comparative studies on effector cell diversity in the cellular immune response to murine sarcoma virus (MSV)-induced tumors in mice. J. Immunol. 112, 1477–1487.

Schirrmacher, V., Rubin, B., and Pross, H. (1974). Cytotoxic immune cells with specificity for defined and soluble antigens. V. Analysis of the interaction of antibody with the cytotoxic effector cells in immune and non-immune spleen cells. J. Immunol. 112, 2219–2226.

Strom, T. B., Garovoy, M. R., Carpenter, C. B., and Merrill, J. P. (1973). Microtubule function in immune and non-immune lymphocyte mediated cytotoxicity. Science 181, 171–173.

Trinchieri, G., De Marchi, M., Mayr, W., Savi, M., and Ceppellini, R. (1973). Lymphocyte antibody lymphocytolytic interaction (LALI) with special emphasis on HL-A. Transplant. Proc. 5, 1631–1646.

Wunderlich, J. R., Rosenberg, E. B., and Conolly, J. M. (1971). Human lymphocyte dependent cytotoxic antibody and mechanisms of target cell destruction *in vitro*. *Progr. Immunol.* **1**, 473–481.

Yust, I., Wunderlich, J. R., Mance, D. L., and Terry, W. D. (1974). Identification of lymphocyte-dependent antibody in sera from multiply transfused patients. *Transplantation* **18**, 99–107.

Short-Term ^{51}Cr-Release Tests for Direct Cell-Mediated Cytotoxicity: Methods, Clinical Uses, and Interpretations

J. WUNDERLICH

Immunology Branch, National Cancer Institute, Bethesda, Maryland

I. Introduction

The clinical usefulness of rapid ^{51}Cr-release tests for direct cell-mediated cytotoxicity has been evaluated in this chapter. The nature of these tests, their limitations, and several clinical applications are presented. A

133

review of the literature is not intended. Rather, selected studies have been used to illustrate particular concepts. To this end, preference has been given to clinical material as opposed to more basic studies in animal model systems. Readers are referred elsewhere for a more general understanding of the various and numerous uses of *in vitro* tests for direct cell-mediated cytotoxicity (Perlmann and Holm, 1969; Bloom, 1971; Möller, 1973; Cerottini and Brunner, 1974; Hellström and Hellström, 1974).

II. Pathways for Direct Cell-Mediated Cytotoxicity

There are three primary populations of cytotoxic cells as detected *in vitro* (Fig. 1). First, sensitized cytotoxic thymus-derived lymphocytes can injure target cells upon direct contact (Cerottini *et al.*, 1970). Thymus-derived lymphocytes can also release soluble, nonspecific toxins (Shacks *et al.*, 1973). Second, armed macrophages injure specific target cells upon contact (Evans and Alexander, 1972; Lohmann-Matthes and Fischer, 1973); activated by antigen contact, armed macrophages also injure target cells nonspecifically (Evans and Alexander, 1972). Arming of macrophages is provided by a cell-free product of antigen-stimulated

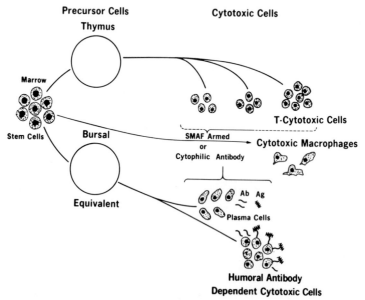

Fig. 1. Different populations of cytotoxic cells. Ab, antibody; Ag, antigen; SMAF, specific macrophage-arming factor.

T lymphocytes, or by direct contact of macrophages with sensitized T cells. A mechanism by which activated macrophages may destroy tumor cells has also been proposed by Hibbs (Hibbs et al., 1972; Hibbs, 1974). Finally, normal nonthymus-derived lymphoid cells (including macrophages) in cooperation with humoral antibody can injure target cells. Only certain subclasses of lymphoid cells and antibody participate in this type of cytotoxicity, also referred to as antibody-dependent, cell-mediated cytotoxicity; the reader is referred elsewhere for additional details (Cerottini and Brunner, 1974).

Direct cell-mediated cytoxicity is an operational term. The rapid (arbitrarily 10 hours or less) direct cell-mediated cytotoxicity tests, to date, have been reported to detect primarily T-cell-mediated cytotoxicity (Cerottini and Brunner, 1974). In these assays, target-cell injury by attacking cells occurs in the absence of added humoral antibody or complement. Cell-free mediators of cytotoxicity have not been detected. In contrast, longer-term tests have been reported to detect several cytotoxic pathways (Lamon et al., 1973).

III. Methodology

The technique most commonly used to detect rapid direct cell-mediated cytotoxicity involves release of ^{51}Cr from damaged target cells. In humans, cells to be tested for cytotoxic activity (effector or attacking cells) are usually prepared from anticoagulated peripheral blood by centrifuging cells layered on Ficoll–Hypaque (FH) (Thorsby and Bratlie, 1970). Red cells, granulocytes, and some monocytes pass through FH; other leukocytes remain at the interphase. Other procedures that have been useful include settling peripheral blood in plasmagel or dextran to diminish the red cell content (Wunderlich et al., 1972) and incubating FH-prepared leukocytes on nylon with 5–10% serum to remove platelets, monocytes, contaminating polymorphonuclear cells, and most B cells (Wisloff and Froland, 1973; Greaves and Brown, 1974). Incubating FH-prepared leukocytes on nylon with 100% autologous serum removes platelets, monocytes, and polymorphonuclear cells; minimal selective loss of B lymphocytes occurs (Dickler, 1974). Both Ficoll (Yu et al., 1974) and bovine serum albumin (Geha et al., 1973) gradients have been used to separate classes of leukocytes and to separate live from dead cells. Other cell separation techniques that are of interest include separation of T and B lymphocytes on the basis of sheep red blood cell rosette formation with subsequent fractionation (O'Toole et al., 1974; Greaves and Brown, 1974), passage of nonimmunoglobulin-bearing cells through antiimmunoglobulin columns (Schlossman and Hudson, 1973), adherence of Fc receptor-bearing cells to antibody-coated target cells (Kedar *et al.*, 1974), adherence of presensitized or sensitized cells to specific target cells (Brondz and Goldberg, 1970; Golstein *et al.*, 1971; Lonai *et al.*, 1972) and depletion of lymphocyte subclasses with specific antisera and complement. Some of these techniques have been demonstrated in animal-model systems, but they should be applicable to human material. Each cell separation procedure being used for the first time to prepare attacking cells must be used with some caution, since cytotoxic effector cells may be functionally inactivated by the procedure but not damaged as determined by dye exclusion.

The preceding techniques are also used to prepare target cells from peripheral blood. In addition, residual contaminating red cells are frequently removed from the target cell preparation by lysis with distilled water or an ammonium chloride buffer (Boyle, 1968). Mitogen-transformed lymphocytes are more sensitive to immune damage than nontransformed lymphocytes, so prestimulation with mitogens (Miggiano *et al.*, 1972) is often used in preparation of lymphocyte target cells. Tissue culture lines are also used as target cells. Ideally, target cells which are trypsinized during the preparation procedure should be given time to regenerate surface antigens prior to use in the cytotoxicity assay. This can be accomplished by incubating trypsinized cells in spinner culture conditions (overnight is usually adequate) followed by ^{51}Cr labeling and addition of target cells to the assay. Alternatively, trypsinized cells which are normally adherent to glass and plastic can be labeled immediately with ^{51}Cr and then aliquoted to dishes that will be used in the cytotoxicity assay (Yust *et al.*, 1973). After overnight incubation in media, cells have usually attached to the bottom surface of the vessels and have regenerated antigens damaged by the trypsin. Media are then discarded, and attacking cells are added to the adherent, ^{51}Cr-labeled, target cells.

A wide variety of vessels have been used for coincubation of attacking and target cells. They include Leighton tubes (Brunner *et al.*, 1968), petri dishes (Canty and Wunderlich, 1970), test tubes (Garovoy *et al.*, 1973), and microtiter plate wells (Menard *et al.*, 1972; Smith, 1973; Steele *et al.*, 1973). Cytotoxic activity in test tubes or microwells is improved by low-speed centrifugation (50 g for 5 minutes) at the beginning of the incubation. Most incubations are carried out in a bicarbonate-buffered tissue culture media under a 37°C, CO_2–air atmosphere. Nonbicarbonate-buffered media also suffice for cell-mediated cytotoxicity (Wunderlich *et al.*, 1973). The optimal incubation time depends on the type of target cell and the cytotoxic activity of attacking cells. Incubation times have ranged from less than an hour to more than 24 hours. The longer time periods permit more target cell damage by immune cells, but the spontaneous leakage of ^{51}Cr from target cells incubated with normal lymphoid cells or media alone also increases. In addition, longer incubation periods appear to detect more cytotoxic pathways and allow *in vitro* differentiation of attacking and target cells (see below).

Several factors affect concentrations of attacking and target cells which are chosen for cytotoxicity assays. The percentage of attacking cells which are actually cytotoxic is not known, since adequate plaquing assays specific for cytotoxic cells (analogous to the Jerne plaquing assay for humoral antibody-forming cells) are not available. Thus ideal attacking to target cell ratios may vary for each experimental system, and we can consider the problem only in general terms. Initially, as the concentration of attacking cells increases, more target cell damage occurs; eventually cell overcrowding occurs with consequent little gain in cytotoxicity. Relatively high ratios of attacking to target cells (A:T ratios approximately >50:1) are used if availability of target cells is limited (a frequent problem with human studies), if the assay is being compared to a different type of cytotoxicity test which traditionally uses low numbers of target cells, if cytotoxic cell activity is particularly weak, or if the investigator wishes to express results in the form of a parallel-line assay (Fig. 2A). Alternatively, high concentrations of target cells (A:T ratios approximately <5:1) are used if the investigator wishes to express results in the form of a slope-ratio assay (Fig. 2B). With the

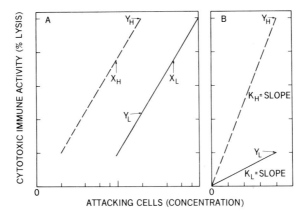

Fig. 2. Parallel-line (A) and slope-ratio (B) assays for determination of cytotoxic immune cell activity. Y_H and Y_L refer to cytotoxic activities associated with two different sources of attacking cells ("high" and "low" cytotoxic activity) tested at the same concentration. X_H and X_L refer to the concentrations of attacking cells from two different sources required to cause a common level of cytotoxicity.

latter procedure, the percentage of total target cells immunologically injured is low; immune activity however, is a linear function of the attacking cell concentration. In the parallel line assay, which in cytotoxicity tests requires plotting immune activity versus log of attacking cell concentration, relative immune activities of two different populations of attacking cells are determined not by the ratio of activities at a fixed attacking cell concentration (Y_H/Y_L in Fig. 2A), but rather by the ratio of attacking cells required to cause a given percentage of lysis (X_L/X_H in Fig. 2A). In the slope-ratio assay, relative immune activities are determined by relative slopes of the two functions (K_H/K_L in Fig. 2B) or by the ratio of activities at a fixed attacking cell concentration (Y_H/Y_L in Fig. 2B). Readers should consult more detailed sources to understand qualifications and limitations of slope-ratio and parallel-line assays (Finney, 1964). It is important to note that many clinical studies have used high A:T ratios and have compared attacking cells from different sources at a fixed attacking cell concentration. As noted above, results of these studies do not permit meaningful quantitative comparison of immune activities (Y_L versus Y_H in Fig. 2A), because immune cells are not saturated with targets. Only qualitative comparisons are valid in these cases.

Two different procedures have been used to calculate immune activity: Test-Control/Max-BG versus Test-Control/Max-Control. "Test" represents the ^{51}Cr released from target cells incubated with immune cells. "Control" represents ^{51}Cr released from target cells incubated in media alone or with nonimmune cells. "Max" represents the maximal amount of releasable ^{51}Cr in the target cells. "BG" refers to background counts detected by the gamma counter. When spontaneous release of label is high, the latter equation increases the calculated value for immune activity. At present neither theoretical considerations nor experimental data favor using only one method of calculation, and both procedures are commonly used (Stulting and Berke, 1973).

IV. Examples of Clinical Applications

Although *in vitro* tests for cell-mediated cytotoxicity have been used widely in clinical studies (see Introduction and References), rapid tests for direct cell-mediated cytotoxicity have had limited use. Consequently, few studies are referred to here in order to illustrate clinical applications.

A. Transplantation Immunity

Patients awaiting organ transplantation have been tested for rapid direct cell-mediated cytotoxicity against cells from potential donors. Garovoy and his colleagues (1973) evaluated 25 patients who were potential renal allograft recipients. Peripheral blood cells were used as attackers and targets in 4-hour assays. Eleven of the patients had positive cell-mediated immunity toward donors against whom complement-dependent antibody tests were negative. Of particular interest is their observation that three patients had rejection episodes following transplantation with kidneys from donors against whom cellular immunity, but not complement-dependent, humoral immunity was observed.

In their evaluation of six patients who were potential renal allograft recipients, Lightbody and Rosenberg (1974) identified two patients who had positive cell-mediated cytotoxicity tests against one or more potential donors. Humoral immunity (complement- or cell-dependent) was also noted in each of these cross matches. Furthermore, humoral (complement- or cell-dependent), but not cellular, immunity against potential donors was found in the other four patients. In this study, 4-hour tests for direct cell-mediated cytotoxicity appeared less useful than tests for cell-dependent and complement-dependent cytotoxic antibody. Differences between the Garovoy and Lightbody studies could represent different patient populations and/or different techniques.

B. Virus Resistance

Sensitized lymphocytes can operate against virus infections in several different ways. Upon contact with antigen they can release lymphokines, such as lymphotoxin, leukotactic factors, and interferon. They also can directly destroy virus-infected cells, as demonstrated by *in vitro* cytotoxicity tests. Labowskie and his colleagues (1974), for example, found that lymphocytes from patients with previous measles infections (rubeola) damaged measles-infected HeLa target cells, but not uninfected HeLa target cells, in 18-hour ^{51}Cr-release cytotoxicity tests. Lymphocytes from normal donors failed to injure infected target cells. Similar findings have occurred with studies of patients with previous histories of rubella infections (Steele *et al.*, 1973). Evidence for cytotoxic lymphocyte responses against virus-related antigens in animal model systems has been recently reviewed (Blanden, 1974; Doherty and Zinkenagel, 1974; Cole and Nathanson, 1974).

C. Autoimmunity

Cytotoxic lymphocytes may have a role in generation of autoimmune disease. Podleski (1972) has demonstrated that lymphocytes from certain patients with Hashimoto's thyroiditis were cytotoxic within 9 hours for target cells to which human thyroglobulin or microsomal antigen from thyrotoxic thyroid glands was chemically coupled. This study also illustrates a useful technique. The target cell itself was simply a reaction indicator. The relevant antigens were attached to the target cell surface prior to addition of attacking cells (Henney, 1970). Patients' lymphocytes were not toxic for uncoated target cells, and lymphocytes from normal donors were minimally toxic for antigen-coated target cells.

D. TUMOR IMMUNITY

Cytotoxic cells which react with tumor-associated antigens have been demonstrated in a wide variety of tumor models (Hellström and Hellström, 1974). Most of the reported assays with human material involve lengthy incubation periods, during which non-T lymphoid cells can play a prominent role in target-cell destruction (O'Toole et al., 1974). Relatively short ^{51}Cr-release assays have demonstrated T-cell-mediated cytotoxicity against tumors in rodent models (Cerottini and Brunner, 1974). Cellular immunity against human tumors, however, has rarely been studied using rapid cytotoxicity assays. One study of interest involved genotypically identical twins, one of whom had leukemia. Rosenberg and his colleagues (1972) used fresh leukemic cells as targets and lymphocytes from the healthy twin, family members, and unrelated donors as attackers in 4-hour cytotoxicity tests. Lymphocytes from 20 individuals were cytotoxic for target cells from the leukemic twin, but not for target cells from the normal identical twin. Reactivity against target cells from the normal twin, but not from the leukemic twin, was not seen. The results suggest that normal donors may have been presensitized against a common leukemia-associated antigen.

V. Interpretive Limitations

Interpretation of results from *in vitro* tests for direct cell-mediated cytotoxicity in terms of clinical relevance is subject to numerous limitations. The effect of these limitations, discussed below in greater detail, is that cytotoxicity may be seen *in vitro* albeit absent *in situ*, and cytotoxicity may be undetectable *in vitro* although present *in situ*.

A. ATTACKING CELL SOURCE

Most clinical studies involving *in vitro* tests for direct cell-mediated cytotoxicity have been limited to peripheral blood as a source of effector cells. In rodent models, detection of effector cell activity depends greatly upon which portion of the lymphon is tested. In a single host, cytotoxic activity may be present in one portion of the lymphon yet absent in another area (Berke *et al.*, 1972; Cerottini and Brunner, 1974). Maturation rates of cytotoxic cells and migration of cells determine whether cytotoxic cells will be detected in a particular segment of the lymphon. Local maturation rates are affected by a complex variety of factors including local concentrations of antigens, responder cells, helper or suppressor cells, blocking factors and hormones. In human testing it is also likely that cytotoxic lymphocytes could be absent in peripheral blood but present at the graft or tumor site. On the other hand, the presence of cytotoxic lymphocytes in peripheral blood does not guarantee the presence of cytotoxic cells at the reaction site.

B. ATTACKING CELL PREPARATION

Loss of suppressor regulatory factors while preparing effector cells for *in vitro* assays may release cytotoxic activity not present *in situ*. Extensive washing of attacking cells may remove humoral blocking factors. Purification of T lymphocytes as attacking cells may remove non-T cells that suppress effector cell activity.

Indiscriminate purification of attacking cells may also result in loss of cytotoxic activity. Methods for purifying human T cells have been oriented toward normal, resting-stage T cells. Differences between normal and cytotoxic T cells (size, density, stickiness, surface receptors) could result in loss of cytotoxic cells during preparation of "pure" T cells. Various cell purification procedures may nonspecifically inactivate or destroy cytotoxic cells. Consequently, as in any purification procedure, it is prudent to monitor cell recovery and biological activity in both the discarded and saved cell fractions.

C. TARGET CELL SOURCE

Target cells of human origin, which are used for *in vitro* detection of cytotoxic cells, are usually mitogen-transformed peripheral blood lymphocytes or tissue-culture lines. Such cells are sensitive to immune damage, and spontaneous leakage of radioactive label such as ^{51}Cr is relatively low. Moreover, unlike the natural target cells *in situ*, they are not coated with antibody against surface antigens, a situation that may block direct cell-mediated cytotoxicity by presensitized lymphocytes. Although tissue-culture lines and mitogen-transformed lymphocytes are sensitive indicators for the presence of cytotoxic cells, they are imperfect replacements for the relevant target cells *in situ*. Cytotoxic cells that are detected by lysis of artificial target cells *in vitro* may not be capable of damaging more resistant natural target cells *in vivo*. Furthermore, tissue-culture cells may have been infected with virus *in vitro* or may otherwise express antigens not present on the natural target cells *in situ*. If the host has been independently immunized against the "irrelevant" antigens, cytotoxic cell activity may be seen *in vitro*.

Another concern regarding target cells involves comparison of cytotoxic cell activity against two different sources of target cells, one of which is the test target and the other a control. When immune cells preferentially damage the test target relative to the control, the test target may simply be more susceptible to damage by any toxic agent. Approaches to this problem include the use of a cytotoxicity inhibition test (de Landazuri and Herberman, 1972a) or of immune cells reactive with antigens present on both test and control target cells, which could reveal nonspecifically different susceptibilities to damage.

D. ISOTOPE RELEASE AS A MEASURE OF CELL-MEDIATED CYTOTOXICITY

Detection of target cell injury by isotope release, such at ^{51}Cr, has inherent limitations. Prominent examples are that the assay will not detect immune stimulation of target cell multiplication, the assay will not detect inhibition of target cell growth as opposed to lysis, the assay may not be long enough to reveal target cell injury, and isotope leakage may not always represent a lethal change in target-cell membrane permeability. Immune cell stimulation of tumor cell growth *in vivo* has been reported by Prehn (1972); an *in vitro* analog of this phenomenon, like inhibition of target cell growth in the absence of lysis, requires assays capable of detecting increases in the number of target cells. Correlation of changes in cell-membrane permeability or transport mechanisms with cell "injury" involves self-evident assumptions. Consequently, each *in vitro* model of cell-mediated cytotoxicity derived from ^{51}Cr release assays is bolstered by parallel but independent evidence for target cell damage.

E. *In Vitro* MATURATION OF CELLS DURING CYTOTOXIC ASSAYS

Noncytotoxic precursors of cytotoxic effector cells are capable of *in vitro* maturation. If maturation occurs within the duration of the cytotoxicity test, then cytotoxic activity not present *in vivo* may be found *in vitro*. The general consequences of this phenomenon are outlined in Fig. 3. The purpose of this simplified scheme is to show a wave of precursor cells which matures into cytotoxic cells with passage of time and under the influence of ancillary factors, such as antigen, helper cells, and blocking factors. If the wave moves rapidly and its forward wall is steep, cytotoxic activity which is absent *in situ* could develop *in vitro*. One might expect the wave to progress from noncytotoxic precursor cells to cytotoxic cells with similar speed *in situ*. The arrangement of ancillary maturation factors (noted above) *in vitro*, however, may be ·such that maturation inhibited *in vivo* can progress rapidly in a privileged *in vitro* environment. Rapid ^{51}Cr-release cytotoxicity tests lasting 10 hours or less have not yet been reported to permit adequate time for *in vitro* generation of cytotoxic cells from partially matured precursor cells (b to c in Fig. 3). If maturation of cytotoxic cells is considered to include deblocking (de Landazuri and Herberman, 1972b), then rapid *in vitro* "maturation" is a particular concern. Deblocking maturation, as opposed to cell differentiation requiring cell division, may occur within hours.

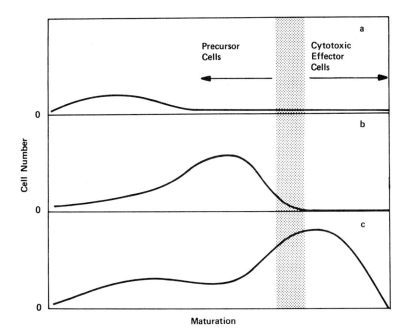

Fig. 3. Maturation of cytotoxic cells. Maturation of cells moves from left to right. Panels a, b, and c represent cell populations at different stages of maturation.

F. Detection of Multiple Cytotoxic Pathways

Earlier, several independent pathways for cell-mediated cytotoxicity were described. Clearly, a negative test for rapid direct cell-mediated cytotoxicity (assumed here to reflect sensitized T-cell activity), does not negate the possibility that other cell-mediated cytotoxic pathways are active in the patient. In addition, instances may arise in which rapid direct cell-mediated cytotoxic assays detect highly active non-T-cell-mediated cytotoxicity (Hibbs *et al.*, 1972; Lohmann-Matthes *et al.*, 1972). More definitive association of cytotoxic activity with T lymphocytes requires selective purification of attacking cells and demonstration that T lymphocytes are indeed mediating cytotoxic activity.

G. Diagnosis

Detection of cell-mediated cytotoxicity *in vitro* can be important for diagnosing the presence of a cellular immune response in the host, even if the response is immature or blocked so that cytotoxic cells do not exist *in situ*. Under these circumstances any manipulation of the *in vitro* test that will improve detection of sensitized cells would be appropriate. Such manipulations would include removal of suppressor factors from the attacking cell population, permitting *in vitro* maturation of effector cells and use of target cells which are highly sensitive to immune damage. It is highly important to note that such manipulations are intended only to distinguish between the normal, nonimmunized patient (Fig. 3a) and the sensitized patient with sensitization representing either partial (Fig. 3b) or more complete (Fig. 3c) maturation of sensitized cells to cytotoxic effector cells. For reasons discussed above, results of such tests would not necessarily be expected to correlate with the clinical status of the patient. The clinical status should reflect the presence of cytotoxic cells only if the cytotoxic cells are active *in situ* and are present in sufficient numbers at the relevant site.

VI. Some Future Applications

Isolation of lymphoid effector cells from reactive sites, including tumors and allografts, is technically feasible at the present time. Mechanical or enzymic dispersion of cells followed by gradient purification (see Section III) often yields viable lymphoid cells satisfactory for use in cytotoxicity assays. Thus, questions relating to the presence of cytotoxic cells at the reactive site can be approached. Target cells for these assays will initially be lymphoid cells or tissue culture lines. If problems accounting for rapid spontaneous leakage of ^{51}Cr from other types of target cells are solved, natural target cells more relevant to the *in situ* reaction will be used.

As currently used, rapid tests for direct cell-mediated cytotoxicity detect primarily cytotoxic cells as opposed to their precursors. It is also possible, however, to monitor development of human cytotoxic cells *in vitro* (Miggiano *et al.*, 1972), either from normal nonsensitized cells or partially matured cells. *In vitro* sensitization techniques permit investigators to search for factors, humoral or cellular, that might inhibit development of cytotoxic cells. *In vitro* sensitization against transplantation antigens has also demonstrated distinct roles for various classes of antigens, "lymphocyte defined" and "serologically defined," which stimulate development of cytotoxic cells (Eijsvoogel *et al.*, 1972; Bach *et al.*, 1973). Thus, the complex array of factors that enter into production of human cytotoxic cells should be better understood in the near future.

Adaptation of techniques for *in vitro* sensitization against transplantation antigens to sensitization against tumor-associated antigens offers great opportunity for studying the cytotoxic cell response to tumor-associated antigens (Golub *et al.*, 1972) and for passive immunotherapy. Regarding the latter point, *in vitro* sensitization allows an optimal immune response, because factors not easily controlled *in situ* can be manipulated *in vitro*. These factors include responder-stimulator cell ratios, helper-suppressor cell ratios, humoral blocking or stimulating factors and hormones.

Rapid detection of cytotoxic immunity against infectious organisms, which are not directly suitable for ^{51}Cr-release assays, may be possible by using indicator target cells or infected host cells as targets. As mentioned earlier, indicator target cells are coated with relevant soluble antigens before exposure to cytotoxic cells. Also noted earlier, virus-infected cells are excellent targets for detecting cytotoxic cells and virus-associated antigens. Cells infected with parasites may also provide satisfactory target cells for detecting cytotoxic host cells (Mauel and Behin, 1974).

VII. Concluding Comments

Awareness of different pathways for cytotoxic cellular immune responses has had a great impact on understanding the host response to allografts, tumors, infections, and autoantigens. Each of these pathways is in some way unique in its maturation or its effector stage; this in turn means that each pathway most likely has some unique aspects regarding its role in a particular disease, its responsiveness to natural amplifying or suppression factors, and its susceptibility to various drugs. The nature of the cytotoxic human T-lymphocyte response, one of the major pathways, is thus an important area of study. The present chapter discussed use of the rapid ^{51}Cr-release test for human direct cell-mediated cytotoxicity. In animal models this test measures primarily T-cell-induced cytotoxicity. The validity of this approximation in human studies remains to be determined. Other methods for measuring cell-mediated cytotoxicity *in vitro* will probably also detect cytotoxic T cells. Further studies utilizing anti-T-cell reagents or T-cell purification procedures will clearly lead to more definitive evaluation of the role of cytotoxic T cells in human immune responses.

Acknowledgments

Drs. Arnold Eggers, Richard Hodes, and Hillel Koren contributed many helpful comments. Preparation of the manuscript by Marilyn Schoenfelder is gratefully acknowledged.

References

Bach, F. H., Segall, M., Zier, K. S., Sondel, P. M., and Alter, B. J. (1973). Cell mediated immunity: Separation of cells involved in recognitive and destructive phases. *Science* **180**, 403–406.

Berke, G., Sullivan, K. A., and Amos, B. (1972). Rejection of ascites tumor allograft. I. Isolation, characterization, and in vitro reactivity of peritoneal lymphoid effector cells from BALB/c mice immune to EL4 leukosis. *J. Exp. Med.* **135**, 1334–1350.

Blanden, R. V. (1974). T cell response to viral and bacterial infection. *Transplant. Rev.* **19**, 56–88.

Bloom, B. R. (1971). In vitro approaches to the mechanism of cell-mediated immune reactions. *Advan. Immunol.* **13**, 101–208.

Boyle, W. (1968). An extension of the ^{51}Cr-release assay for the estimation of mouse cytotoxins. *Transplantation* **6**, 761–764.

Brondz, B. D., and Goldberg, N. E. (1970). Further in vitro evidence for polyvalent specificity of immune lymphocytes. *Folia Biol.* (*Prague*) **16**, 20–28.

Brunner, K. T., Mauel, J., Cerottini, J.-C., and Chapuis, B. (1968). Quantitative assay of the lytic action of immune lymphoid cells on ^{51}Cr-labeled allogenic target cells in vitro. Inhibition by isoantibody and by drugs. *Immunology* **14**, 181–196.

Canty, T. G., and Wunderlich, J. R. (1970). Quantitative in vitro assay of cytotoxic cellular immunity. *J. Nat. Cancer Inst.* **45**, 761–772.

Cerottini, J.-C., and Brunner, K. T. (1974). Cell mediated cytotoxicity, allograft rejection and tumor immunity. *Advan. Immunol.* 18, 67–123.

Cerottini, J.-C., Nordin, A. A., and Brunner, K. T. (1970). Specific *in vitro* cytotoxicity of thymus-derived lymphocytes sensitized to alloantigens. *Nature (London)* 228, 1308–1309.

Cole, G., and Nathanson, N. (1974). Lymphocytic choriomeningitis. Pathogenesis. *Prog. Med. Virol.* 18, 94–110.

de Landazuri, M. O., and Herberman, R. B. (1972a). Specificity of cellular immune reactivity to virus-induced tumors. *Nature (London), New. Biol.* 238, 18–19.

de Landazuri, M. O., and Herberman, R. B. (1972b). In vitro activation of cellular immune response to gross virus-induced lymphoma. *J. Exp. Med.* 136, 969–983.

Dickler, H. B. (1974). Studies of the human lymphocyte receptor for heat-aggregated or antigen-complexed immunoglobulin *J. Exp. Med.* 140, 508–522.

Doherty, P. C., and Zinkernagel, R. M. (1974). T cell-mediated immunopathology in viral infections. *Transplant. Rev.* 19, 89–120.

Eijsvoogel, V. P., du Bois, M. J. G. J., Melief, C. H., de Groot-Kooy, M. L., Koning, L., van Leeuwen, A., van Rood, J. J., du Toit, E. D., and Schellekens, P. T. A. (1972). Position of a locus determining mixed lymphocyte reaction (MLR) distinct from the known HLA loci and its relationship to cell mediated lympholysis (CML). *In* "Histocompatibility Testing" (P. I. Terasaki, ed.,), pp. 501–508. Munksgaard, Copenhagen.

Evans, R., and Alexander, P. (1972). Mechanism of immunologically specific killing of tumor cells by macrophages. *Nature (London)* 236, 168–170.

Finney, D. J. (1964). "Statistical Method in Biological Assay." Hafner, New York.

Garovoy, M. R., Zschaeck, D., Strom, T. B., Franco, V. Carpenter, C. B., and Merrill, J. P. (1973). Direct lymphocyte-mediated cytotoxicity as an assay of presensitization. *Lancet* 1, 573–576.

Geha, R. S., Rosen, F. S., and Merler, E. (1973). Identification and characterization of subpopulations of lymphocytes in human peripheral blood after fractionation on discontinuous gradients of albumin. The cellular defect in X linked agammaglobulinemia. *J. Clin. Invest.* 52, 1726–1734.

Golstein, P., Svedmyr, E. A. J., and Wigzell, H. (1971). Cells mediating specific *in vitro* cytotoxicity. I. Detection of receptor-bearing lymphocytes. *J. Exp. Med.* 134, 1385–1402.

Golub, S. H., Svedmyr, E. A., Hewetson, J. F., and Klein, G. (1972). Cellular reactions against Burkitt lymphoma cells. III. Effector cell activity of leukocytes stimulated *in vitro* with autochthonous cultured lymphoma cells. *Int. J. Cancer* 10, 157–164.

Greaves, M. F., and Brown, G. (1974). Purification of human T and B lymphocytes. *J. Immunol.* 112, 420–423.

Hellström, K. E., and Hellström, I. (1974). Lymphocyte-mediated cytotoxicity and blocking serum activity to tumor antigens. *Advan. Immunol.* 18, 209–277.

Henney, C. S. (1970). A cytolytic system for the *in vitro* detection of cell-mediated immunity to soluble antigen. *J. Immunol.* 105, 919–927.

Hibbs, J. B. (1974). Heterocytolysis by macrophages activated by Bacillus Calmette-Guerin: Lysosome exocytoxis into tumor cells. *Science* 184, 468–471.

Hibbs, J. B., Lambert, L. H., and Remington, J. S. (1972). Possible role of macrophage mediated nonspecific cytotoxicity in tumor resistance. *Nature (London)* 235, 48–50.

Kedar, E., de Landazuri, M. O., and Bonavida, B. (1974). Cellular immunoadsorbents: A simplified technique for separation of lymphoid cell populations. *J. Immunol.* **112,** 1231–1243.

Labowskie, R. J., Edelman, R., Rustigian, R., and Bellanti, J. A. (1974). Studies of cell-mediated immunity to measles virus by a vitro lymphocyte-mediated cytotoxicity. *J. Infec. Dis.* **129,** 233–239.

Lamon, E. W., Wigzell, H., Klein, E., Andersson, B., and Skurzak, H. M. (1973). The lymphocyte response to primary Moloney sarcoma virus tumors in BALB/c mice. Definition of the active subpopulations at different times after infection. *J. Exp. Med.* **137,** 1472–1493.

Lightbody, J. J., and Rosenberg, J. C. (1974). Antibody-dependent cell-mediated cytotoxicity in prospective kidney transplant recipients. *J. Immunol.* **112,** 890–896.

Lohmann-Matthes, M. L., and Fischer, H. (1973). T-cell cytotoxicity and amplification of the cytotoxic reaction by macrophages. *Transplant. Rev.* **17,** 150–171.

Lohmann-Matthes, M. L., Schipper, H., and Fischer, H. (1972). Macrophage-mediated cytotoxicity against allogeneic target cells *in vitro. Eur. J. Immunol.* **2,** 45–49.

Lonai, P., Wekerle, H., and Feldman, M. (1972). Fractionation of specific antigen-reactive cells in an *in vitro* system of cell-mediated immunity. *Nature (London), New Biol.* **235,** 235–236.

Mauel, J., and Behin, R. (1974). Cell-mediated and humoral immunity to protozoan infections (with special reference to leishmaniasis). *Transplant. Rev.* **19,** 121–146.

Menard, S., Pierotti, M., and Colnaghi, M. (1972). A ^{51}Cr microtest for cellular immunity. *Transplantation* **14,** 155–158.

Miggiano, V. C., Bernoco, D., Lightbody, J., Trinchieri, G., and Ceppellini, R. (1972). Cell-mediated lympholysis *in vitro* with normal lymphocytes as target: Specificity and cross reactivity of the test. *Transplant. Proc.* **4,** 231–237.

Möller, G., (1973). "Effector Cells in Cell Mediated Immunity," *Transplantation Reviews,* Vol. 17. Munksgaard, Copenhagen.

O'Toole, C., Stejskal, V., Perlmann, P., and Karlsson, M. (1974). Lymphoid cells mediating tumor specific cytotoxicity to carcinoma of the urinary bladder. *J. Exp. Med.* **959,** 457–466.

Perlmann, P., and Holm, G. (1969). Cytotoxic effects of lymphoid cells in vitro. *Advan. Immunol.* **11,** 117–185.

Podleski, N. K. (1972). Cytotoxic lymphocytes in Hashimoto thyroiditis. *Clin. Exp. Immunol.* **11,** 543–548.

Prehn, R. T. (1972). The immune reaction as a stimulator of tumor growth. *Science* **176,** 170.

Rosenberg, E. B., Herberman, R. B., Levine, P. H., Halterman, R. H., McCoy, J. L., and Wunderlich, J. R. (1972). Lymphocyte cytotoxicity reactions to leukemia-associated antigens in identical twins. *Int. J. Cancer* **9,** 648–658.

Schlossman, S. F., and Hudson, L. (1973). Specific purification of lymphocyte populations on a digestible immunoabsorbent. *J. Immunol.* **110,** 313–315.

Shacks, S. J., Chiller, J., and Granger, G. A. (1973). Studies on *in vitro* models of cellular immunity: The role of T and B cells in the secretion of lymphotoxin. *Cell. Immunol.* **7,** 313–321.

Smith, R. W. (1973). ^{51}Cr release microassays for histocompatibility antigens on normal and malignant cells. *Transplantation* **16,** 246–249.

Steele, R. W., Hensen, S. A., Vincent, M. M., Fuccillo, D. A., and Bellanti, J. A.

(1973) A ^{51}Cr microassay technique for cell-mediated immunity to viruses. *J. Immunol.* 110, 1502–1510.

Stulting, R. D., and Berke, G. (1973). The use of ^{51}Cr release as a measure of lymphocyte-mediated cytolysis *in vitro*. *Cell. Immunol.* 9, 474–476.

Thorsby, E., and Bratlie, A. (1970). A rapid method for preparation of pure lymphocyte suspensions. *In* "Histocompatibility Testing" (P. I. Terasaki, ed.), pp. 655–658. Munksgaard, Copenhagen.

Wisloff, F., and Froland, S. S. (1973). Antibody-dependent lymphocyte-mediated cytotoxicity in man: No requirement for lymphocytes with membrane-bound immunoglobulin. *Scand. J. Immunol.* 2, 151–157.

Wunderlich, J. R., Rogentine, G. N., Jr., and Yankee, R. A. (1972). Rapid in vitro detection of cellular immunity in man against freshly explanted allogeneic cells. *Transplantation* 13, 31–37.

Wunderlich, J. R., Martin, W. J., and Macdonald, J. (1973). Functional efficiency of antitumor cytotoxic lymphoid cells. *Isr. J. Med. Sci.* 9, 317–323.

Yu, D. T. Y., Peter, J. B., Paulus, H. E., and Nies, K. M. (1974). Human lymphocyte subpopulations. Study of T and B cells and their density distribution. *Clin. Immunol. Immunopathol.* 2, 333–342.

Yust, I., Wunderlich, J. R., Mann, D. L., and Buell, D. N. (1973). Cytotoxicity mediated by human lymphocyte-dependent antibody in a rapid assay with adherent target cells. *J. Immunol.* 110, 1672–1681.

Lymphocyte Transformation *in Vitro* in Response to Mitogens and Antigens[1]

SUSANNA CUNNINGHAM-RUNDLES, JOHN A. HANSEN, and BO DUPONT

Clinical Immunology Laboratory, Memorial Sloan-Kettering Cancer Center, New York, New York

[1] Original work reported in this chapter has been supported in part by the American Cancer Society, U.S. Public Health NIH-CA08748-0851, NCI Program Project Grant CA 17404-01-02, and the Zelda Weintraub Fund. We thank Joan Feld for excellent technical assistance and John W. Hadden for critical reading of the manuscript.

151

I. Introduction

When normal human lymphocytes are isolated from peripheral blood and incubated in tissue culture medium with small amounts of a number of substances including plant lectins, microbial products, and some inorganic molecules, they transform into blast cells that proliferate by undergoing mitosis. This proliferative phase of culture may last for some days before culture growth plateaus and finally declines. Both the proportion of the initial population that undergoes blast transformation and the kinetics of the mitotic response that follows are characteristic for the particular type of lymphocyte stimulant that is used to initiate the reaction. Chemical differences in the binding reaction, the specificity of certain binding cells, and ensuing cell-triggering form the molecular basis of this difference between stimulants.

In vitro transformation of human lymphocytes can be induced by at least four different types of stimulants: (1) the nonspecific mitogens, which include the plant lectins and certain microbial products (phytohemagglutinin, pokeweed mitogen, concanavalin A, staphylococcal filtrate, etc.), (2) the specific antigens that stimulate lymphocytes from presensitized donors, (3) allogeneic lymphocytes, and (4) antiimmunoglobulin antibodies. The first two types of stimulants will be discussed in this chapter.

The ability of the mammalian lymphocyte to respond to the extracts of several plants and to microbial metabolites by undergoing mitotic proliferation is a distinctive characteristic, which has increasingly been shown to reflect both the immunological status and the immune potential of the whole organism.

Lymphocyte transformation is conveniently measured by the incorporation of radioactive thymidine into the DNA of dividing cells. The rate and amount of isotope incorporated, expressed as counts per minute (cpm), is a reflection of the strength of response and is directly related to the number of cells responding. Other parameters of lymphocyte response can also be measured, e.g., incorporation of amino acids into protein, amino acid transport, enzyme synthesis, RNA synthesis, and membrane changes. Lymphocyte transformation may also lead to secretion of lymphokines, e.g., blastogenic factor, migration inhibition factor, and interferon; however, elaboration of lymphoid products may occur in the absence of proliferation.

In this chapter, lymphocyte transformation will be discussed in relation to the proliferative response as measured by the rate of incorporation of radioactive thymidine. The differences between antigen-induced and mitogen-stimulated lymphocyte transformation will be explored both in relation to our present understanding of lymphocyte transformation as a biological phenomenon and as a tool for the clinical evaluation of primary and secondary deficiency diseases. A specific methodology suitable for obtaining and evaluating such data for the clinical application of *in vitro* lymphocyte transformation will be presented.

II. Lymphocyte Activation: Specific or Nonspecific

The substances that can induce lymphocyte transformation have been classified as specific or nonspecific depending upon whether or not response to the stimulus requires prior exposure of the cell donor to the stimulant. In man, this usually means that an *in vivo* primary response has occurred. In experimental animal model systems, this is referred to as the requirement for presensitization. The clonal selection theory (Burnet, 1959) implies that during ontogenetic development each lymphocyte becomes committed to respond to a specific antigen. Since the responding population for any specific antigen is at most a few cells, proliferation would be based on clonal expansion. Biochemical exploration of lymphocyte response has necessitated the use of quantitative techniques, which are not necessarily sensitive enough to prove or disprove this theory at the present time. In addition, the discovery of functional subclasses of lymphocytes, e.g., helper cells, killer cells, suppressor cells, which participate in the generation of the immune response make it seem most probable that clonal restriction is only one aspect of a complex biological phenomenon.

Cells that interact in a specific way with antigen are sometimes referred to an *antigen-binding cells.* Some, but not all, of these cells will be stimulated to undergo blastogenesis and may be referred to as *antigen-reactive cells* (ARC).

Kinetic analysis of mitogen- and antigen-induced lymphocyte transformation has proven to be of major empirical value in discriminating between the two types of stimulators. The magnitude of mitogenic response is greater than that of antigenic response. Since the proportion of the lymphocyte population that participates is greater, mitogens induce an earlier peak response, which can be quantitated as incorporation of radioactive thymidine or by microscopic examination of the number of blast cells (Ling and Husband, 1964; Jimenez *et al.*, 1970). Figure 1 illustrates the typical response of a normal cell donor to mitogens and antigens. Substances that induce *in vitro* proliferation without the cell donor's having been previously sensitized are considered to have the capacity to react in a relatively nonspecific way with many different lymphocyte clones. Since a large number of clones respond to this type of stimulus, mitogens are often referred to as polyclonal activators.

Response to antigen implies prior immunization. Common microbial

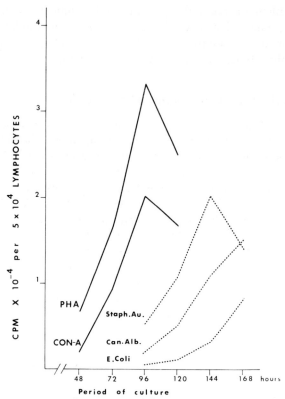

Fig. 1. Time sequences for mitogen and antigen response. Data obtained from microtiter culture of normal donor lymphocytes with mitogens and antigens. Cultures were harvested on several days as shown, and the time courses obtained are characteristic for these stimulants. CON-A, concanavalin A; PHA, phytohemagglutinin; E. Coli, *Escherichia coli;* Can. Alb., *Candida albicans;* Staph. Au., *Staphylococcus aureus.*

antigens may be ubiquitous in the environs of the organism, and even for rare antigens it may be difficult to exclude the possibility of a primary exposure. Also human cord blood lymphocytes can be shown to possess some reactivity to a number of antigens. Prior immunization may have occurred in newborn infants, since the human placenta is permeable to albumins, globulins, and viruses. In addition, cross-reacting specificities may exist between sensitizing molecules and essential determinants on test substances which themselves have molecular heterogeneity. Purification of test substances in at least one instance (Plate and Amos, 1971a,b) has led to the isolation of an antigenlike lymphocyte stimulant from a more heterogeneous mitogenlike activator.

A. Mitogens: Nonspecific Inducers of Lymphocyte Transformation

The capacity of extracts made from plants to cause lymphocytes to grow and divide in culture was first recognized by Hungerford *et al.* in 1959. The extract of the red kidney bean (*Phaseolus vulgaris*) used in this experiment is called phytohemagglutinin (PHA) because of its red cell agglutinating properties. The stimulatory capacity of PHA was confirmed by Nowell (1960). Lymphocytes isolated from a number of sources, i.e., from peripheral blood, lymph nodes, spleen, and thoracic duct, were subsequently shown to be capable of mitogenic response. A number of other plant substances, including concanavalin A (Con A) extracted from jack beans, wax bean glycoprotein, and pokeweed mitogen (PWM), have been characterized and shown to possess this kind of lymphocyte-stimulating activity. Similar effects have been observed with streptolysin S and staphylococcal filtrate. A representative list of mitogens appears in Table I. Nonspecific stimulation of lymphocytes may also be achieved to a lesser extent by some proteolytic enzymes, by divalent cations such as zinc and mercury, and by sodium periodate.

The ability of the phytomitogens to initiate lymphocyte transformation was recognized long before the purification was undertaken. The phyto-

TABLE I

Mitogens

Name	Characteristics
Phytohemagglutinin, PHA (*Phaseolus vulgaris*)	Mitogenic and cell wall agglutinating properties; PHA-M is impure extract, PHA-P is partially purified and heterogeneous; PHA-H: erythroagglutinin with mitogenic properties; PHA-L: mitogenic, no agglutinating properties; protein and carbohydrate
Concanavalin A, Con A (*Canavalia ensiformis*)	Mitogenic and cell wall agglutinating properties; protein
Lentil mitogen (*Lens culinaris*)	Mitogenic with weak agglutinating properties; similar to Con A; protein and carbohydrate
Pokeweed mitogen, PWM (*Phytolacca americana*)	Little agglutinating activity; mitogenic; glycoprotein
Staphylococcal filtrates (*Staphyloccocus aureus*)	Soluble diffusible mitogens produced by all strains of *S. aureus*
Streptolysin S (B-hemolytic streptococci)	Filtrate activity distinct from hemolysin
Endotoxins, LPS (*Serratia marcesens, Escherichia coli, Proteus vulgaris, Shigella flexneri*)	Lipopolysaccharide with endotoxin activity, mitogenic for mouse spleen cells (B cells), little effect on man, rabbit

hemagglutinins have now been shown to be proteins containing carbohydrates in varying amounts except for Con A, which contains no carbohydrate. Several phytomitogens contain separable leukoagglutinating and erythroagglutinating components, both types of which can stimulate lymphocytes. Molecular analysis of PHA by Weber (1969) demonstrated that the leukoagglutinating property and the lymphocyte-stimulating property occupy different sites on the same molecule. Lymphocyte-stimulating capacity could be abolished without affecting the agglutinating property, but agglutination was found to be necessary for cell activation. This may imply that the leukoagglutinating activity reflects the ability of the molecule to attach to the lymphocyte, and may promote lymphocyte transformation by increasing cell-to-cell contact and effective cell density.

Although the precise relationship between lymphocyte activation by mitogens and lymphocyte function *in vivo* is not yet understood, there is a remarkable correlation between the loss or the decrease of *in vitro* lymphocyte response to mitogens and a number of primary and secondary immunodeficiency diseases. Anergy to skin-testing antigens and allergens can be paralleled by loss of normal PHA response. This relationship between *in vitro* responsiveness has been demonstrated in sarcoidosis (Hirschorn *et al.*, 1964), Hodgkin's disease (Hersh and Oppenheim, 1965), and ataxia telangiectasia (Leikin *et al.*, 1966) among other diseases.

B. ANTIGENS: SPECIFIC INDUCERS OF AN IMMUNE REACTION

In 1963 Pearmain *et al.* reported that the lymphocytes of tuberculin-positive individuals transformed *in vitro* in the presence of the purified protein derivative obtained from tuberculin (PPD) whereas the lymphocytes of tuberculin-negative individuals failed to transform. The strength of the skin test response has been found to correlate well with the degree of lymphocyte transformation (Miller and Jones, 1973). High dose stimulation with tuberculin, however, may cause lymphocytes from skin test-negative donors to respond (Nilsson, 1972).

Specific transformation of presensitized cells has similarly been obtained with antigens in a number of animal studies. Whereas PHA stimulates rabbit spleen cells and peripheral leukocytes to divide (Harris and Littleton, 1966; Sabesin *et al.*, 1965) without the animal's having been immunized previously, stimulation with heterologous proteins or sheep red cells does require previous immunization with the stimulating antigen. Oppenheim *et al.* (1967) similarly demonstrated transformation to PPD and to guinea pig albumin-orthanilic acid with lymphocytes that had been taken from guinea pigs preimmunized with the same antigen. Nonimmunized guinea pigs did not respond. Germfree, colostrum-deprived piglets respond to the mitogen streptococcal pyrogenic exotoxin, but not to lipopolysaccharide (LPS), keyhole limpet hemocyanin (KLH), or sheep red blood cells (Kim, 1975).

Viral antigens have been somewhat less extensively investigated than bacterial antigens, although transformation with vaccinia (Matsaniotis and Tsenghi, 1964; Sarkany and Caron, 1966) and poliomyelitis vaccine (Elves, 1963) were among the earliest reports of antigen-induced lymphocyte transformation. In some instances, the addition of live virus (rubella, Newcastle disease, polio, and influenza) to human lymphocyte cultures depresses lymphocyte transformation. Olsen *et al.* (1968) have demonstrated impaired DNA, RNA, and protein synthesis in measles-infected lymphocytes following stimulation with PHA or PWM. This experimental situation has been viewed as an *in vitro* mimic of congenital rubella, where a lack of response to PHA has often been correlated with clinically identifiable infection. In addition, Smithwick and Berkovich (1966) observed depressed response to PPD *in vitro* with lymphocytes taken from children with measles and active tuberculosis. Virus-induced suppression may result from cell surface changes induced by replicating virus within the cell. Thompson *et al.* (1973) have demonstrated lymphocyte activation of fresh cells from donors by their own lymphocytes infected in short-term cultures by adenovirus type 2, influenza, and herpes simplex type 1. Viral replication does not always produce suppression and may occur simultaneously with transformation (e.g., parainfluenza). Inactivation of viruses alone does not always permit lymphocyte transformation. Antigen preparation (and hence antigen presentation) must be determined for each system (Simons and Fitzgerald, 1968; Smith *et al.*, 1973; Graziano *et al.*, 1975). The specificity of virus-induced lymphocyte transformation has been established in a number of instances. Herpes simplex (type 1) will stimulate the lymphocytes of individuals having histories of repeated herpetic infections (Russell, 1974; O'Reilly and Lopez, 1975). The specificity of lymphocyte responses to herpes simplex antigen can be demonstrated in experimental animals. Rabbits which have been preimmunized with herpes simplex have been shown to respond to herpes, but not to vaccinia. The reciprocal experiment yielded equivalent results (Rosenberg *et al.*, 1972). The use of specific antigens in clinical assessment of immune deficiencies has particular application in cases where disease-specific or disease-related antigens may be developed. Such antigens [e.g., herpes virus in herpetic infections (O'Reilly and Lopez, 1975), paramyxoviruses in multiple sclerosis (Cunningham-Rundles *et al.*, 1976)] may reveal specific immune deficiencies in otherwise immunocompetent individuals. Table II lists antigens that are commonly used in immune response studies.

TABLE II
Antigens

Name	Characteristics
Candida albicans	*C. albicans* (A) grown on Sabouraud agar for 48 hours extracted by sonication; the supernatant following ultracentrifugation is used
Escherichia coli	Whole "heat-inactivated" late log phase *E. coli*, 10^9 cells/ml, isolated from normal donors
Staphylococcus aureus	Prepared as for *E. coli*
Purified protein derivative (PPD)	Acetone and ether-dried preparation of human tuberculin, commercial
Streptokinase/streptodornase (SK/SD)	Commercial enzyme preparation from *Streptococcus* dialyzed against phosphate-buffered saline
Tetanus toxoid	Commercial vaccine preparation
Mumps	Commercial skin test antigen dialyzed against phosphate-buffered saline
Viral antigens including measles, parainfluenza, cytomegalovirus, adenovirus, and poliovirus	Commercially available as complement fixation antigens with control antigen from uninfected cells; some require additional concentration and/or inactivation

C. Changes in *in Vitro* Lymphocyte Responses during *in Vivo* Immunization

The small lymphocyte plays a key role in cell-mediated reactions as shown by the passive transfer of delayed hypersensitivity reactions to nonsensitized recipients (Mitchison, 1955). Mills (1966) demonstrated delayed hypersensitivity in guinea pigs sensitized with extremely small amounts of egg albumin. Skin tests in such animals revealed no Arthus reactivity, but weak to moderately strong delayed hypersensitivity reactions appeared 2 weeks after immunization. Serum antibody titers were negligibly low. Lymphocytes from presensitized animals transformed in culture when challenged with this antigen. On the other hand, animals immunized intravenously had strong Arthus reactions, high serum antibody titers, and no *in vitro* lymphocyte transformation. Other workers have demonstrated that the transformation phenomenon is initiated by the immunizing conjugate only; antigenic recognition will not take place in the presence of a hapten conjugated to an indifferent carrier, although antibodies directed against the hapten alone are clearly synthesized. The presence of the hapten may, however, somewhat inhibit the response to the conjugate. This could imply competition for an antigenic site (Oppenheim *et al.*, 1967; Dutton and Bulman, 1964). Similar results have been observed by Spitler *et al.* (1970) with specific peptides of tobacco mosaic virus protein, where carrier specificity was shown to be required for lymphocyte transformation but not for the elicitation of delayed skin reactions.

Curtis *et al.* (1970) utilized an antigen prepared from the murine keyhole limpet (keyhole limpet hemocyanin, KLH) to investigate *in vitro* correlation with primary *in vivo* antigenic immunization in man. Increases in *in vitro* antigen stimulation were observed 7 days after immunization. Positive antibody titer was also evident. During the early period following immunization, strong increases in response were observed with increasing antigen concentrations whereas at later times strong transformation was observed with lower concentrations of antigen. The primary response has also been studied by Andersen *et al.* (1971a,b) using killed *Brucella abortus* Bang as the antigen. Donors were patients with a variety of disorders selected for their initial lack of reactivity to *Brucella.* Considerable variation was observed among the responders. One group showed a maximal response between day 6 and day 9 and decreased response by day 15. Another group showed increasing response until day 6. After day 6, response remained constant and did not increase. Finally, a third group showed increasing response throughout the period of observation. Antibody formation did not parallel lymphocyte transformation. The finding common to both these studies is that lower concentrations of antigen are more effective in stimulating lymphocytes after the initial period of primary induction. This may reflect a process of differentiation within lymphocyte subclasses that participate in the response and may indicate the production of cells with increasing receptor affinity for antigen.

III. Characteristics of the Reaction

A. Morphological and Metabolic Changes in the Transformed Cell

The addition of phytomitogens to human lymphocytes *in vitro* initiates a series of morphological changes that can be observed by light microscopy, histochemistry, and electron microscopy. Most of the lymphocytes in peripheral blood are in a resting phase characterized by sparse, finely granular cytoplasm, a few, large mitochondria, and scattered ribosomes. The Golgi apparatus is not well developed (Inman and Cooper, 1963). The nuclei contain coarse, closely packed heterochromatin and some euchromatin. The comparative morphology of T and B cells is currently being investigated, and one report (Sun-Lin *et al.*, 1973) indicates that B cells may have a more complex villous surface than T cells, which are smaller and smoother. PHA stimulation initiates a graded series of changes that produces a large population of blast cells. Morphological changes are detectable by 24 hours of culture with PHA. Cell size increases, euchromatin content of the nucleus increases, and nucleoli appear. A few blast cells are visible. A large proportion of the lymphocyte population is activated by 48 hours. Yoffey *et al.* (1965) characterized three types of blast cells. The functional meaning of this characterization is not known at present. By 72 hours large blast cells are common. Differences in PWM- and PHA-stimulated lymphocytes were described by Chessin *et al.* (1966) and Douglas (1972), and a distinct cell type characteristic for this stimulant was proposed. After 7–10 days in culture, this cell type has undergone extensive development of rough surface endoplastic reticulum and is morphologically indistinguishable from the plasma cell.

Lymphocyte stimulation is initiated by the attachment of the stimulating substance to the outer cell membrane. Mitogens and antigens have been shown to have receptors on the plasma membrane (Nossal and Ada, 1971; Allan *et al.*, 1971; Coombs *et al.*, 1970; Rabellino *et al.*, 1971; Wigzell and Andersson, 1969). The primary candidate for B-cell antigen receptor has been surface immunoglobulin; however, much clarification of this question is still required (see Table III). The recognition process of T lymphocytes, which may also bear immunoglobulin on their surfaces (Marchalonis, 1975), remains to be elucidated.

Early events in lymphocyte stimulation have been studied primarily by means of mitogens, since quantitative stimulation is needed to make these studies feasible. Removal of Con A from the cell surface by a specific inhibitor (α-methyl-D-mannoside) abolishes the mitogenic responses (Andersson *et al.*, 1972). A number of reports have suggested that affinity of mitogen binding is equal for lymphocytes of differing responsiveness (Stobo *et al.*, 1972; Skoog *et al.*, 1974; Inbar *et al.*, 1973; Powell and Leon, 1970; Wang *et al.* 1971). Similar work has been presented by Ozato *et al.* (1975), who have suggested that the inhibition of Con A binding to mouse thymocytes by PHA-P may occur either by means of competition for the same binding site or by conformational alteration of closely related binding sites. Subsequent to mitogen binding, a number of membrane changes occur, including enhanced uptake of amino acids (Mendelsohn *et al.*, 1971; Van den Berg and Betel, 1971), potassium (Quastel and Kaplan, 1970), calcium (Whitney and Sutherland, 1973), and sugars and nucleosides (Peters and Hansen, 1971a,b). The intracellular level of cyclic GMP increases (Hadden *et al.*, 1972). Endocytosis is stimulated (Hirschorn *et al.*, 1968). Membrane phospholipid metabo-

TABLE III

MODELS FOR B-CELL ACTIVATION

	I[a] One nonspecific signal	II[b] Pattern of antigen stimulation	III[c] Two signal
Receptor site	Non-Ig receptor not clonally distributed	Ig receptor	Ig receptor
Mechanism of triggering stimulation	Nonspecific polyclonal activation; signal is quantifiable, below threshold no response	Multivalent antigen; binding is required; spacing of antigen matrix is critical	Antigen binds to Ig receptor (signal 1) and second signal is generated by associative antibody binding to an antigen molecule bound by B-cell receptor. Signal 2 requires T cell, T-cell product, or macrophage
Mechanism of inducing tolerance	Beyond zone of stimulation, higher threshold above which paralysis ensues	High zone tolerance induced by high antigen concentration via lattice immobilization	Signal 1 occurs without signal 2
Prediction	B cells cannot be activated by thymus-dependent antigens and haptens	Epitope density is critical and bears quantitative relationship to stimulation and tolerance	Inductive signal includes paralytic signal. Reaction is antigen specific and implies that new B cells specific for self and/or foreign antigens are continuously generated

[a] Coutinho et al., 1975; Coutinho and Möller, 1974.
[b] Feldman et al., 1975; Diener and Feldman, 1972.
[c] Bretscher and Cohn, 1970; Schrader, 1973.

lism changes, and the incorporation of long-chain fatty acids into phospholipid lecithin have been reported (Kay, 1968; Resch and Ferber, 1972). Increased uptake of small molecules, which seems to be a primary response of the activated lymphocyte, will occur in the presence of high doses of mitogen that are toxic to later events. With the exception of Ca^{2+} uptake, where mitogen probably acts to increase carrier affinity for this ion, lymphocyte stimulation raises V_{max} (maximal velocity) without affecting K_m (concentration of substrate where velocity is $\frac{1}{2} V_{max}$ for the various uptake systems. This would tend to suggest that activation specifically affects uptake either by causing an increase in carrier molecules or by increasing the rate of uptake rather than by nonspecific loosening of the membrane. Inhibition of K^+ uptake by ouabain blocks protein synthesis but permits the early increase in RNA synthesis (Kay, 1972; Quastel and Kaplan, 1968). Many of the early transport activities are dependent upon Na^+ increase (Kay, 1973). Similarly, Ca^{2+} uptake is essential for lymphocyte stimulation. The relationship between the early phase of membrane activation and subsequent internal events is not clear at the present time. Studies in which the hypothesis that lymphocyte stimulation might be regulated by increases in the level of adenyl cyclases has been tested have yielded somewhat conflicting data, but current evidence does not support such a relationship (Webb *et al.*, 1973; Novogrodsky and Katchalski, 1970; Hadden *et al.*, 1972). The concentration of cyclic GMP, initially much lower than that of cyclic AMP, has been reported by Hadden *et al.* (1972) to increase between 10- and 20-fold within 20 minutes of the addition of Con A or PHA to lymphocytes. This nucleotide may therefore have a direct regulatory role in lymphocyte stimulation. The nature of gene activation that must occur during lymphocyte stimulation is not yet understood. Present failure to detect new species of RNA (Neiman and MacDonnell, 1971) has suggested that gene activation may be quite selective and need not evoke general derepression of the genome. Reported changes in cell deoxyribonucleoprotein (DNP) following activation include increased availability of DNA phosphate groups for binding to acridine orange (Killander and Rigler, 1965) and decreased interaction of histone basic groups with DNA phosphates (Zetterberg and Auer, 1969). The relationship of these observed nuclear changes to gene activation has been complicated by a number of facts including the following ones: (1) granulocytes undergo similar changes when incubated with PHA but do not divide; (2) acridine orange binding may occur at 4°C (Darzynkiewicz *et al.*, 1969); and (3) acridine orange binding may reflect cell concentration (Auer *et al.*, 1970) but not increased binding sites (Traganos *et al.*, 1976).

RNA synthesis begins to increase soon after mitogen stimulation (Cooper and Rubin, 1965; Hausen *et al.*, 1969). The overall increase in RNA synthesis is about two-fold (Cooper, 1972) by 20 hours after PHA stimulation. Both informational (messenger RNA and high molecular weight RNA) and structural RNA (ribosomal and transfer) increase. Informational RNA has a high turnover rate and consequently accounts for a greater proportion of total new synthesis. Measurement of RNA accumulation by flow cytofluorimetry, in which the fluorescence of individual cells may be quantified, has been used to measure lymphocyte stimulation (Braunstein *et al.*, 1976) and may permit fine resolution of responding cells into proliferative and nonproliferative subclasses.

The rate of protein synthesis increases by 3 hours after PHA stimulation (Ahern and Kay, 1975) and increases linearly between 3 and 12 hours. This is accompanied by an increase in active ribosomes and may indicate an increase in the rate of initiation of translation. The studies of Waithe *et al.* (1975) have indicated that stimulated lymphocytes may have changing requirements for amino acids during stimulation and that this may reflect underlying regulatory patterns during the cell cycle. Table IV summarizes some of the principal biochemical events that occur during lymphocyte transformation.

Biochemical differentiation of antigen-induced lymphocyte stimulation compared to mitogen-initiated response has been elusive. Cooper and Rubin (1966) found that stimulation of human lymphocytes by PHA produced a large fraction of nonribosomal RNA (6–20 S) whereas antigen (streptolysin 0) stimulated cultures produced precursor (45 S) ribosomal RNA as the single largest accumulated class. Lucas *et al.* (1971) demonstrated that inorganic phosphate is incorporated into different classes of phospholipids when cells are stimulated with streptokinase/streptodornase or PHA than when they are stimulated by tetanus toxoid.

Control of lymphocyte transformation may well occur at the level of the receptor binding reaction and lead in every effective interaction to essentially the same set of biochemical events. Different subpopulations of lymphocytes, as discussed below, have been shown to respond differently to the same stimulus and may provide the key to regulation.

B. The Response of Lymphocyte Subpopulations

A critical issue in evaluating lymphocyte stimulation *in vitro* is the evaluation of different responding lymphocyte subpopulations. The development of immunological techniques for estimating the percentage of thymus-dependent T lymphocytes and bursa-equivalent or bone marrow-derived B lymphocytes in a given population of lymphocytes has made evaluation of this question possible. B lymphocytes are defined as lymphocytes carrying membrane-bound immunoglobulins. These cells can be demonstrated with direct immunofluorescent technique.

Radioimmunoelectrophoretic experiments have demonstrated that only a small amount of immunoglobulin is synthesized and secreted by peripheral blood lymphocytes cultured in the presence of PHA (Ling *et al.*, 1965). This amount is negligible when compared to control culture synthesis. In contrast to this, a small number of lymphocytes cultured with

TABLE IV

SUMMARY OF MAJOR BIOCHEMICAL EVENTS DURING LYMPHOCYTE STIMULATION

Event	Stimulant[a]	Time of occurrence	Characteristic
Increase in K^+ influx	PHA	2–3 Min	Increase in rate and magnitude; essential for mitosis
Increase in Ca^{2+} uptake	PHA	30 Min to 1 hr	Required for mitosis
Increase in cyclic adenosine 3′,5′-monophosphate (cAMP)	PHA	5–10 Min	cAMP rapidly accumulates and is then degraded
Increase in cyclic 3′,5′-guanosine monophosphate (cGMP)	PHA, Con A	Within 20 min	Tenfold increase that returns to resting levels at 30 min
Increased incorporation of phosphate into phosphatidylinositol	PHA or SK/SD	3–30 Min	Enhanced turnover rather than *de novo* synthesis
Increase in glucose uptake	PHA	1–3 Min	Flow rate in both directions is increased; i.e., uptake is by facilitated diffusion
Increase in endocytosis	PHA	2–4 Hr	Internalization of plasma membrane allowing enhanced entry of small molecules
Acetylation of arginine-rich histones	PHA	15–30 Min	A possible signal for increase in RNA synthetic activity
Increase in RNA synthesis	PHA	15–30 Min	All forms of RNA (mainly heterogeneous nuclear) ↑4× after 20 hr of PHA treatment
Redistribution of hydrolases from the lysosomal granule	PHA	2–3 Hr	β-Glucuronidase and acid phosphotase become solubilized
Increase in lactic pyruvate and decrease in ATP and ADP ↓ Increase in ATP, ADP, glucose 1,6-diphosphate, and 2,3-phosphoglycerate	PHA	2 Hr or less	This increase in anerobic glycolysis is followed by induction of aerobic glycolysis and occurs in the early induction phase before the onset of DNA synthesis

[a] PHA, phytohemagglutinin; Con A, concanavalin A; SK/SD, streptokinase/streptodornase.

TABLE IV (*Continued*)

Event	Stimulant[a]	Time of occurrence	Characteristic
↑ Amino acid uptake	PHA	After 30 min	Amino acids that enter via Na$^+$-dependent transport system show increased uptake
Increased specific activity of uridine kinase, cytidine kinase, RNA polymerase I, DNA polymerase, thymidine kinase, ornithine decarboxylase, S-adenosylmethionine decarboxylase	PHA	Maximum levels 24–72 hr	Probably related to DNA and RNA synthesis
Increased incorporation of amino acids into protein	PHA	2–3 Hr	This includes many cytoplasmic structures and enzymes. Prior to mitosis, DNA polymerase activity is enhanced
DNA synthesis	PHA	24–36 Hr	Usually measured by incorporation of labeled thymidine, accompanied by increased phosphorylation of histones

PWM or PPD were shown by Greaves and Roitt (1968) to synthesize immunoglobulins. The number of immunoglobulin-positive blasts described in this study corresponded to the proportion of cells having a well-developed rough-surfaced endoplastic reticulum (the cell type described by Douglas in 1972). The concept that T cells respond to PHA and that T and B cells respond to PWM has been established in animal model systems, notably the chicken (Meuwissen *et al.*, 1969) and the mouse (Andersson *et al.*, 1972). The selectivity of the response in mice depends upon the degree of T- and B-cell separation, culture conditions, the particular stimulant chosen, and the source of the tissue (see Table V). Thymus and spleen cells of adult mice respond well to Con A. The strongest PHA responses have been obtained with blood and lymph node lymphocytes (Stobo, 1972; Greaves and Janossy, 1972). Lymphocytes from congenitally athymic (nude) mice which lack T cells do not re-

TABLE V

SPECIFICITY OF THE RESPONDING POPULATION[a]

Stimulant (mitogen)	T cells		B cells	
	Man	Mouse	Man	Mouse
PHA	PBL[b]	PBL[b]	PBL[b] (slight)	None
	Tonsil	Thymocyte	Tonsil[b] (15 % max)	
	Spleen	(variable)	Spleen[b] (slight)	
		Lymph node		
Soluble Con A	PBL[b]	PBL	—	None
		Thymocyte		
		Spleen		
		Lymph node		
Bound Con A	None	No response	—	Spleen
PWM	PBL (moderate)	Thymocytes	PBL (slight)	Spleen
	Tonsil	Pure T	Tonsil (slight)	Pure B
	Spleen (slight)	Spleen	Spleen	
LPS, Escherichia coli	—	None	Spleen (weak)	Spleen
				Pure B
LPS, Serratia marcesens	None	Thymocyte (slight)	Spleen (weak)	Spleen Pure B
Staphyloccocal endotoxin B	PBL[b]	—	Spleen (weak) PBL (weak)	—

[a] PHA, phytohemagglutinin; Con A, concanavalin A; PWM, pokeweed mitogen; LPS, lipopolysaccharides; PBL, peripheral blood lymphocytes.

[b] Mixed T and B culture.

spond to Con A and PHA. Both B and T cells do bind Con A and PHA, however, so that lack of receptors cannot be the basis of this differential response (Shortman et al., 1973). Mixed populations of T and B cells respond differently to Con A and PHA than do "pure" T and B cells, where indirect stimulation of B cells has been observed. This activation of B cells may be mediated by soluble factors from T cells (Andersson et al., 1972).

Studies with human lymphocyte T and B cell responses to mitogens have depended upon the development of marker systems and cell separation techniques. Greaves et al. (1974a,b) have demonstrated the selective stimulation of T and B lymphocytes by mitogens by using cell surface markers. Tonsillar T cells responded to PHA and PWM. B cells were not activated by PHA and only slightly by PWM. In contrast, in mixed B and T cell cultures, as much as 15% of the PHA-activated lymphoblasts were B cells. T cells also predominated in the reaction to PWM in mixed-cell culture of tonsillar lymphocytes. Peripheral blood lymphocytes gave comparable results. Spleen cell cultures showed a different response pattern.

In mixed T and B cell culture, B cells predominated in the PWM response. Evidence for B-cell stimulation by PHA (Phillips and Roitt, 1973) was neither obtained nor fully excluded in these studies. Table V summarizes current knowledge of T and B cell responses in man and mouse. Since a specific B-cell stimulant is not presently available, the ability of the B cell to proliferate in response to stimulation has not been fully assessed.

Analysis of lymphocyte transformation in man in response to PWM has been useful in differentiating among several immunodeficiencies characterized by reduced or absent immunoglobulin synthesis. Wu *et al.* (1973) demonstrated that lymphocytes from patients with Bruton's sex-linked agammaglobulinemia synthesized DNA in response to PWM in culture, but failed to show any increase in immunoglobulin synthesis in contrast to normals. This is consistent with the absence of B lymphocytes in the disease. In addition, these workers demonstrated that the lymphocytes of two patients with nearly normal levels of membrane-bound immunoglobulin, but having reduced circulating immunoglobulins, showed proliferation in response to PWM in culture in the absence of increased immunoglobulin synthesis. In contrast, a number of patients with a deficiency in circulating IgA and normal numbers of B lymphocytes responded in culture to PWM not only with DNA synthesis, but also with increased immunoglobulin synthesis and secretion. These data indicate that defects in B-lymphocyte differentiation may occur at more than one stage of development and imply the possibility of blocks in the regulation of immunoglobulin synthesis as well as blocks in secretion.

The response of lymphocyte subpopulations to antigens has not yet been analyzed and remains to be explored.

IV. Regulation of the Reaction

A. The Kinetics of Proliferation in Lymphocyte Cultures

Since the spontaneous initiation of DNA synthesis in many lymphocyte populations is quite low, measurement of DNA synthesis following lymphocyte stimulation by mitogens and antigens has found wide application in the quantitation of this phenomenon. Radioactive thymidine (either ^3H or ^{14}C) is not a direct precursor for lymphocyte DNA synthesis (thymidine nucleotides are made from ribonucleotides) and is normally employed in pulse-labeling of lymphocyte cultures at concentrations that do not saturate the internal pool (Schellekens and Eijsvoogel, 1968;

Sample and Chrétien, 1971). Therefore, rate of incorporation of labeled thymidine measures the relative rate of DNA synthesis among different cultures. Empirical evidence has indicated that this parameter correlates closely with blastogenesis. Total incorporated radioactive thymidine increases in proportion to the number of mitoses present in culture and, therefore, quantitatively reflects the vigor of the reaction. Since thymidine is degraded at 37°C, cultures are usually pulse labeled, and the data obtained reflect synthesis during the labeling period.

The proliferative response induced by any lymphocyte stimulant is a concentration-dependent phenomenon. For most stimulants, antigenic or mitogenic, suboptimal, optimal, and supraoptimal doses can be defined. Within that part of the dose-response curve that reflects suboptimal lymphocyte stimulation, the proliferative response is approximately proportional to the concentration of the stimulant. Since the number of responding cells for any specific antigen is limited, maximal peak response is later and of less magnitude than that observed for mitogens. Although mitotic figures may appear in antigen-stimulated cultures as early as those in mitogen-stimulated cultures, the peak of thymidine incorporation occurs later than that obtained for mitogens. This may imply that secondary recruitment is an essential component for the quantitative expression of antigenic stimulation.

The cellular mechanism responsible for the graded response to increasing stimulant concentration is not known. Ling (1971) has proposed two alternative theories to explain this phenomenon: (1) the number of responding lymphocytes is proportional to the concentration of the stimulant; (2) the number of responding lymphocytes is always the same for any given stimulant, but the time spent in compartment(s) of the cell cycle can vary according to stimulant concentration. In addition, Lohrmann et al. (1974) have proposed that the time required for responsive cells to enter the cell cycle from the resting state may occur at different time intervals (see Fig. 2). They studied this problem in synchronized lymphocyte cultures in which mitosis was blocked by colchicine. This method permitted a direct study of the number of cells responding to any given strength of stimulant and also of the time at which newly responding cells enter the division cycle for the first time. The duration of the total cell cycle (see Fig. 2) was found not to vary, being about 14 hours, regardless of the type or strength of the stimulant. The DNA synthetic phase, S, varied between 7 and 9 hours, but did not correlate with stimulant concentration. The first colchicine-arrested metaphases were observed at 11 hours, giving an average G_2 of about 3 hours; G_1 was estimated at 2 hours from these data. When PHA was the stimulant, first-generation responders appeared between 28 and 40 hours

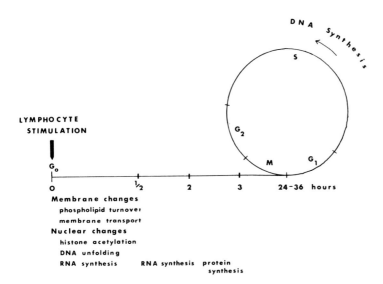

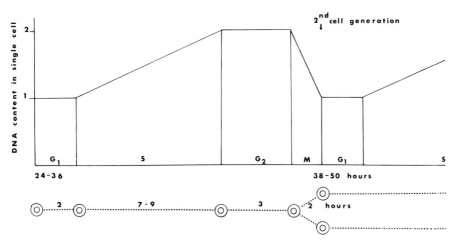

Fig. 2. Cellular and kinetic events following lymphocyte activation. A few representative biochemical changes are shown as they relate to cells entering the cell cycle for the first time. Kinetic data are from Lohrmann *et al.* (1974).

after stimulation. The highest number of first-generation responders entered the division cycle during the first 12-hour period. The number of cells showing proliferative response for the first time directly increased with increasing PHA stimulation until virtually all those cells capable of response had entered division.

Mitogenic response as measured by DNA synthesis was shown to be regulated, therefore, by the number of cells entering first division and the time required for entrance. The cell cycle itself appeared to be relatively constant.

These data are directly paralleled by the work of Gunther and Wang (1974) in which the kinetics of cellular proliferative response following Con A stimulation were investigated in mouse spleen cells. The competitive inhibitor α-methyl-D-mannoside (αMM) was added to cultures at various times after Con A stimulation. During increasing periods of exposure to Con A the percentage of blast cells and radioactive thymidine uptake increased in parallel while total radioactive uptake per cell remained constant. After 20 hours of preexposure to Con A, αMM could no longer inhibit stimulation. These data are consistent with the possibility that different lymphocytes require different induction periods to be stimulated.

The cell cycle times for second and subsequent divisions have usually been found to be shorter than that of the first division. Although few mitoses are found in PHA-stimulated cells before 48 hours, the majority of cells are in second division metaphase by 72 hours (Sasaki and Norman, 1966). Similar observations have been made for lymphocytes stimulated with antigens (Marshall *et al.*, 1969).

B. The Interaction of Mitogens and Antigens with the Cell Surface

The initial and critical event in lymphocyte stimulation by both specific and nonspecific binding molecules or ligands is their attachment to the appropriate lymphocyte receptor. The phenomenon of dose-dependent response to mitogens may suggest that individual cell activation is not an all-or-none phenomenon, but that weaker stimulation may result in an extended G_1 (Ling and Kay, 1975). Alternatively, subpopulation heterogeneity and/or lymphocyte-macrophage interactions may affect the binding reaction.

When stimulation of lymphocytes requires presensitization, it may be presumed that the stimulant interacts with a specific cell surface receptor. The situation is not as clear with regard to mitogens. The plant lectins, some of which stimulate lymphocytes, also have receptors that agglutinate erythrocytes and leukocytes. Both Con A- and lentil mitogen-induced lymphocyte stimulation and erythroagglutination can be blocked by mannose, glucose, and αMM (Powell and Leon, 1970; Young *et al.*, 1971). PHA erythroagglutination is blocked by αMM but not by mannose or glucose, and lymphocyte stimulation is only slightly inhibited

(Lindahl-Kiessling and Peterson, 1969). Although these observations have been interpreted to indicate that sugars may competitively inhibit lectin binding with oligosaccharide receptors, the binding sites themselves are more probably of greater complexity. Other glycopeptides isolated by Kornfeld and Kornfeld (1969), which are stronger inhibitors of lymphocyte stimulation, block lymphocyte activation by PHA, Con A, and lentil mitogen.

The length of time during which the lymphocyte culture is exposed to the stimulant has been demonstrated to be a critical factor in the regulation of the reaction. A study of Kay (1970) in which PHA was removed by washing indicated that activation becomes rapidly independent of the presence of PHA. In these experiments, lymphocyte activation was maximal after exposure of lymphocytes for 20 minutes to PHA. Even suboptimal concentrations were effective within 2 hours. However, activation did not become totally refractory to inhibition by anti-PHA for 6 hours after the initiation of stimulation. Lower concentrations of stimulant required longer periods of exposure in culture to have an equivalent stimulatory effect upon the lymphocytes. Weber et al. (1975) have confirmed that addition of antimitogen antisera to lymphocyte cultures removes the mitogen from the cell surface. Preactivation of lymphocytes by limited contact with mitogen was found to alter cells so that rapid stimulation by a second, different mitogen could be obtained. This effect was found to be specific for pairs of mitogens and suggests that different mitogens may react with the cell surfaces of lymphocytes in essentially different ways. Similar evidence for preactivation of lymphocytes by mitogens has been obtained by Sell et al. (1975) for rabbit lymphocytes. Lymphocyte activation by the nonspecific mitogens may therefore be affected by previous cell surface events.

Inhibition as well as stimulation may be mediated through specific cell surface interactions. Wang et al. (1975) have demonstrated that a dimeric derivative of Con A, succinyl Con A, while equally as mitogenic as the parent compound, shows no high dose inhibition. The unimodal dose response curve of native Con A, which is tetrameric, could also be enhanced by a phorbol ester. The response to dimeric Con A could also be enhanced, but the dose curve continued to have saturation kinetics. Similar data has been obtained by Hadden et al. (1975), and the conclusion of both studies is that high dose inhibition is regulated by a specific cell surface signal.

The differential interaction of different mitogens with the surface of lymphocytes may be considered as a function of subpopulation differences Touraine et al. (1975) have demonstrated that the T-cell population may be divided into functional subsets. Human peripheral blood lymphocytes were stimulated with PHA, and the responding population was subsequently ablated (by addition of the thymidine analog 5-bromo-2'-deoxyuridine); restimulation with Con A was ineffective. By contrast, Con A stimulation did not totally deplete the lymphocyte population of cells able to respond to PHA. At least 50% of the PWM response was found to be independent of either PHA or Con A prestimulation. Allogeneic stimulation was not ablated by any mitogen tested.

Lymphocyte activation may be influenced by the structure of the mitogen. B cells have been shown to be activated either indirectly via T cells, T-cell products, or macrophages or directly by some stimulants (see Table III for summary of models for B cell activation). Greaves and Bauminger (1972) have demonstrated that lymphocyte transformation can be obtained with mouse lymphocytes stimulated by PHA and PWM covalently linked to Sepharose beads. They used both T cells and B cells in separated cell preparations as well as T- and B-cell mixtures. Although T cells responded more effectively to soluble PWM, B cells and T- and B-cell mixtures showed enhanced response with insoluble PWM. In distinct contrast to the lack of response of B cells to soluble PHA, Sepharose-bound PHA produced marked stimulation of these cells. Purified B cells were found to be capable of transforming in the presence of PHA bound to the beads. Similar results have been obtained in mice with Con A cross-linked to the bottom of petri dishes by Andersson *et al.* (1972).

These data demonstrate that under a rather specific condition B cells can in fact be induced to proliferate in culture with Con A and PHA. The fact that they do not normally do so may indicate that a sufficient number of antigen receptors per unit cell surface may not be available on this cell type. The effect of linking mitogens to a fixed substrate may effectively serve to concentrate the receptors around the mitogen. Soluble mitogen would be expected to suppress activation if this were true. This has been verified experimentally for Con A. The stimulation of B cells by polymerized flagellin and pneumococcal polysaccharide may occur similarly.

The fact that bound PHA may stimulate lymphocytes suggests that internalization of the stimulant cannot be a prerequisite for cell activation. Lindahl-Kiessling and Mattsson (1971) have shown that washed PHA-treated cells will stimulate untreated cells whereas little stimulation is effected by the filtrate alone. Since this event can be inhibited by N-acetylgalactosamine as can PHA activation, it is assumed that PHA is tightly bound to the cell surface and that secondary activation occurs via cell-to-cell contact. In this case, PHA may be acting as a ligand between cells. The operation of a nonspecific blastogenic factor in mitogen-stimulated cultures has also been demonstrated to be unlikely by Jones (1972) since specific antisera effectively abolished the stimulating activity of supernatants from Con A- and PHA-stimulated cultures.

The antigen-responsive lymphocyte population has been regarded as a series of lymphocyte clones, each of which arose in response to an original antigenic stimulus. Therefore the population of cells for any particular antigenic stimulus is both small and specific. Subpopulation response to different antigens has been studied in situations where response to one antigen has been abrogated either spontaneously during the acute phase of infection, or artificially, in culture by the addition of DNA synthetic inhibitors, such as bromodeoxyuridine, to antigen-stimulated cultures. Kreth *et al.* (1970) observed the effect of a course of fibrinolytic therapy with the streptococcal antigen streptokinase on patients with occlusive vascular disease. Patients exhibiting pretherapy *in vitro* sensitivity to streptokinase were rendered temporarily negative by treatment. Patients who were nonresponsive to streptokinase prior to therapy developed sensitivity after the conclusion of treatment. Stimulation of lymphocytes by phytohemagglutinin or by tuberculin was not affected during or after therapy. If two different antigens stimulate two different clones of presensitized lymphocytes, it should follow that stimulation with the same two immunizing antigens should produce an additive effect. Zoshke and Bach (1970) and Ling and Husband (1964) have reported this effect for mumps, streptokinase/streptodornase, tetanus toxoid, PPD, and smallpox. Lazda and Baram (1974) achieved a similar discrimination of responding populations with PHA and antigen stimulation in the monkey. Increased stimulation was observed when antigen and PHA were added simultaneously to cultures.

Clonal proliferation alone is probably insufficient to account for lymphocyte activation by antigens. In addition to subpopulations of lymphocytes that are capable of responding to the stimulating antigen directly, there may be a larger pool of not fully differentiated lymphocytes that respond to activated lymphocytes or to the products of activated lymphocytes.

Secondary recruitment, which may occur by means of the release of a nonspecific activating substance from activated lymphocytes, has been reported for antigens (Gordon and Mac Lean, 1965; Wolstencroft and Dumonde, 1970). Schellekens and Eijsvoogel (1971) have presented evidence consistent with a possible secondary and nonspecific recruitment under certain culture conditions. They demonstrated that the effect of decreasing the sediment surface area in antigen-stimulated cultures is increased stimulation. The effect was complete at 24 hours and did not occur with PHA. This phenomenon of enhanced stimulation secondary to increased cell proximity can be considered as evidence for recruitment in antigenic stimulation. The regulation of such a mechanism under physiological conditions is, however, unknown.

Since mitogens, antigens, and lymphocyte populations are all heterogeneous, the complexity of their interactions will require much further clarification with purified reagents and defined subpopulations before the relationship of these events to immune recognition and immune response may be understood.

V. Lymphocyte Transformation *in Vitro* in Clinical Immunology

The observation that lymphocyte transformation *in vitro* does not occur in some patients with severe immunodeficiencies when their lymphocytes are stimulated by mitogens or antigens suggests that this laboratory test in some way reflects functional immunological phenomena. Data from *in vitro* lymphocyte transformation studies are now regularly included as an essential part of the immunological evaluation of a patient. Standardized laboratory techniques and standardized criteria for interpretation, however, have not been developed. In order to make possible a direct comparison of data obtained in different laboratories, some consistency in methodology is being developed. Most lymphocyte transformation *in vitro* is now being performed in microtiter plates using a small number of cells ($2 \times 10^4 \rightarrow 2 \times 10^5$) per well after isolation from blood by centrifugation on Ficoll-Isopaque density gradients.

A. Technique for Lymphocyte Culture

The methodology and the technical guidelines given in the following paragraphs have been in use in our laboratories for the past three years. These procedures are used in a number of other laboratories, and the results obtained are comparable.

1. Culture Medium Source

RPMI 1640 with 25 mM HEPES buffer is supplemented with heparin (10 IU/ml, preservative free), penicillin (10 IU/ml), streptomycin (10 μg/cc), and glutamine (0.23 mg/ml).

Serum is collected under sterile conditions from nontransfused, healthy, young male blood donors without regard to ABO blood grouping. Clot formation is allowed for a few hours, then the serum is separated by centrifugation, which is repeated three times. Serum may be stored temporarily at 4°C but should be frozen at −70°C for longer storage. Individual units of serum are frozen until pooling. A single batch of serum is prepared by pooling the serum from 1 unit of blood from at least 15 different donors. After pooling, the serum is filtered through 2 Millipore filters (1.2 and 0.8 μm), aliquoted, and frozen again to −70°C. The use of routine blood bags and transfer packs allows for sterile conditions throughout the bleeding, clotting, separation, temporary storage, centrifugation, and pooling processes.

2. Blood Sampling

Whole-blood samples can be collected with anticoagulants, or blood can be defibrinated. The preferred anticoagulant is heparin, but ACD or EDTA can also be used. The clot from defibrinated blood should be removed promptly. If any blood samples are not to be processed within an hour, we routinely dilute them with equal volumes of tissue culture medium containing antibiotics. When heparinized blood is used, the tissue culture medium is supplemented with heparin to avoid clumping of platelets and cells. Diluted blood can be shipped or stored at room temperature for up to 24 hours.

3. Isolation of Lymphocytes

The generally accepted method for separation of lymphocytes consists of centrifugation of diluted whole or defibrinated blood or of resuspended buffy coat cells on a Ficoll-Isopaque density gradient (Boyum, 1968). The Ficoll-Isopaque suspension is mixed to a final density of 1.077 gm/ml. Whole blood is diluted with an equal volume of culture medium or with Hanks' Balanced Salt Solution, or, if buffy coat cells are used, these are resuspended to the equivalent volume of whole blood. The diluted or resuspended blood cells are then layered directly on Ficoll-Isopaque in sterile centrifuge tubes. We use 4 ml of Ficoll-Isopaque in a 12- or 15-ml plastic centrifuge tube. After centrifugation at 400 g for 30 minutes, erythrocytes and polymorphonuclear leukocytes pass through to the bottom of the gradient. The mononuclear leukocytes and platelets layer out in the interphase between the plasma medium layer on top and the Ficoll-Isopaque layer below. Mononuclear cells are removed from each tube with a sterile Pasteur pipette, and all mononuclear cells from each individual are pooled. The pooled cell suspension is resuspended in at least 3 times its volume with medium or Hanks' Balanced Salt Solution and then washed at least twice to remove anticoagulant, plasma, and Ficoll-Isopaque. The addition of a small amount of pooled human serum (5–10%) to the washing solution may help protect against cell loss. If heparinized blood is used, heparin should also be present in the tissue culture medium used for washing.

4. Cell Counting

The mononuclear fraction from the Ficoll-Isopaque density gradient contains lymphocytes and monocytes. If anticoagulated blood was used, this fraction will also contain platelets. In order to standardize the number of responding cells per culture, the approximate number of lymphocytes must be known. This can be accomplished either microscopically by using a hemacytometer and a dye, such as Crystal violet, or it may be done automatically with a Coulter counter and a size distribution analyzer to determine the fraction of typical lymphocytes, but excluding the larger monocytes from the count. Periodic checks of aliquots from cell suspensions with vital dyes, such as trypan blue, is advisable.

5. Period of Culture

Mitogen-stimulated cultures are usually cultured for 96 hours, whereas antigen-stimulated cultures are incubated for 120–144 hours.

6. Pulse Labeling

The lymphocyte transformation is quantitated by pulse-labeling during the last 24 hours of culture with ^{14}C- or ^{3}H-labeled thymidine. The exogenic thymidine concentration should be no less than 3 μg/ml (Schellekens and Eijsvoogel, 1968).

7. Conditions of Lymphocyte Culture: Cell Concentration, Volume, and Geometry

The concentration of cells, the volume of the culture, and the geometry of the tissue culture tube or microtiter plate are important factors that will affect cell metabolism, proliferation, and kinetics of in vitro transformation. Ideally, all responding lymphocytes of a stimulated culture should remain within exponential growth phase during the period of labeling. Each laboratory, must therefore, perform a series of experiments to define precisely the characteristics of their own individual lymphocyte culture system. These experiments should include: (1) time-course ex-

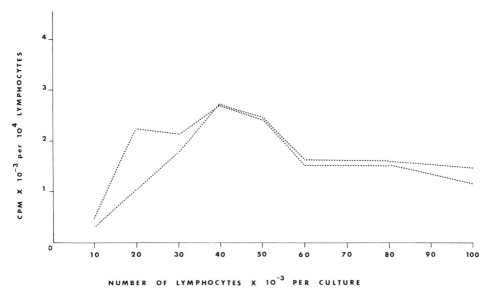

Fig. 3. Effect of varying cell number on response to *Staphylococcus aureus* anti-gen. Data presented are for 6-day microtiter cultures labeled between day 5 and day 6. Two dilutions of *S. aureus* antigen (1:10 and 1:20) are shown. Typical curves obtained with one cell donor are represented.

periments for both strongly and weakly responding cells; (2) dose re-sponse curves with mitogens and antigens for both strongly and weakly responding cells; (3) standardization of the amount and specific activity of radioactive thymidine added to the cultures; and (4) selection of an optimal period of time for thymidine labeling. If a flat-bottom microtiter plate system is used, the optimal cell number per well is 1 to 1.5×10^5 lymphocytes. If the round-bottom microtiter plate system is used, 5×10^4 lymphocytes per well is optimal. In Fig. 3 the incorporation of [^{14}C]thymidine in lymphocytes stimulated with *Staphylococcus aureus* antigen is shown after labeling from 120 hours to 144 hours of culture in round-bottom microtiter plates. The data are expressed as counts per minute incorporated per 10^4 lymphocytes. The efficiency of the labeling is optimal with a cell number of 4×10^4 to 6×10^4 lymphocytes per well. Comparable data can be obtained with mitogens and in mixed lymphocyte culture (DuBois *et al.*, 1974).

8. *Harvest of Cultures*

Lymphocyte cultures performed in microtiter plates can be conveniently harvested with a multisample harvesting machine (Hartzman *et al.*,

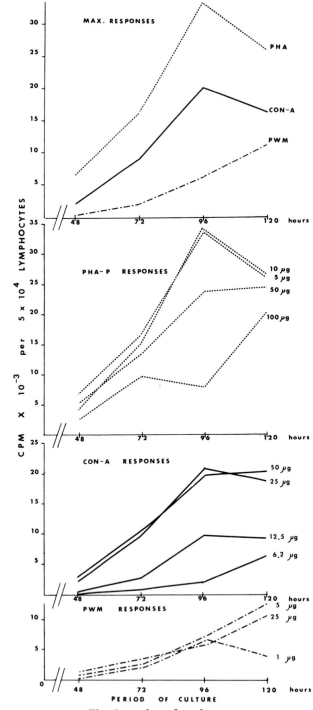

Fig. 4. See legend on facing page.

1971). In essence, cells are aspirated with distilled water and then collected and washed on small glass-fiber filter papers. Dried filter papers are transferred to scintillation vials for determination of the amount of radioactive thymidine incorporation.

B. Selection of Mitogens and Antigens for Clinical Use

The selection of mitogens and antigens for lymphocyte transformation *in vitro* may vary according to the questions and problems the investigator is studying. A specific antigen may be of special interest for the immunological analysis of one patient, but not be of general value in the routine laboratory. We have selected a panel of mitogens and antigens which routinely gives a standardized result in normal individuals. Basically, a panel for routine testing should be able to reveal abnormal results in patients with primary and secondary immunodeficiencies. *In vitro* stimulation with other specific antigens are included in some patients or in the analysis of some special problem.

1. Selection of Mitogens

For practical clinical use we have selected the three common plant mitogens: phytohemagglutinin (PHA-P), concanavalin A (Con A), and pokeweed mitogen (PWM). Dose-response curves are performed with each of the three mitogens. A typical pattern of response is illustrated in Fig. 4. Appropriate dilutions of each mitogen are made from commercial stock, and aliquots are frozen until used. For PHA-P, six dilutions are made with a final dose of mitogen per culture of 50, 12.5, 4.2, 2.1, 1.0, and 0.5 μg. For Con A the dose per culture is: 50, 25, 6.2, 1.6, 0.4, and 0.1 μg. PWM is used in the amount of 25, 5, and 1 μg per culture. A dose-response curve for each set of mitogen dilutions is obtained with normal lymphocytes prior to use in the routine assay. The dilutions are selected so as to cover the response range from maximal to threshold response in normal individuals. As shown in Fig. 4, the response to PHA is usually a little greater than the response to Con A (70–100% of PHA response),

Fig. 4. Dose-response curves for mitogens. The kinetics of response to three mitogens are shown for different concentrations of the respective stimulants as indicated. In addition, maximum responses for the noted mitogens are mutually compared (top graph) so that the kinetics of relative response may be observed. PHA, phytohemagglutinin; PHA-P, partially purified, heterogeneous PHA; Con-A, concanavalin A; PWN, pokeweed mitogen.

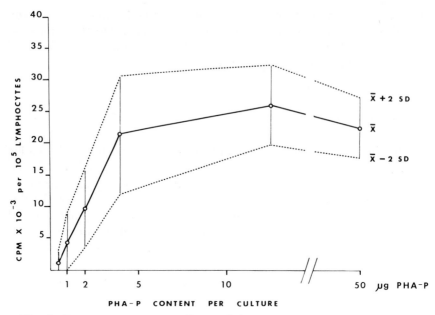

Fig. 5. Dose titration to partially purified, heterogeneous phytohemagglutinin (PHA-P) for normal controls. Data are complied from daily assays over a 3-month period.

and the response to PWM is considerably lower (20–70% of PHA response). Figure 5 demonstrates the combined PHA-P dose-response curves performed on lymphocytes obtained from 36 normal blood donors. The culture system used was the flat-bottom microtiter plate with 10^5 lymphocytes per well. Labeling was performed from 72 hours to 96 hours of culture with [^{14}C]thymidine. The results are given as the mean response to each dose of PHA in cpm ± 250. Abnormal dose responses to mitogens may be seen in some patients with immunodeficiencies (Hosking *et al.*, 1971).

2. Selection of Antigens

For routine testing of specific lymphocyte response *in vitro* we have selected three common microbial antigens for stimulation: antigenic extracts from a pool of common *Escherichia coli* strains, antigenic extracts from a pool of common *Staphylococcus aureus* strains, and antigens from *Candida albicans*. The *E. coli* and *S. aureus* preparations are crude whole-cell suspensions while the *C. albicans* antigen is derived from the supernatant of broken-cell ultracentrifuged *C. albicans* suspensions (Axelsen, 1971).

These antigen preparations were first produced for lymphocyte transformation *in vitro* in collaboration with Dr. Klaus Jensen, Dr. Niels Axelsen, and Dr. Vagn Andersen of the Staten Serum Institute and University of Copenhagen, Denmark. Subsequently, similar preparations were made in other laboratories and results were similar. The method as modified by us for preparing these antigens follows.

Escherichia coli antigen is prepared from *E. coli* strains isolated from the stools of 8–10 normal individuals. Each strain is purified and grown separately in enriched medium to late log or early stationary phase. Cultures are combined following harvesting by centrifugation and are washed twice in phosphate-buffered saline. Two types of antigen preparations may be made from these cultures:

1. Whole-cell preparation. The cultures are incubated at 70°C for 30 minutes, counted, and diluted to 10^9 cells/ml in RPMI 1640 with 40 units of penicillin and streptomycin per milliliter and frozen at -70°C.

2. Sonic extract. The cell suspension is diluted in phosphate-buffered saline to an optical density of 0.4 (Lumetron colorimeter, $\lambda = 490$) and sonicated at 4°C for 15 minutes. The sonicate is centrifuged at 8000 g for 20 minutes. The supernatant is decanted and frozen at -70°C.

Staphylococcus aureus antigen is prepared from multiple isolates from normal individuals. The method of preparation follows that outlined above for *E. coli* antigen.

Candida albicans antigens is prepared from common *Candida albicans* isolates. A culture aliquot is streaked for single colonies on Sabouraud's dextrose agar. Then single colonies are resuspended and grown on Sabouraud plates at 37°C for 48 hours. The cultures are combined and washed twice in phosphate-buffered saline, resuspended (1 gm wet weight per 2 ml), and sonicated for 1 hour at 4°C. The sonicate is then centrifuged at 100,000 g for 1 hour. The supernatant is decanted and frozen at -70°C.

Antigens such as purified protein derivative (PPD) for mycobacterium tuberculi or the streptococcal extracts containing streptodornase (SK/SD) can be used as specific antigens. These two antigens may be useful in determining sensitization or level of reactivity against the respective microbial agent.

C. PRESENTATION, TREATMENT, AND EVALUATION OF DATA

The conventional way to quantify lymphocyte transformation *in vitro* is to perform pulse-labeling with ^{14}C- or ^{3}H-labeled radioactive thymidine. The degree of lymphocyte transformation or response will then be measured as counts per minute of ^{14}C or ^{3}H incorporated in the DNA of the proliferating lymphocytes (see Fig. 1).

In order to evaluate the response to a given mitogen or antigen the degree of transformation in unstimulated cultures is compared to the degree of transformation in stimulated cultures.

There is a considerable variation from day to day and between different individuals in the counts per minute obtained in the unstimulated cultures. Many of the factors involved in determining the level of the unstimulated control value are unknown. One important factor is the subjectivity involved in the definition of which cells to count when the cell count in the mononuclear cell suspension used for the cultures is made.

All counts (cpm) are initially corrected for the background counts. The test results are then expressed in different ways: (1) Net cpm. The cpm in the stimulated culture minus the cpm in the unstimulated culture. (2) Stimulation ratio (SR). The SR is defined as the ratio of the cpm in a stimulated culture to the cpm in the unstimulated culture.

The SR is very sensitive to the variation in the cpm in the unstimulated control cultures. The variation in unstimulated cultures from day to day, from individual to individual, and from disease to disease, will sometimes make comparison of data, when expressed as SRs, difficult.

Evaluation of SRs when the cpm in the unstimulated control cultures are excessively high or low must be performed with caution.

In Fig. 6 is shown the variations in SR obtained with PHA-P and the antigens from *C. albicans, E. coli, S. aureus*, PPD, and SK/SD over a period of 7–9 months with lymphocytes obtained from one normal individual. This individual showed positive delayed hypersensitivity upon skin testing with SK/SD and with PPD.

Figure 5 demonstrates that the net counts per minute obtained in PHA-P dose-response experiments in normal donors also vary with maximum responses between 17,000 and 30,000 cpm (cultures labeled with [^{14}C]thymidine). Similar curves can be obtained with mitogens other than PHA. The variation in SR obtained with the antigen panel applied to normal blood donors is shown in Fig. 7. This figure demonstrates that the SR varies to the same extent among normal donors as the SR varies in repeated testings of the same donor (Fig. 6). However, the lymphocytes of normal blood donors always show a positive response to the *C. albicans, E. coli*, and *S. aureus* antigen when a SR > 3 is considered a positive response. If the individual is sensitized to PPD and SK/SD, the *in vitro* lymphocyte response to these antigens will also be positive whereas nonsensitized lymphocytes do not respond with SR larger than 2 to these antigens.

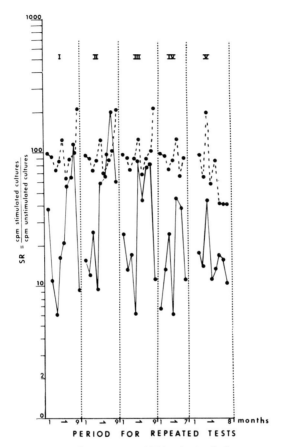

Fig. 6. Variation in stimulation ratio (SR) obtained from repeated testings of the same donor. ———, Antigen; ---, phytohemagglutinin. Panel I, *Candida albicans*, antigen; II, *Escherichia coli* antigen; III, *Staphylococcus aureus* antigen; IV, purified protein derivative antigen; V, streptokinase/streptodornase antigen.

The following conclusions can be made for evaluation of the *in vitro* lymphocyte transformation data obtained in a flat-bottom microtiter plate system with 10^5 lymphocytes per well and labeling of mitogen-stimulated cultures from 72 to 96 hours of culture and of antigen-stimulated cultures from 120 hours to 144 hours of culture:

1. The maximum response to the optimal PHA-P concentration should be at least 17,000 cpm.

2. The response to optimal concentrations of Con A and PWM should not be larger than the response to PHA.

3. Normal lymphocytes always respond *in vitro* to a crude extract from

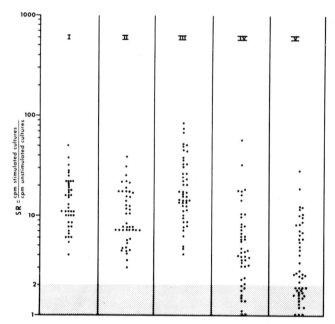

Fig. 7. Variation in stimulation ratio (SR) obtained among normal controls. Data are shown as maximum response of each donor to multiple dilutions of the indicated stimulants. Panel I, *Candida albicans* antigen; II, *Escherichia coli* antigen; III, *Staphylococcus aureus* antigen; IV, purified protein derivative antigen; V, streptokinase/streptodornase antigen.

C. albicans, *E. coli*, and *S. aureus*. A positive response is defined as SR > 3.

4. Repeated responses to these antigens with SR between 2 and 3.5 is an indication of some immunodeficiency and should be further explored by additional and extended studies.

The application of these criteria to data obtained from studies of patients is permitted only if the patient's lymphocytes are studied in parallel with lymphocytes obtained from normal individuals and if these control cells fulfill the four criteria.

D. Evaluation of Immune Deficiency

The thorough evaluation of any patient's immunobiological status requires comprehensive *in vivo* and *in vitro* testing. Humoral immunity is evaluated by qualitative determination of serum immunoglobulin levels and the secretory IgA level. The presence of specific antibodies can be determined or specific humoral responses can be measured by immunizing and then testing for the specific antibody response (i.e., against mumps vaccine, tetanus toxoid, pneumococcal polysaccharides, etc.). The phagocytic system is evaluated by testing neutrophile or monocyte chemotaxis, phagocytosis, and killing of bacteria or yeast. The complement system is evaluated by determining total hemolytic complement or by functionally or immunochemically quantifying specific complement components. The *in vivo* evaluation of cell-mediated immunity is done by testing for delayed hypersensitivity responses to intradermal antigens or by inducing delayed hypersensitivity responses with chemical allergens, such as dinitrochlorobenzene (DNCB). The identification of lymphocytes and lymphocyte subpopulations (T cells, B cells, K cells) can be performed by direct identification of certain lymphocyte surface markers.

As indicated previously, the evaluation of *in vitro* lymphocyte function can be performed by studying several different phenomena. Lymphocyte transformation and proliferation, secretion of certain lymphokines, changes in DNA synthesis, changes in protein synthesis, changes in the membrane transport of ions, and changes in membrane configuration or fluidity are all measurable parameters of lymphocyte response. The major goal in defining the significance of these functional indicators is to relate them to specific immune responses. The interpretation of these observations in the definition of the immune status of a patient is largely empirical.

Congenital immunodeficiency disease and malignant disease of the lymphoid system have provided essential models for analyzing the state of immune function in different pathological conditions (Good, 1973; Hansen and Good, 1974). Indeed, the biological significance of lymphocyte transformation *in vitro*, in response to both mitogens and antigens, has been established largely by tests carried out in patients with different forms of immune deficiency disease (Dupont and Good, 1975). In most patients with X-linked agammaglobulinemia, a disease severely affecting the precursor of normal B cells, lymphocyte transformation *in vitro* following stimulation with PHA is normal (Bach *et al.*, 1968). In patients with the DiGeorge syndrome, a disease of abnormal thymus development associated with deficiencies in cell-mediated immunity, lymphocytes do not respond to PHA (Lischner *et al.*, 1967). Following the transplantation of fetal thymus to patients with DiGeorge syndrome, the deficiencies in cell-mediated immunity become normalized, and lymphocytes again respond to PHA (Cleveland *et al.*, 1968). In children born with severe combined immune deficiency (SCID), the function of both the T- and B-cell systems are defective, and severe lymphopenia may be present. These children are deficient in both humoral and cellular immunity, and death usually occurs in infancy from fungal or viral infection (Good, 1973). Generally, the few lymphocytes that may be collected from such children do not respond to mitogens or antigens *in vitro* (Bach *et al.*, 1968). The cells from some of these children, however, do respond *in vitro* to stimulation with allogeneic cells in the mixed lymphocyte culture reaction (Meuwissen *et al.*, 1968; Greenberg *et al.*, 1969). Following immunobiological reconstitution of patients with SCID by allogeneic bone marrow transplantation, the combined immune deficiency is corrected, and the responses of lymphocytes *in vitro* are restored (Gatti *et al.*, 1968; Buckley, 1971). An example of lymphocyte transformation studies in a patient with SCID before and after bone marrow transplantation is shown in Fig. 8.

A more complex pattern of abnormalities can be seen in some of the other congenital immunodeficiency diseases. Children with the Wiskott-Aldrich syndrome are known for their characteristic triad of bleeding (secondary to thrombocytopenia), eczema, and repeated episodes of infection to a wide variety of microbials. In spite of generally normal numbers of B cells and normal levels of immunoglobulin, these children have depressed specific antibody responses to most antigens and almost no response to polysaccharide antigens (Blaese *et al.*, 1968, 1975; Cooper *et al.*, 1968). Skin testing reveals anergy to many antigens (Blaese *et al.*, 1968). Lymphocyte transformation in response to nonspecific mitogens including PHA, PWM, staphylococcal filtrate, and Con A are vari-

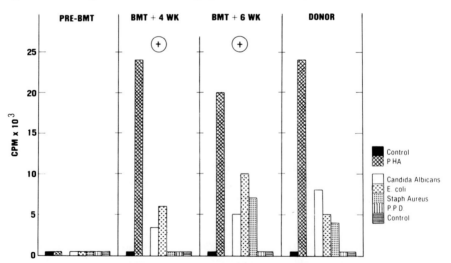

Fig. 8. Effect of allogeneic bone marrow transplant (AMT) at 4 and at 6 weeks in patient with severe combined immunodeficiency on lymphocyte transformation (Biggar *et al.*, 1974). Figure redrawn with permission from *Clin. Immunol. Immunopath.*

able from near normal to markedly depressed (Oppenheim *et al.*, 1970). Lymphocyte responses to specific antigens (streptolysin O, SK/SD, *Candida*, diphtheria, and tetanus toxoid) and to allogeneic cells (MLC) are markedly reduced or absent (Spitler *et al.*, 1972; Blaese *et al.*, 1975). Hodgkin's disease has been one of the most important models for studying acquired immunodeficiency (Hansen and Good, 1974). In the first systematic analysis of patients with Hodgkin's disease, Schier showed that skin test reactions to tuberculin, mumps, *Candida*, and *Trichophyton* were negative, even while some patients were found to have a normal humoral response following vaccination with mumps virus (Schier *et al.*, 1956). This defect in delayed hypersensitivity has subsequently been shown to represent a broadly based deficiency of cellular immunity, which may involve anergy to many antigens, prolongation of skin allograft survival (Kelly *et al.*, 1958), resistance to immunization with Bacillus Calmette-Guérin (BCG) (Sokal and Primikirios, 1961), and resistance to induction of delayed hypersensitivity using the potent chemical allergens dinitrofluorobenzene (DNFB) (Good *et al.*, 1962) and dinitrochlorobenzene (DNCB) (Aisenberg, 1962). Patients with Hodgkin's disease also show abnormal lymphocyte transformation *in vitro* to PHA, PPD, and vaccinia antigens (Aisenberg, 1965; Sartoris *et al.*, 1965; Hersh and Oppenheim, 1965).

Some controversy has existed, however, about whether these defects of cellular immunity in Hodgkin's disease represent a primary part of the pathophysiology of the malignant process or some secondary complication of an advancing disease that leads to severe lymphocyte depletion. When newly diagnosed untreated patients were studied, some investigations suggested that delayed hypersensitivity reactions and PHA response might be normal in patients with limited, or clinical stage I, disease (Brown *et al.*, 1967; Corder *et al.*, 1972). Using a panel of specific microbial antigens to stimulate lymphocyte *in vitro*, we were able to show significant abnormalities in responsiveness among patients with stage I disease (Hansen *et al.*, 1974).

Further studies using a more sensitive technique for DNCB testing showed that a quantitative deficiency in DNCB response also occurs in early untreated stage I Hodgkin's disease (Eltringham and Kaplan, 1973; Case *et al.*, 1976). Levy and Kaplan (1974) measured protein synthesis in lymphocytes stimulated by PHA and found abnormal dose-response curves in patients with stage I disease. We have studied lymphocyte responses of 52 untreated patients with Hodgkin's disease, using graded doses of PHA to stimulate in a microculture method (Case *et al.*, 1976). The mean maximum response of the control group was 25,691 cpm, and the mean response for patients with stage I was significantly less than the

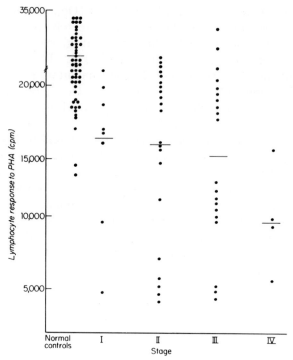

Fig. 9. Relationship of maximum lymphocyte response to phytohemagglutinin (PHA) in counts per minute (cpm) to stage (mean response for concurrent controls, 25,691) (Case *et al.,* 1976). Reprinted by courtesy of J. P. Lippincott from *Cancer* (in press).

control group $(p < 0.01)$ (see Fig. 9). There appears to be a trend toward decreased responses in the advanced stages, although the difference in mean response between each stage is not statistically significant.

Assessment of the immunological status of patients with disease of the lymphoid system sometimes cannot be made by testing of blood lymphocytes alone. An interesting example was a patient with lymphocytic lymphoma and a pleural effusion containing small lymphocytes (Hansen *et al.,* 1974). The blood lymphocyte response to PHA was very low, and to specific antigens and allogeneic cells (MLC) it was absent. Pleural effusion lymphocytes, however, responded normally *in vitro* with brisk responses to PHA, antigens, and MLC. Immunofluorescence for immunoglobulin-bearing cells revealed expansion of a monoclonal population in the blood, but a normal distribution of cells in the pleural effusion. This case demonstrates that a perturbation in the circulation of lymphocytes may lead to redistribution of functional populations (ecotaxopathy).

A possible abnormal distribution of lymphocytes in patients with Hodgkin's disease was examined by de Sousa *et al.* (1976). Lymphocytes were isolated from blood and from surgically biopsied spleen and liver, as well as from involved and uninvolved lymph nodes of children with Hodgkin's disease. The deficiency of normal mitogen responses in blood and involved lymph nodes did not necessarily indicate an overall depletion of competent cells, but rather seemed to reflect an abnormal accumulation of responsive cells in the spleen. In one patient, who was a stage IA and treated with only local radiotherapy to the cervical region, repeat evaluation 3 months following splenomectomy revealed that the number of circulating lymphocytes, the proportion of circulating T cells, and the *in vitro* response to PHA were markedly increased. The accumulation of cells in the spleen does not necessarily result from a splenic abnormality or presence of tumor, but may result from changes in the lymphocyte or lymphocyte membrane. These findings indicate the difficulties and limitations of studying the immune system through only one compartment, such as the circulating lymphocyte. Complete evaluation of lymphoproliferative disorders may require simultaneous study of tissue from several selected sites.

E. Evaluation of Immunotherapy by Longitudinal Testing of Lymphocyte Function

In addition to being a help in the diagnosis of both congenital and acquired immunodeficiency disease, and the evaluation of immune pathology in lymphoproliferative disorders, clinical testing of lymphocyte function is of increasing importance in the evaluation of immune therapy. In the treatment of some immune deficiency diseases, or in the immune therapy of cancer patients, an objective measure of response to therapy is often lacking. Multiple different immune potentiators, including transfer factor, levamisole, BCG, pertussis, or poly I.C., are utilized in clinical trials. Some reliable and objective measure of change in immune function or responsiveness is greatly needed.

Although the introduction of micromethods for lymphocyte transformation allows repeated study of the same patient, requiring from 2 to 10×10^6 lymphocytes for each comprehensive test, several technical limitations have made longitudinal studies difficult to perform. Lymphocyte transformation *in vitro* requires tissue culture for 4–7 days and utilizes different biological materials. Standardization of mitogens, antigens, and serum supplements requires pooling, and freezing of large numbers of aliquots.

The major problems in performing longitudinal studies have been interexperimental and day-to-day variations. *In vitro* lymphocyte responses of a normal donor to mitogen or antigen can vary significantly when fresh bleedings are made over several days. If aliquots of cells from each bleeding are cryopreserved under the right conditions and then thawed and tested simultaneously, the interexperimental variation seen previously between each sample decreases remarkably, and the responses of one individual appear to be quite uniform (Jewett et al., 1976). Cryopreservation of lymphocytes for longitudinal studies will be useful in the study of patients with minimal immune deficiencies and in the evaluation of any immune therapy that requires a sensitive methodology.

References

Ahern, T., and Kay, J. E. (1975). *Exp. Cell Res.* **92**, 513–518.

Aisenberg, A. C. (1962). *J. Clin. Invest.* **41**, 1964–1970.

Aisenberg, A. C. (1965). *Nature (London)* **205**, 1233–1234.

Allan, D., Auger, J., and Crumpton, M. J. (1971). *Exp. Cell Res.* **66**, 362–368.

Andersson, J., Sjöberg, O., and Möller, G. (1972). *Transplant. Rev.* **11**, 131–171.

Andersen, V., Söberg, M., and Sörensen, S. F. (1971a). *Acta Pathol. Microbiol. Scand., Sect. B* **79**, 489–494.

Andersen, V., Söberg, M., and Sörensen, S. F. (1971b). *Acta Pathol. Microbiol. Scand., Sect. B* **79**, 495–501.

Auer, G., Zetterberg, A., and Killander, D. (1970). *Exp. Cell Res.* **62**, 32–38.

Axelson, N. H. (1971). *Infect. Immun.* **4**, 525–527.

Bach, F. H., Meuwissen, H. J., Albertini, R. J., and Good, R. A. (1968). *Birth Defects, Orig. Artic. Ser.* **4**, 245.

Biggar, W. D., Park, B. H., Dupont, B., and Good, R. A. (1974). *Clin. Immunol. Immunopath.* **2**, 501–509.

Blaese, R. M., Strober, W., Brown, R. S., and Waldmann, T. A. (1968). *Lancet* **1**, 1056–1060.

Blaese, R. M., Strober, W., and Waldmann, T. A. (1975). *Birth Defects, Orig. Artic. Ser.* **11**, 250–254.

Böyum, A. (1968). *Scand. J. Clin. Lab. Invest.* **21**, Suppl. 97, 31–50.

Braunstein, J. D., Good, R. A., Hansen, J. A., Dupont, B., Sharpless, T. K., and Melamed, M. R. (1976). *J. Histochem. Cytochem.* **24**, 378–382.

Bretscher, P., and Cohn, M. (1970). *Science* **169**, 1042.

Brown, R. S., Haynes, H. A., Foley, H. T., Goodwin, H. A., Berard, C. W., and Carbone, P. P. (1967). *Ann. Intern. Med.* **67**, 291–302.

Buckley, R. H. (1971). *Prog. Immunol., Int. Congr. Immunol., 1st, 1971* pp. 1061–1080.

Burnett, F. M. (1959). "The Clonal Selection Theory of Acquired Immunity." Vanderbilt Univ. Press, Nashville, Tennessee.

Case, D. C., Jr., Hansen, J. A., Corralles, E., Young, C. W., Dupont, B., Pinsky, C. M., and Good, R. A. (1976). *Cancer* (in press).

Chessin, C. M., Börjeson, J., Welsh, P. D., Douglas, S. D., and Cooper, H. L. (1966). *J. Exp. Med.* **124**, 873–884.

Cleveland, W. W., Fogel, B. J., Brown, W. T., and Kay, H. E. M. (1968). *Lancet* **2**, 1211–1214.

Coombs, R. R. A., Garner, B. W., Janeway, C. A., Jr., Wilson, A. B., Gell, P. G. H., and Kelus, A. S. (1970). *Immunology* **18**, 417–429.

Cooper, H. L. (1972). *Transplant. Rev.* 11, 3–38.

Cooper, H. L., and Rubin, A. D. (1965). *Blood* 25, 1014–1027.

Cooper, H. L., and Rubin, A. D. (1966). *Science* 152, 516–518.

Cooper, M. D., Chase, H. P., Lawman, J. T., Krivit, W., and Good, R. A. (1968). *Am. J. Med.* 44, 499–513.

Corder, M. P., Young, R. C., Brown, R. S., and DeVita, V. T. (1972). *Blood* 39, 595–601.

Coutinho, A., and Möller, G. (1974). *Scand. J. Immunol.* 3, 321.

Coutinho, A., Gronowicz, E., and Möller, G. (1975). *Scand. J. Immunol.* 4, 89.

Cunningham-Rundles, S., Dupont, B., Posner, J. B., Hansen, J. A., and Good, R. A. (1976). *Acta Neurol. Scand.* 53, Suppl. (in press).

Curtis, J. E., Hersh, E. M., Harris, J. E., McBride, C., and Freireich, E. J. (1970). *Clin. Exp. Immunol.* 6, 473–491.

Darzynkiewicz, Z., Boland, L., and Ringertz, N. R. (1969). *Exp. Cell Res.* 55, 120–123.

de Sousa, M., Yang, M., Lopes-Corrales, E., Tan, C., Dupont, B., and Good, R. A. (1976). *Hum. Pathol.* (in press).

Diener, E., and Feldman, M. (1972). *Transplant. Rev.* 8, 76.

Douglas, S. D. (1972). *Transplant. Rev.* 11, 39–59.

DuBois, R., Meinesz, A., Bierhorst-Eijlander, A., Groenewoud, M., Schellekens, P. T. A., and Eijsvoogel, V. P. (1974). *Tissue Antigens* 4, 458–468.

Dupont, B., and Good, R. A. (1975). *Birth Defects, Orig. Artic. Ser.* 11, 377–379.

Dutton, R. W., and Bulman, H. N. (1964). *Immunology* 7, 54–64.

Eltringham, J. R., and Kaplan, H. S. (1973). *Natl. Cancer Inst., Monogr.* 36, 107–115.

Elves, M. W. (1963). *Lancet* 1, 806–807.

Feldman, M., Howard, J. G., and Desaynard, C. (1975). *Transplant. Rev.* 23, 78.

Gatti, R. A., Meuwissen, H. J., Allen, H. D., Hong, R., and Good, R. A. (1968). *Lancet* 2, 1366–1369.

Good, R. A. (1973). *Harvey Lect.* 67, 1–107.

Good, R. A., Kelly, W. D., Rötstein, J., and Varco, R. L. (1962). *Prog. Allergy* 6, 275.

Gordon, J., and MacLean, L. D. (1965). *Nature (London)* 208, 795–796.

Graziano, K. D., Ruckdeschel, J. C., and Mardiney, M. R. (1975). *Cell. Immunol.* 10, 347–359.

Greaves, M. F., and Bauminger, S. (1972). *Nature (London), New Biol.* 235, 67–69.

Greaves, M. F., and Janossy, G. (1972). *Transplant. Rev.* 11, 87–130.

Greaves, M. F., and Roitt, I. M. (1968). *Clin. Exp. Immunol.* 3, 393–412.

Greaves, M. F., Janossy, G., and Doenhoff, M. (1974a). *J. Exp. Med.* 140, 1–17.

Greaves, M. F., Janossy, C., and Doenhoff, M. (1947b). *Nature (London)* 248, 698–701.

Greenberg, A. H., Ray, M., and Tsai, Y. T. (1969). *J. Pediatr.* 75, 95–103.

Gunther, C. R., and Wang, J. L. (1974). *J. Cell Biol.* 62, 366–377.

Hadden, J. W., Hadden, E. M., Haddox, M. K., and Goldberg, N. D. (1972). *Proc. Natl. Acad. Sci. U.S.A.* 69, 3024–3027.

Hadden, J. W., Hadden, E. M., Sadlik, S. R., and Coffey, B. G. (1975). *Proc. Natl. Acad. Sci. U.S.A.* 73, 1717–1721.

Hansen, J. A., and Good, R. A. (1974). *Hum. Pathol.* 5, 567–599.

Hansen, J. A., Bloomfield, C. D., Dupont, B., Gajl-Peczalska, K. J., Kiszkiss, D., and Good, R. A. (1974). *Proc. Leukocyte Cult. Conf., 8th, 1973* pp. 119–123.

Harris, G., and Littleton, R. J. (1966). *J. Exp. Med.* **124**, 621–634.

Hartzman, R. J., Segall, M., Bach, M. L., and Bach, F. L. (1971). *Transplantation* **11**, 268–273.

Hausen, P., Stein, H., and Peters, H. (1969). *Eur. J. Biochem.* **9**, 542–549.

Hersh, E. M., and Oppenheim, J. J. (1965). *N. Engl. J. Med.* **273**, 1006–1012.

Hirschorn, K., Schreibman, R. R., Bach, F. H., and Siltzbach, L. E. (1964). *Lancet* **2**, 842–843.

Hirschorn, R., Brittinger, G., Hirschorn, S., and Weissman, G. (1968). *J. Cell Biol.* **37**, 412–423.

Hosking, C. S., Fitzgerald, M. G., and Simons, M. J. (1971). *Clin. Exp. Immunol.* **9**, 467–476.

Hungerford, D. A., Donally, A. J., Nowell, P. C., and Beck, S. (1959). *Am. J. Hum. Genet.* **11**, 215–236.

Inbar, M., Ben-Bassett, H., and Sachs, L. (1973). *Exp. Cell Res.* **76**, 143–151.

Inman, D. R., and Cooper, E. H. (1963). *J. Cell Biol.* **19**, 441–452.

Jewett, M. A. S., Gupta, S., Hansen, J. A., Cunningham-Rundles, S., Siegal, F. P., Good, R. A., and Dupont, B. (1976). In preparation.

Jimenez, L., Bloom, B. R., Blume, M. R., and Oettgen, H. F. (1970). *J. Exp. Med.* **133**, 740–749.

Jones, G. (1972). *Clin. Exp. Immunol.* **12**, 403–417.

Kay, J. E. (1968). *Nature (London)* **219**, 172–173.

Kay, J. E. (1970). *Exp. Cell Res.* **58**, 185–187.

Kay, J. E. (1972). *Exp. Cell Res.* **71**, 245–247.

Kay, J. E. (1973). *Scand. J. Immunol.* **2**, 86.

Kelly, W. D., Good, R. A., and Varco, R. L. (1958). *Surg., Gynecol. Obstet.* **107**, 565–570.

Killander, D., and Rigler, R. (1965). *Exp. Cell Res.* **39**, 701–704.

Kim, Y. B. (1975). In "Immunodeficiency in Man and Animals" (D. Bergsma, R. A. Good, and G. Finstad, eds.), pp. 549–557. Sinauer Assoc., Sunderland, Massachusetts.

Kornfeld, S., and Kornfeld, R. (1969). *Proc. Natl. Acad. Sci. U.S.A.* **63**, 1439–1446.

Kreth, H. W., Thiessen, G., and Deicher, H. (1970). *Clin. Exp. Immunol.* **7**, 109–114.

Lazda, V. A., and Baram, P. (1974). *J. Immunol.* **112**, 1705–1717.

Leikin, S. L., Bazelon, M., and Park, B. H. (1966). *J. Pediatr.* **68**, 477–479.

Levy, R., and Kaplan, H. S. (1974). *N. Engl. J. Med.* **290**, 181–185.

Lindahl-Kiessling, K., and Mattsson, A. (1971). *Exp. Cell Res.* **65**, 307–312.

Lindahl-Kiessling, K., and Peterson, B. D. A. (1969). *Exp. Cell. Res.* **55**, 85–87.

Ling, N. R. (1971). "Lymphocyte Stimulation," 1st ed., p. 181. North-Holland Publ., Amsterdam.

Ling, N. R., and Husband, E. M. (1964). *Lancet* **1**, 363–365.

Ling, N. R., and Kay, J. E. (1975). "Lymphocyte Stimulation," 2nd ed., Chapter 9. North-Holland Publ., Amsterdam.

Ling, N. R., Spicer, E., James, K., and Williamson, N. (1965), *Br. J. Haematol.* **11**, 421.

Lischner, H. W., Punnett, H. H., and DiGeorge, A. M. (1967). *Nature (London)* **214**, 580–589.

Lohrmann, H.-P., Graw, C. M., and Graw, R. G. (1974). *J. Exp. Med.* **139**, 1037–1048.

Lucas, D. O., Shohet, S. B., and Merler, E. (1971). *J. Immunol.* **106**, 768–772.

Marchalonis, J. J. (1975). *Science* **190**, 20–29.

Marshall, W. H., Valentine, F. T., and Lawrence, H. S. (1969). *J. Exp. Med.* 130, 327–344.

Matsoniotis, N. S., and Tsenghi, L. J. (1964). *Lancet* 1, 989.

Mendelsohn, J., Skinner, A., and Kornfeld, S. (1971). *J. Clin. Invest.* 50, 818–826.

Meuwissen, H. J., Bach, F. W., Hong, R., and Good, R. A. (1968). *J. Pediat.* 72, 177–185.

Meuwissen, H. J., Van Alten, P. A., and Good, R. A. (1969). *Transplantation* 7, 1–11.

Miller, S. D., and Jones, H. E. (1973). *Am. Rev. Respir. Dis.* 107, 530–538.

Mills, J. A. (1966). *J. Immunol.* 97, 239–247.

Mitchison, N. A. (1955). *J. Exp. Med.* 102, 157–177.

Neiman, P. E., and MacDonnell, D. M. (1971). *Proc. Leucocyte Cult. Conf.*, 5th, 1970 p. 61.

Nilsson, B. S. (1972). *Cell. Immunol.* 3, 493–500.

Nossal, G. J. V., and Ada, G. L. (1971). "Antigens, Lymphoid Cells and the Immune Response." Academic Press, New York.

Novogrodsky, A., and Katchalski, E. (1970). *Biochim. Biophys. Acta* 215, 291–296.

Nowell, P. C. (1960). *Cancer Res.* 20, 462–466.

Olsen, G. B., Dent, P. B., Rawls, W. E., Smith, M., Montgomery, J., Melnick, J., and Good, R. A. (1968). *J. Exp. Med.* 128, 47–68.

Oppenheim, J. J., Wolstencroft, R. A., and Fell, P. G. H. (1967). *Immunology* 12, 89–102.

Oppenheim, J. J., Blaese, R. M., and Waldmann, T. A. (1970). *J. Immunol.* 104, 835–844.

O'Reilly, R. R. J., and Lopez, C. (1975). *Fed. Proc., Fed. Am. Soc. Exp. Biol.* 34, 947.

Ozato, K., Ebert, J. D., and Adler, W. H. (1975). *J. Immunol.* 115, 339–344.

Pearmain, G., Lycette, R. R., and Fitzgerald, D. H. (1963). *Lancet* 1, 637–638.

Peters, J. H., and Hansen, P. (1971a). *Eur. J. Biochem.* 19, 502–508.

Peters, J. H., and Hansen, P. (1971b). *Eur. J. Biochem.* 19, 509–513.

Phillips, B., and Roitt, I. M. (1973). *Nature (London) New Biol.* 241, 254–256.

Plate, J. M., and Amos, B. (1971a). *Cell. Immunol.* 1, 476–487.

Plate, J. M. and Amos, B. (1971b). *Cell. Immunol.* 1, 488–499.

Powell, A. E., and Leon, M. A. (1970). *Exp. Cell Res.* 62, 315–325.

Quastel, M. R., and Kaplan, J. G. (1968). *Nature (London)* 219, 198.

Quastel, M. R., and Kaplan, J. G. (1970). *Exp. Cell Res.* 63, 230–233.

Rabellino, E., Colon, S., Grey, H. M., and Unanue, E. R. (1971). *J. Exp. Med.* 133, 156–168.

Resch, K., and Ferber, E. (1972). *Eur. J. Biochem.* 27, 153–161.

Rosenberg, G. L., Farber, P. A., and Notkins, A. L. (1972). *Proc. Natl. Acad. Sci. U.S.A.* 69, 756–760.

Russell, A. S. (1974). *J. Infect. Dis.* 129, 142–146.

Sabesin, S. M., Maglio, M. T., and Isselbacher, K. J. (1965). *Fed. Proc., Fed. Am. Soc. Exp. Biol.* 24, 304.

Sample, W. F., and Chrétien, P. B. (1971). *Clin. Exp. Immunol.* 9, 419–427.

Sarkany, I., and Caron, G. A. (1966). *Br. J. Dermatol.* 78, 352–354.

Sartoris, S., Cavallero, P., Pegororo, L., Vernano, F., and Fazio, M. (1965). *Panminerva Med.* 7, 370–372.

Sasaki, M. S., and Norman, A. (1966). *Nature (London)* 210, 913–914.

Schellekens, P., T. A., and Eijsvoogel, V. P. (1968). *Clin. Exp. Immunol.* 3, 571–584.

Schellekens, P. T. A., and Eijsvoogel, V. P. (1971). *Clin. Exp. Immunol.* 8, 187–194.

Schier, W. W., Roth, A., Ostroff, G., and Schrift, M. H. (1956). *Am. J. Med.* **20**, 94–99.

Schrader, J. W. (1973). *J. Exp. Med.* **138**, 1466.

Sell, S., Sheppard, H. W., Jr., and Redelman, D. (1975). *Exp. Cell Res.* **90**, 309–316.

Shortman, K., Burd, W. J., Cerottini, J. C., and Brunner, K. T. (1973). *Cell. Immunol.* **6**, 25–40.

Simons, M. J., and Fitzgerald, M. G. (1968). *Lancet* **2**, 937–940.

Skoog, V. T., Weber, T. H., and Richter, W. (1974). *Exp. Cell Res.* **85**, 339–350.

Smith, K. A., Chess, L., and Mardiney, M. R. (1973). *Cell. Immunol.* **8**, 321–327.

Smithwick, E. M., and Berkovich, S. (1966). *Proc. Soc. Exp. Biol. Med.* **123**, 266–270.

Sokal, J. E., and Primikirios, N. (1961). *Cancer* **14**, 597–607.

Spitler, L., Benjamini, E., Young, J. D., Kaplan, H., and Fudenberg, H. H. (1970). *J. Exp. Med.* **131**, 133–148.

Spitler, L. E., Levin, A. S., Stiles, D. P., Fudenberg, H., Pirofsky, B., August, C. S., Stiehm, E. R., Hitzig, W. H., and Gatti, R. A. (1972). *J. Clin. Invest.* **51**, 3216–3224.

Stobo, J. D. (1972). *Transplant. Rev.* **11**, 60–88.

Stobo, J. D., Rosenthal, A. S., and Paul, W. E. (1972). *J. Immunol.* **108**, 1–17.

Sun-Lin, P., Cooper, A. G., and Wortis, H. H. (1973). *N. Engl. J. Med.* **289**, 548–551.

Thompson, E., Lewis, C. M., and Pegrum, G. D. (1973). *Br. Med. J.* **4**, 709–711.

Touraine, J. L., Touraine, F., Hadden, J. W., Hadden, E. M., and Good, R. A. (1975). *Int. Arch. Allergy Appl. Immunol.* (in press).

Traganos, F., Darzynkiewicz, Z., Sharpless, T., and Melamed, M. R. (1976). *J. Histochem. Cytochem.* **24**, 40–48.

Van den Berg, K. J., and Betel, I. (1971). *Exp. Cell Res.* **66**, 257–259.

Waithe, W. I., Dauphinais, C., Hathaway, P., and Hirschorn, K. (1975). *Cell. Immunol.* **17**, 323–334.

Wang, J. L., Cunningham, B. A., and Edelman, G. M. (1971). *Proc. Natl. Acad. Sci. U.S.A.* **68**, 1130–1134.

Wang, J. L., McClain, D. A., and Edelman, G. M. (1975). *Proc. Natl. Acad. Sci. U.S.A.* **72**, 1917–1921.

Webb, D. B., Stites, D. P., Perlman, J. D., Luong, D., and Fudenberg, H. H. (1973). *Biochem. Biophys. Res. Commun.* **53**, 1002–1008.

Weber, T. H. (1969). *Scand. J. Clin. Lab. Invest., Suppl.* **117**.

Weber, T. H., Skoog, V. T., Mattsson, A., and Lindahl-Kiessling, K. (1975). *Exp. Cell Res.* **85**, 351–361.

Whitney, R. B., and Sutherland, B. M. (1973). *J. Cell. Physiol.* **82**, 9–20.

Wigzell, H., and Andersson, B. (1969). *J. Exp. Med.* **129**, 23–36.

Wolstencroft, B. A., and Dumonde, D. C. (1970). *Immunology* **18**, 599.

Wu, L. Y. F., Lawton, A. R., Greaves, M. F., and Cooper, M. D. (1973). *Proc. Leukocyte Cult. Conf., 7th, 1972* pp. 485–500.

Yoffey, J. M., Winter, C. C., Osmond, D. G., and Meek, E. S. (1965). *Br. J. Haematol.* **11**, 488–497.

Young, W. M., Leon, M. A., Takahashi, T., Howard, I. K., and Sage, H. J. (1971). *J. Biol. Chem.* **246**, 1596–1601.

Zetterberg, A., and Auer, G. (1969). *Exp. Cell Res.* **56**, 122–126.

Zoshke, D. C., and Bach, F. H. (1970). *Science* **170**, 1404–1406.

Products of Activated Lymphocytes

ROSS E. ROCKLIN[1]

Department of Medicine, Robert B. Brigham Hospital,
Harvard Medical School, Boston, Massachusetts

I. Introduction

The best screening procedure to evaluate cellular hypersensitivity or immunity at present is still the delayed (24–48 hour) skin test. One or more positive responses to environmental antigens, such as tuberculin purified protein derivative (PPD), *Candida,* streptokinase-streptodornase (SK-SD), or other fungal antigens and/or the ability to be actively sensitized to new antigens, such as keyhole limpet hemocyanin or dinitrochlorobenzene, indicates that the cellular immune system is basically intact in that individual. The presence of cutaneous anergy, i.e., the failure to develop positive skin tests to environmental antigens or be sensitized to new antigens, was formerly thought to represent solely a defect in cellular immune function. However, on the basis of much *in vivo* and *in vitro* experimentation, we now know that cutaneous anergy may result

[1] Recipient of a Research Career Development Award AI-70796.

195

from lesions other than those involving lymphocyte function. For example, a defect in macrophage function, the clotting system, skin or subcutaneous tissue, the microvasculature, or the inflammatory response in general may result in cutaneous anergy. The *in vitro* tests that measure lymphocyte and macrophage function, which is the subject of this report, are of particular use in the evaluation of the patient with cutaneous anergy. These tests can, in the latter patient, define the lymphoid or nonlymphoid nature of the defect in cellular immunity.

The *in vitro* tests which measure lymphocyte function all have as a common feature the detection of cell activation. The methods that detect lymphocyte activation currently in the use include the measurement of cellular proliferation (DNA synthesis), the elaboration of biologically active mediators (lymphokines), and direct lymphocyte-mediated cytotoxicity. This report describes several assay systems currently employed to detect the production of lymphocyte mediators.

When lymphocytes are stimulated *in vitro* by mitogens, such as phytohemagglutinin (PHA) or concanavalin A (Con A), as well as by antigens, such as PPD, *Candida*, or SK-SD, they release a variety of biologically active materials. A number of these mediators are listed in Table I. As can be seen, these factors affect the function of a number of cells, including macrophages, neutrophils, basophils, eosinophils, lymphocytes, and other cell types. The production of mediators by lymphoid cells after immunologically specific stimulation may serve as a means of communication between sensitized lymphocytes, macrophages, and other cells involved in the cellular immune reaction. Furthermore, they may serve as biological amplifiers, recruiting and perhaps activating other inflammatory cells at the reaction site. Exactly how many chemically distinct substances are present and how many are necessary for the generation of a cellular immune response is not known. Because of the space limitation and the fact that many of these activities have not been well characterized, much less used as clinical tools, only some of the better understood mediators and their assay systems will be mentioned.

II. Cell Migration Inhibition System

The antigen-induced inhibition of cell migration has been used as an *in vitro* correlate of cellular immunity for many years after its original description by Rich and Lewis (1932). The development of the capillary tube technique by George and Vaughan (1962) has greatly facilitated a resolution of its mechanism and has led to the recent progress in the mediator field. Studies by David and David (1973) and by Bloom (1971)

TABLE I
PRODUCTS OF ACTIVATED LYMPHOCYTES

I. Mediators affecting macrophages
   A. Migration-inhibitory factor (MIF)
   B. Macrophage-activating factor (indistinguishable from MIF)
   C. Macrophage-aggregation factor (MAF) (? same as MIF)
   D. Factor causing disappearance of macrophages from peritoneum (? same as MIF)
   E. Chemotactic factor for macrophages
   F. Antigen-dependent MIF
II. Mediators affecting neutrophil leukocytes
   A. Chemotactic factor
   B. Leukocyte inhibitory factor (LIF)
III. Mediators affecting lymphocytes
   A. Mitogenic factors
   B. Antibody-enhancing factors
   C. Antibody-suppressing factors
   D. ? Chemotactic factor
IV. Mediators affecting eosinophils
   A. Chemotactic factor[a]
   B. Migration-stimulation factor
V. Mediators affecting basophils
   Chemotactic augmentation factor
VI. Other cells
   A. Cytotoxic factors—lymphotoxin
   B. Growth-inhibitory factors
      1. Clonal inhibitory factor
      2. Proliferation-inhibitory factor
   C. Osteoclast-activating factor (OAF)
VII. Skin reactive factor
VIII. Interferon
IX. Immunoglobulin

[a] Requires antigen–antibody complexes.

have revealed that sensitized lymphocytes produce a soluble factor, migration-inhibitory factor (MIF), which inhibits the migration of peritoneal exudate cells obtained from normal guinea pigs. MIF is produced by lymphocytes after incubation with specific antigen and is not found in the cell-free supernatants of lymphocytes cultured either in the absence of antigen or in the presence of unrelated antigen. Antigen-induced production of MIF is closely associated with the presence of *in vivo* cellular hypersensitivity to the same antigen and is independent of concomitant antibody production.

Presently, two *in vitro* cell migration systems are widely used to study cellular hypersensitivity in man. In one, guinea pig macrophages or human monocytes serve as indicator cells, and their migration has been

TABLE II

CELL MIGRATION SYSTEMS[a]

I. Direct (one-step)
   A. Lymph node or spleen explants (animal)
   B. Peritoneal exudate cells (many animal species)
      1. Capillary tubes
      2. Agarose drops
   C. Human lymphocytes mixed with exudate cells
      1. Capillary tubes
      2. Electrophoretic field
   D. Human buffy-coat leukocytes
      1. Capillary tubes
      2. Agar plates
II. Indirect (two-step)
   A. Culture human lymphocytes separately to produce mediators (MIF and LIF)
   B. Assay culture supernatants on indicator cells (capillary tube, agar)
      1. Peritoneal exudate cells
      2. Human buffy-coat leukocytes
      3. Human monocytes
      4. Human PMN leukocytes

[a] MIF, migration inhibitory factor; LIF, leukocyte inhibitory factor; PMN, polymorphonuclear.

shown to be inhibited by MIF. In the other system, human buffy-coat leukocytes serve as indicator cells, and their migration is inhibited by a leukocyte-inhibitory factor (LIF). We have recently shown that LIF is distinct from MIF by virtue of its size and its ability to inhibit the migration of human polymorphonuclear (PMN) leukocytes but not guinea pig macrophages or human monocytes.

Two assay methods can be used to measure cell migration: an indirect method (two-step) and a direct method (one-step). The various assay systems are shown in Table II. With the indirect method, lymphocytes are first cultured separately with antigen to produce the mediator, which is later assayed on autologous or homologous indicator cells that have been placed in capillary tubes, on agar plates, or in agarose drops. The area of migration is measured at 18–24 hours later, and the inhibition of migration is calculated by comparing the area of migration in the presence of antigen to that in the absence of antigen (Fig. 1). In the direct procedure, lymphocytes and indicator cells are cultured together. The mediator is produced locally subsequent to exposure of the lymphocytes to antigen and inhibition of migration of the indicator cells measured at 18–24 hours. For both systems, 20% inhibition or greater is usually statistically significant and indicative of MIF or LIF production. Occasionally, less than 20% migration inhibition is statistically significant and may indicate a positive response. MIF and LIF production correlates

SKIN TEST	NO ANTIGEN	PPD	SKSD

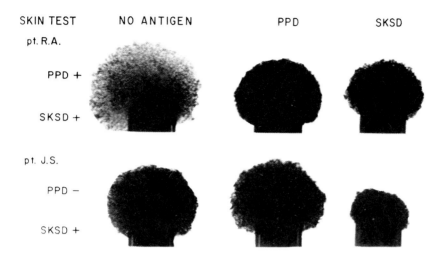

pt. R.A.

PPD +

SKSD +

pt. J.S.

PPD −

SKSD +

Fig. 1. Effects of supernatants taken from lymphocyte cultures of patients RA and JS on normal guinea pig macrophages in capillary tubes. Note that RA was tuberculin purified protein derivative (PPD) positive, streptokinase-streptodornase (SK-SD) positive and migration-inhibitory factor (MIF) was produced to both antigens, whereas JS was PPD negative, SK-SD positive and MIF was produced only in response to SK-SD. (From Rocklin *et al.*, 1970b. *J. Immunol.* **104,** 95. © 1970 The Williams & Wilkins Co., Baltimore.)

qualitatively well with cutaneous cellular hypersensitivity in the host but not quantitatively. That is, the amount of inhibition of migration does not correlate wih the size of the delayed skin test (Fig. 2).

The advantage of the indirect method is that it permits dissection of the cellular immune response. One can assess separately the ability of the patient's lymphocytes to elaborate MIF or LIF if normal indicator cells are provided. One can additionally assess whether the patient's indicator cells—monocytes or PMN leukocytes—respond to autologous or homologous mediator preparation or both. The disadvantage with this assay is that it requires large amounts of blood from patients and is time-consuming (takes 3 days to perform). Moreover, because of the 10–20% incidence of false negative results, a negative response should be repeated in an individual patient to confirm the findings. However, false positive results generally do not occur if the proper antigen controls are included in the experiments.

The advantage of the direct assay over the indirect method is that it requires less time to perform, requires fewer cells (if a microassay system is used), and can give an answer in 18 hours. The main disadvantage of this technique is that negative results may be difficult to interpret. No

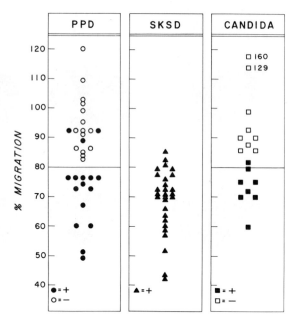

Fig. 2. Correlation of delayed hypersensitivity *in vivo* and *in vitro* using tuberculin purified protein derivative (PPD), streptokinase-streptodornase (SK-SD), and *Candida* as antigens. Filled symbols represent skin test-positive individuals; open symbols represent the skin test negatives. A line could be drawn at 80% migration which separated the skin test negatives from the majority of skin test positives. (From Rocklin *et al.*, 1970b. *J. Immunol.* **104**, 95. © 1970 The Williams & Wilkins Co., Baltimore.)

inhibition of migration may result from a lymphocyte defect (lack of mediator production), absence of sensitivity to the antigen, or a failure of the indicator cell to respond to the mediator. Distinguishing between these possibilities is quite important in evaluating patients with cutaneous anergy who may have more than one defect.

Thus, the direct migration test is a useful screening test to assess mediator production in patients. One or more positive response to antigens may be taken to mean intact cellular immunity. A negative response, however, would require the use of the indirect technique to pinpoint the defect precisely.

Migration inhibition may occur independently of MIF or LIF. Inhibition may result from such nonspecific means as antigen toxicity, alkaline pH, and serum factors or by antigen–antibody complexes. This latter mechanism is of particular interest since cytophilic antibody present on the surface of PMN leukocytes may interact with particulate antigen and inhibit cell migration. Therefore, some caution should be exercised in the interpretation of results derived from migration tests. If the proper

TABLE III

COMPARISON OF THE PROPERTIES OF HUMAN AND
GUINEA PIG MIGRATION-INHIBITORY FACTOR (MIF)[a]

Property	Human MIF$_{SK-SD}$	Guinea pig MIF$_{OCB-BGG}$
Temperature 56°C	Stable	Stable
Approximate MW determined by gel filtration	23,000	35,000–55,000[b]
Disc electrophoresis	Albumin	Prealbumin
Isopycnic centrifugation on CsCl	Protein	Denser than protein
Neuraminidase	Resistant	Sensitive
Chymotrypsin	Sensitive	Sensitive

[a] From Rocklin, 1974a. *J. Immunol.* **112,** 1461. © 1974 The Williams & Wilkins Co., Baltimore.

[b] Guinea pig MIF$_{Con A}$: MW 23,000–55,000; guinea pig MIF$_{PPD}$: MW 23,000.

controls have not been carried out, one might not be justified in attributing the inhibition to LIF or MIF.

We have previously shown that antigen-induced human MIF is a protein having a molecular weight of 23,000. By contrast, guinea pig MIF is slightly larger (25,000–55,000) and behaves like an acidic glycoprotein (Table III). Recently, experiments have been carried out to determine the characteristics of human LIF. A study comparing the physicochemical properties, as well as the effects of enzymic treatment on both mediators, is summarized in Table IV. Both factors appear to have properties similar to those of proteins; LIF, but not MIF, is an esterase.

Studies have only recently been carried out to examine the important question of which cell types (thymus-derived, or T cells, and bone marrow-derived, or B cells) produce MIF and LIF. The availability of

TABLE IV

COMPARISON OF THE PROPERTIES OF HUMAN MIGRATION-INHIBITORY FACTOR
(MIF) AND LEUKOCYTE-INHIBITORY FACTOR (LIF)[a]

Treatment	Human MIF	Human LIF
Indicator cell	Macrophage or monocyte	Polymorphonuclear leukocyte
Temperature 56°C	Stable	Stable
MW determined by gel filtration	23,000	69,000
Disc electrophoresis	Albumin	Albumin
Isopycnic centrifugation	Protein	Protein
Neuraminidase	Resistant	Resistant
Chymotrypsin	Sensitive	Sensitive
Difluorophosphate	Resistant	Sensitive

[a] From Rocklin, 1974a. *J. Immunol.* **112,** 1461. © 1974 The Williams & Wilkins Co., Baltimore.

a technique that separates lymphocytes into highly purified subpopulations has allowed further study of this problem. Using an immunoabsorbent column technique, Chess, MacDermott, and Schlossman have obtained pure and functionally distinct populations of human T and B lymphocytes. They showed that both T- and B-cell subpopulations proliferate in response to mitogens, such as PHA, Con A, and pokeweed, whereas only T cells respond to soluble or allogeneic antigenic stimuli. In collaboration with the above, Rocklin and David (1974c) have demonstrated that both human T and B blood lymphocytes produce MIF and LIF in response to antigens such as tuberculin PPD, *Candida,* or SK-SD. The elaboration of MIF and LIF by human T and B lymphocytes is antigen specific; that is, each factor is only produced by lymphocytes from donors who have cutaneous delayed hypersensitivity to the various antigens used *in vitro.* Donors lacking cutaneous sensitivity to these antigens did not produce either factor. MIF produced by T and B cells is similar in size, as is LIF produced by T and B cells. Thus, although the production of MIF or LIF correlates with *in vivo* cellular hypersensitivity, the assay cannot be used to measure the function of a particular cell type (T or B).

The migration inhibition assays have been widely used to study lymphocyte responses in patients with depressed cellular immunity, drug hypersensitivity, tissue antigens and in patients with cancer. Only a few instances will be mentioned below. For example, Table V shows a comparison of the results of skin testing, MIF production, and lymphocyte transformation in 131 patients having diseases associated with defective cellular immunity. Sixty-one patients (Hodgkin's disease, sarcoidosis,

TABLE V

CORRELATION BETWEEN SKIN TEST REACTIVITY AND *in Vitro* LYMPHOCYTE FUNCTION IN PATIENTS WITH DEPRESSED CELLULAR IMMUNITY[a]

Patient diagnosis[c]	Skin	MIF[b]	[3H]-Thymidine
Group I(61)			
Hodgkin's, sarcoid, collagen disease	+	+	+
Group II (70)			
(22) Hodgkin's, sarcoid, collagen disease, chronic candidiasis, DeGeorge syndrome	−	−	−
(34) Sarcoid, chronic candidiasis, collagen disease	−	−	+
(14) Hodgkin's, collagen disease	−	+	+

[a] From R. E. Rocklin *et al.,* unpublished data.

[b] Migration-inhibitory factor.

[c] In parentheses, number of cases.

collagen diseases) appeared to have intact cellular immunity at the time of study in that skin tests, MIF production, and proliferative responses to mitogens and antigens were normal. The remaining 70 patients had cutaneous anergy but could be distinguished from one another on the basis of their *in vitro* results. Twenty patients (Hodgkin's disease, sarcoidosis, DiGeorge syndrome, collagen diseases, chronic mucocutaneous candidiasis) had negative MIF tests and proliferative responses and, therefore, appeared to have both a T- and B-lymphocyte defect to account for their anergy. In 34 patients (sarcoidosis, chronic mucocutaneous candidiasis, collagen diseases), there was a dissociation between MIF production and lymphocyte transformation. The former was absent while the latter was normal. There appears to be a partial defect in T- and B-lymphocyte function in these latter patients, i.e., the T- and B-lymphocyte populations that produce MIF are defective while the proliferating T-cell populations are intact. Of particular interest was the finding that 14 patients (Hodgkin's disease, collagen diseases) with cutaneous anergy appeared to have normal lymphocyte function in that mediator production and proliferation were present. A nonlymphoid defect like the ones mentioned earlier might explain the cutaneous anergy in these latter patients. We have observed that in some patients the *in vivo* and *in vitro* responses become progressively impaired with clinical severity. With treatment and clinical improvement, function may return to normal.

Use of the migration inhibition system has provided some insight into the pathogenesis of diseases thought to involve autoimmune mechanisms. One may invoke the participation of cellular immune mechanisms in some groups of patients where specific MIF or LIF responses have been obtained. For example, only lymphocytes from patients with certain forms of glomerulonephritis produce MIF in response to glomerular basement membrane antigens (Fig. 3), and only lymphocytes from patients with the Guillain-Barre syndrome (Fig. 4) produce MIF to peripheral nerve antigens. However, in some instances, a positive result may not be specific for a particular disease. Lymphocytes from some patients with multiple sclerosis produce MIF when challenged by myelin basic protein antigen, but so do lymphocytes from patients with cerebrovascular accidents. These latter results illustrate a shortcoming common to all *in vitro* lymphocyte tests. They do not allow one to distinguish a lymphocyte response that may be important to the pathogenesis of a disease from one that develops as a result of massive tissue injury. Thus, the detection of lymphocyte sensitization by this or other tests should be interpreted with some caution. In contrast to ascertaining pathogenetic significance, these tests may be of considerable value in distinguishing those patients who may develop severe disease. Patients whose lympho-

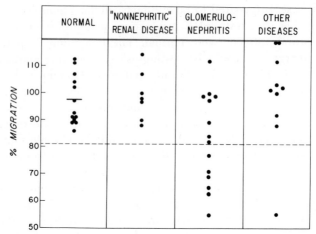

Fig. 3. Response of all patients to glomerular basement membrane antigens. The dotted line at 81% migration represents two standard deviations from the normal mean. Migration-inhibitory factor (MIF) production was primarily observed by lymphocytes from patients with glomerular nephritis. (From Rocklin *et al.*, 1970a.)

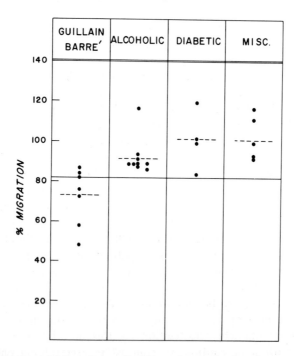

Fig. 4. Migration-inhibitory factor (MIF) production by lymphocytes from patients with peripheral neuropathies to peripheral nervous tissue antigens. Only patients with Guillain-Barre syndrome produced MIF in response to this antigen. (From Rocklin *et al.*, 1971.)

cytes remain sensitized to tissue antigens for long periods of time may go on to develop progressive disease whereas those patients whose lymphocytes become unresponsive by these techniques may have a more benign clinical course.

III. Macrophage Activation by Lymphocyte Mediators

Studies by Mackaness and co-workers (1964) have shown that resistance to infection by facultative intracellular organisms, such as *Listeria monocytogenes*, has an immunological basis, the lymphocyte playing an important role. Macrophages obtained from animals made immune by infection exhibit enhanced function *in vitro*. These cells are more spread out on glass, more adherent, more phagocytic, and show enhanced bactericidal activity even against organisms that are antigenically unrelated to those infecting the host. One might have predicted that lymphocyte mediators would be involved, at least in part, in the activation of macrophages. In fact, several investigators have demonstrated a role for lymphocyte mediators in the *in vitro* activation of normal macrophages. Mooney and Waksman (1970) studied the effect of whole supernatants from stimulated lymphocyte cultures on normal macrophages. These workers found that more cells were adherent to their culture vessel in those dishes which had been incubated with supernatants from antigen-stimulated lymphocytes than the presence of control supernatants. Nathan, Karnovsky, and David (1971), using MIF-rich fractions, showed that normal macrophages could be activated after 72 hours of incubation and observed changes in these cells that were similar in nature to those activated macrophages recovered from immune animals (Fig. 5). These macrophages became more adherent, had enhanced rates of phagocytosis, increased glucose oxidation through the hexose monophosphate shunt pathway, and increased ruffled membrane activity, and were more motile than their control counterparts. Furthermore, Nathan, Remold, and David (1973) have found that the macrophage-activating principle and MIF are indistinguishable from one another.

In animals, peritoneal exudate cells can be used as a source of macrophages, and in man, monocytes can be isolated from the peripheral blood. The monocytes or macrophages are plated to form monolayers and then incubated with control or MIF-containing supernatants for 1–3 days. Activation of the monolayers can be measured in a number of ways. One can determine the amount of cellular protein or DNA content per dish. Data from one study are shown in Table VI. There was a mean increase of 41% and 35% in the adherent cell protein and DNA content, respectively, in monolayers that had been incubated with MIF containing

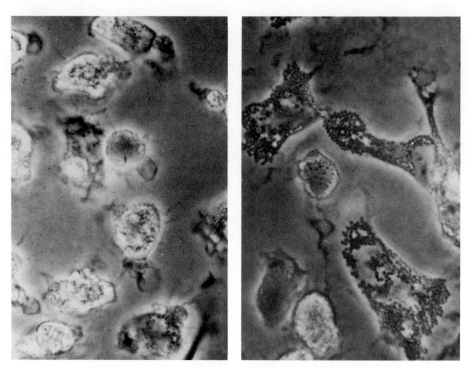

Fig. 5. *Left:* Macrophages that have been incubated with control supernatants. *Right:* Macrophages incubated with migration-inhibitory factor (MIF)-rich fractions. Note that the latter are more spread out. (From Nathan *et al.*, 1971.)

TABLE VI

EFFECT OF SUPERNATANTS ON MONOCYTE ADHERENCE[a]

No. of experiments	Supernatant	(Protein (per dish)	Increase in MIF[b]
	Adherent macrophage protein		
13	MIF	38.7 ± 5.6	$41\%^c$
	Control	27.5 ± 4.8	
	Adherent macrophage DNA		
18	MIF	28.7 ± 2.8	$35\%^c$
	Control	21.3 ± 2.6	

[a] From Rocklin *et al.*, 1974d.
[b] Migration-inhibitory factor.
[c] $P < 0.05$.

supernatants for 72 hours compared to monolayers incubated with control supernatants. The increase in cell adherence was not due to macrophage multiplication. The metabolism of monocyte monolayers can be assessed by pulsing the monolayers with ^{14}C-labeled glucose. After a brief incubation period, the amount of radioactive $^{14}CO_2$ that has been liberated is collected in a filter paper, and the radioactivity is determined by scintillation counting. Greater amounts of $^{14}CO_2$ are produced in dishes preincubated with MIF-containing supernatants than in the monolayers that have been incubated with control supernatants or culture medium (Fig. 6). Phagocytosis can be assessed by exposing the macrophage monolayers to starch particles and then counting the number of particles that have been ingested per cell. Enhanced bactericidal activity of macrophage monolayers can be determined by exposing MIF-rich or control monolayers to various numbers of bacteria and then incubating the monolayers for a short time. The cells are then disrupted, the contents are plated, and the numbers of surviving bacteria in the MIF-rich versus control monolayers are counted.

The ability of lymphocyte mediators to enhance macrophage function *in vitro* has been investigated in some patients with impaired cellular immunity. Thus far, no particular pattern has emerged. Godal and associates have shown that supernatants from mixed lymphocyte reactions are capable of activating blood monocytes from patients with the tuberculoid form of leprosy. No such activation of macrophages was observed in cultures obtained from patients with the lepromatous form of leprosy, where cellular immunity is depressed. In addition, Rocklin *et al.* (unpublished) found that monocytes from anergic patients with sarcoidosis respond normally to MIF-rich supernatants by increased cell adherence.

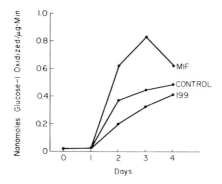

Fig. 6. Effect of migration-inhibitory factor (MIF)-rich and control supernatants and culture medium itself on glucose carbon-1 oxidation by human monocytes. Note that MIF-containing supernatants induce a two fold increase in glucose oxidation on day 3 compared to control supernatants. (From Rocklin *et al.*, 1974d.)

TABLE VII

ACTIVATION OF HUMAN MONOCYTE MONOLAYERS FROM HODGKIN'S DISEASE PATIENTS AND NORMAL SUBJECTS[a]

	Unfractionated supernatant			Sephadex G-100 fraction		
	Control	MIF	MIF/CON	Control	MIF	MIF/CON
Protein/dish						
Patients (7)	29.7 ± 3.1	57.1 ± 13.8	92% increase	30.3 ± 5.5	40.4 ± 7.5	33% increase
Normal subjects (5)	25.3 ± 4.1	40.1 ± 7.2	58% increase	25.9 ± 3.4	36.8 ± 5.5	42% increase
Glucose-1-^{14}C oxidation						
Patients (7)	1.12 ± 0.2	1.46 ± 0.2	30% increase	1.0 ± 0.2	1.31 ± 0.02	31% increase
Normal subjects (7)	1.34 ± 0.2	1.51 ± 0.1	20% increase	1.3 ± 0.2	1.71 ± 0.1	32% increase

[a] From R. E. Rocklin and R. Broulliard, unpublished data.
[b] Values are expressed as mean ± standard error: upper part, in micrograms of protein per dish; lower part, as nanomoles of glucose-1-^{14}C oxidation per milligrams per minute.

Similar results were found in several patients with Hodgkin's disease (Table VII). Further studies are necessary to determine which aspects of monocyte function in particular should be followed in these patients.

IV. Macrophage (Monocyte) Chemotactic Factor

The majority of cells infiltrating the site of a delayed hypersensitivity reaction are rapidly dividing nonsensitive mononuclear cells. Only a few of the infiltrating cells are sensitized lymphocytes. This suggested that antigen-activated lymphocytes might be producing a chemotactic factor that attracts monocytes to the site of reaction. In later studies, Ward, Remold, and David (1969) showed that antigen-stimulated lymphocytes generated a chemotactic substance in the culture fluid. These studies were carried out *in vitro* using Boyden chambers containing an upper and lower compartment separated by a micropore filter. The cell suspension was placed in the upper compartment. The lower compartment contained the test material; either supernatants from control or antigen-stimulated lymphocytes. Chemotactic activity was assessed by counting the number of cells that migrated through the micropore filter toward the lower compartment. A chemotactic index was calculated by subtracting the number of cells migrating through the filter in the presence of control supernatants from the number migrating through in the presence of the supernatant from antigen-stimulated lymphocytes. An index of greater than 50 cells is usually considered a positive response (Fig. 7).

Recent work by Gallin and co-workers (1973) indicate that one can radioactively label the indicator cells with ^{51}Cr and with the use of two filters assess the amount of radioactivity in the lower filter. This latter modification correlates very well with the morphological counting of cells and is more objective.

The production of chemotactic factor is antigen specific. The factor is heat stable after incubation at 56°C for 30 minutes (Table VIII). Studies by Ward, Remold, and David (1970) have revealed that macrophage chemotactic factor has properties similar to those of a protein.

A major problem associated with this technique is the observation that chemotactic activity in the control supernatant may sometimes be very high compared to the chemotactic activity in the supernatant obtained from antigen or mitogen-stimulated cultures. This may result in a low (or negative) chemotactic index and a false negative determination (Table IX). This high level of chemotactic activity in the control supernatant has been accounted for by the method used to isolate the

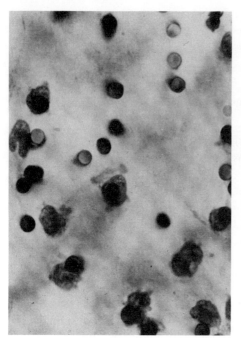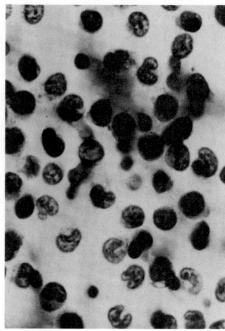

Fig. 7. Left: The number of cells that have migrated through the Millipore filter in the absence of a chemotactic stimulant. *Right:* The number of cells that have migrated through the Millipore filter in the presence of a chemotactic stimulant. (From Snyderman *et al.,* 1972. *J. Immunol.* **108,** 857. © 1972 The Williams & Wilkins Co., Baltimore.)

lymphocytes. It has been suggested by Snyderman *et al.* (unpublished) that the use of the Ficoll–Hypaque gradient technique to purify lymphocyte preparations might be responsible for nonspecifically activating lymphocytes so that they spontaneously release monocyte chemotactic factor.

TABLE VIII

MONOCYTE CHEMOTACTIC FACTOR

Treatment	Guinea pig[a]	Human
Heat	Stable	Stable
Sephadex	35,000–55,000	12,500–25,000
Electrophoresis	Albumin	Albumin
$CsCl_{25}$	1.34	—
Chymotrypsin	Sensitive	Sensitive
Neuraminidase	Stable	—

[a] From David and David, 1973.

TABLE IX
CHEMOTACTIC ACTIVITY OF SUPERNATANTS[a]

Background	Supernatants		Chemotactic index (A-C)
	Control	Active	
<50			
Mean ± SE	33 ± 4.6[b]	178 ± 25.3[b]	146 ± 25.7
>50			
Mean ± SE	102 ± 11.3[c]	115 ± 18.6[c]	34 ± 14.4

[a] From Ward and Rocklin, 1975.
[b] Means statistically different ($P = 0.0005$) by Student t test for paired means.
[c] Means not statistically different.

Therefore, it has been recommended that lymphocytes be separated by other means, such as the use of glass, wool, or cotton columns.

Using a rosette formation technique to purify populations of human T and B lymphocytes, Altman and co-workers have shown that antigen or mitogen-stimulated cultures of enriched T cells elaborate monocyte chemotactic factor. Furthermore, they have demonstrated that mitogen-stimulated B-cell populations also release monocyte chemotactic factor. These results are similar to those reported for MIF production. Thus, the chemotactic assay, like the MIF assay, has been shown to correlate with *in vivo* delayed hypersensitivity but cannot be used as an assay to measure the function of a particular cell type (T or B).

The chemotactic assay has been used to study clinical problems in patients with impaired cellular immunity. Snyderman *et al.* (1973) showed that lymphocytes from a patient with chronic mucocutaneous candidiasis failed to elaborate a lymphocyte-derived chemotactic factor for macrophages. In addition, the patient's monocytes did not respond to preformed monocyte chemotactic factors (lymphocyte-derived or complement-mediated) from a normal individual. Thus, the defect in this patient was at two levels. One defect was demonstrated to be in the lymphocyte because of its inability to produce a chemotactic factor for monocytes (this patient's lymphocytes also did not produce MIF). The other defect was demonstrated by the unresponsiveness of the patient's monocytes to preformed chemotactic stimulants. After the administration of transfer factor, the patient's monocytes were reported able to respond to chemotactic stimulants, although clinically the patient did not improve. Snyderman and co-workers have also demonstrated a monocyte defect in some patients with malignant melanoma. Monocytes from some patients with melanoma did not respond to preformed lymphocyte che-

TABLE X
HUMAN LYMPHOCYTE-INDUCED CHEMOTACTIC FACTOR FOR MONOCYTES[a]

Subjects	Number	Control	Antigen-stimulated	Chemotactic index
Normal	14 (20)[b]	67 ± 9.9	146 ± 16.9	90 ± 19.2
Hodgkin's disease	7 (11)	69 ± 16.4	140 ± 24.2	80 ± 19.3

[a] From P. A. Ward and R. E. Rocklin, unpublished data.
[b] Number in parentheses indicates total number of experiments.

motactic factor or complement-mediated chemotactic factors. After successful treatment of these patients, there was a marked improvement in their monocyte response. In other studies, Rocklin and Ward have shown that lymphocytes from a number of anergic Hodgkin's patients produced as much monocyte chemotactic factor as did cells from normal subjects (Table X). Furthermore, lymphocytes from these patients also produced MIF and incorporated increased amounts of ^{3}H-labeled thymidine in response to mitogens and antigens (Table V).

V. Lymphocyte Mitogenic (Blastogenic) Factors

Studies by Gordon and McClean (1965) as well as by Kasakura and Lowenstein (1967) have shown that supernatants obtained from human mixed lymphocyte cultures contained substances that were mitogenic for cultures of nonrelated lymphocytes. Several investigators have subsequently reported that nonsensitive lymphocytes undergo blast transformation and incorporate increased amounts of ^{3}H-labeled thymidine when cultured in the presence of supernatants from sensitized lymphocytes that have been stimulated by specific antigen. For example, Valentine and Lawrence (1969) found that supernatants from tuberculin-sensitive lymphocytes incubated with PPD cause increased thymidine incorporation by lymphocytes obtained from tuberculin-negative donors. Maini and coworkers (1969) described similar findings with an antigen-induced lymphocyte mitogenic factor (LMF). Janis and Bach (1970) have also shown that supernatants from mixed lymphocyte cultures have mitogenic activity for unrelated lymphocytes and, further, that these supernatants also contain a potentiating activity. That is, the total number of radioactive counts incorporated by unstimulated cells is greater than that produced by medium alone. This potentiating activity could be found in the supernatants from nonstimulated or mitomycin-treated lymphocytes.

LMF may be detected in supernatants of antigen-stimulated cultures after 24–48 hours. These supernatants are diluted with culture medium and then incubated with nonsensitive lymphocytes for approximately 6 days. Cell division and transformation are monitored either by counting transformed cells on stained smears or by measuring the incorporation of ³H-labeled thymidine into cellular DNA. An increase in cell division is usually found in the cultures that have been incubated with supernatants obtained from antigen-stimulated lymphocytes compared to that due to supernatants from unstimulated lymphocytes. LMF activity is customarily expressed as a net increase in counts per minute or as a stimulation index, as shown in Table XI. LMF should be assayed on nonsensitive lymphocytes rather than on lymphocytes from donors sensitive to the antigen used to produce the material. The presence of antigen in the supernatant may trigger the sensitive lymphocytes to divide and obscure some LMF activity.

LMF is nondialyzable and heat stable at 56°C for 30 minutes. It is resistant to treatment with RNase and DNase and has a molecular weight between 25,000 and 55,000. It is not clear at present whether cell division is required for LMF to be generated.

Recent studies by Geha *et al.* (1973) and by Rocklin *et al.* (1974c) have shown that LMF is produced by sensitized T lymphocytes in response to specific antigen. By contrast, B lymphocytes do not produce

TABLE XI

MITOGENIC FACTOR[a]

Supernatant source, PPD[b] positive	T and B cells		T cells		B cells	
	P − R[c]	SI[d]	P − R	SI	P − R	SI
T and B cells						
1	1155[e]	6.3	524	3.4	762	7.7
2	1008	6.3	738	5.4	1497	10.7
T cells						
1	1437	8.5	499	4.1	1373	11.5
2	1598	10.4	1002	8.0	1533	8.3
B cells						
1	50	1.2	42	1.2	68	1.5
2	55	1.2	11	1.1	120	1.6

[a] From Rocklin *et al.*, 1974c.
[b] PPD = tuberculin purified protein derivative.
[c] Cpm Preincubated (P) − Cpm Reconstituted (R) (control).
[d] Stimulation Index = P/R.
[e] Cpm, mean of quadruplicate cultures.

LMF. Furthermore, lymphocytes from patients with X-linked agammaglobulinemia produce normal amounts of LMF despite the fact that they lack detectable B cells. Both cell types, however, respond to LMF by increasing their DNA synthesis.

There is a close correlation between the production of LMF and the proliferative response by an individual's lymphocytes. Since the incorporation of ^{3}H-labeled thymidine is used to detect the effect of LMF on lymphocytes, this is not an unexpected observation. The finding that T cells but not B cells produce LMF, as well as the observation that LMF can be produced in the absence of MIF, suggests that these two factors are distinct. In this regard, it has been shown by Rocklin that lymphocytes from anergic patients with sarcoidosis proliferate normally in response to mitogens and antigens and produce LMF despite the fact that their lymphocytes do not produce MIF.

Mitogenic factors capable of activating or recruiting nonsensitive cells could furnish a mechanism for expanding a cellular reaction and producing greater amounts of other mediators. Alternatively, this material may act with antigen to stimulate cells which are already precommitted or potentially reactive to the antigen that has elicited its production. Furthermore, the observation that only T lymphocytes proliferate directly in response to antigen as well as produce LMF intimately links these two events. It may be that the first stage of proliferation is initiated after T lymphocytes are activated by antigen and release LMF. The second stage would be the nonspecific activation of either T or B lymphocytes by LMF. The cells activated by LMF may then produce mediators and/or secrete antibody.

VI. Cytotoxic Factors (Lymphotoxins)

The production of a soluble cytotoxic material by sensitized lymphocytes following stimulation by specific antigen was initially described by Ruddle and Waksman (1968). They showed that cell-free supernatants obtained from sensitized rat lymph node lymphocytes, which had been stimulated by soluble antigen, killed normal rat embryo fibroblasts. Subsequently, others have described the production of cytotoxic factors from spleen and peritoneal exudate cells from guinea pigs exhibiting delayed hypersensitivity to various antigens. Granger and Williams (1968) first reported the release of lymphotoxic factors by normal lymphocytes stimulated nonspecifically by PHA. Then they showed that lymphocytes from several species produced lymphotoxins.

Several assay systems are currently available to detect the presence of lymphotoxin (LT) in cultures of activated lymphocytes. Control and lymphotoxin-containing supernatants are prepared by incubating lymphocytes in the absence or in the presence, respectively, of a stimulant such as PHA or PPD for 1–2 days. The supernatants are then incubated with the target cells, one of the most susceptible being mouse L cells (fibroblasts). Cytotoxic activity by LT on the mouse L cell can be detected in a number of ways: morphological counting of the viable remaining cells, incorporation of ^{14}C-labeled amino acids into cell protein, release of ^{51}Cr from labeled target cells, or determination of the intracellular potassium by exchange with extracellular ^{86}Rb (Fig. 8).

Each of these assays is attended by some disadvantages. While morphological counting of target cells attached to glass may be thought to represent the actual amount of cell lysis by LT, there is evidence that some cells detach from the glass and are still viable while floating free in the supernatant. The chromium release assay is less sensitive than the

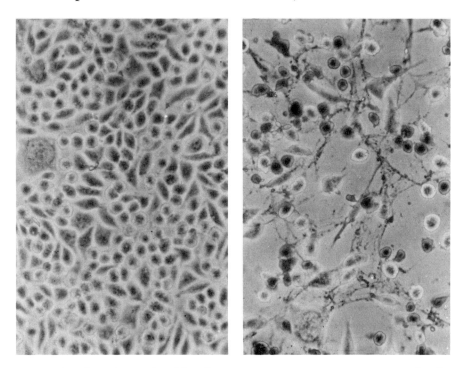

Fig. 8. Effect of control and lymphotoxin-containing supernatants on mouse L-cell monolayers. *Left:* Effect of control supernatants on monolayers. *Right:* Effect of lymphotoxin-containing supernatants on monolayers that have been incubated for 48 hours in the presence of this material. (From Coyne *et al.*, 1973. *J. Immunol.* **110**, 1630. © 1973 The Williams & Wilkins Co., Baltimore.)

above in detecting maximum cell destruction. This can be attributed to the high background release of label from control cultures during the 48 hours of incubation. Since background release increases with time, the chromium assay may be best applicable to short-term experiments where the background release may be low. The release of chromium is independent of cell proliferation and clearly measures cell destruction. Results obtained by using the ^{14}C-labeled amino acid incorporation assay are roughly equivalent to measuring the number of viable cells remaining in monolayers. However, this assay does not measure cell destruction. The latter assay, then, might be used to measure either reduction in cell numbers from cytotoxic reaction or inhibition of cell growth below that of control cultures.

The properties of lymphotoxic factors produced by two species of lymphocytes are shown in Table XII. LT has properties similar to those of a protein. Part of the mechanism by which LT acts on susceptible target cells has recently been elucidated by Jeffes and Granger (1975). The lymphocyte, having been activated by intimate contact with target cell membrane antigens, is induced into LT synthesis. After its secretion, LT binds to the target cell membrane, where it effects target cell lysis by as yet unknown mechanisms. Target cell membrane disruption or physical dislodgement promotes the lymphocytes' release and subsequent cessation of LT secretion. This mechanism would inhibit an indiscriminate wandering of an LT-secreting lymphocyte and prevents nonspecific cell destruction.

The ability of lymphocytes from patients with depressed immunity to produce lymphotoxin has recently been evaluated. It has been found that lymphocytes from patients with Hodgkin's disease, the Wiskott–Aldrich syndrome, and systemic lupus erythematosis are unable to produce lymphotoxin following stimulation by either antigens or mitogens. This behavior correlates with other aspects of lymphocyte function, for example, depressed lymphocyte transformation and absence of MIF pro-

TABLE XII

LYMPHOTOXIN

Treatment	Guinea pig[a]	Human[b]
Heat	Labile	Stable
Sephadex	35,000–55,000	80,000–90,000
Electrophoresis	Albumin	Postalbumin
CsCl$_{25}$	1.34	1.33
Chymotrypsin	Sensitive	—
Neuraminidase	Stable	—

[a] Coyne et al., 1973.
[b] Granger et al., 1968.

duction. The significance of *in vivo* production of lymphotoxin is unclear. It might be related to tumor surveillance, but how it relates to other delayed hypersensitivity reactions (such as the expression of the delayed skin test or resistance to infection) is not now known. Perhaps the absence of LT production in patients with depressed immunity may be related to the high incidence of neoplasms in these patients.

VII. Interferon

While it is well known that many cell types can be induced to produce interferon by viruses, it has been shown that lymphocytes may also produce interferon-like materials when stimulated by various either viral or nonviral inducers. Interferon-like activity can be detected in the culture fluid of both antigen- and mitogen-stimulated cultures of normal lymphocytes. Green *et al.* (1969) found that lymphocytes from tuberculin-sensitive subjects, when incubated *in vitro* with tuberculin PPD, released an interferon-like material which was maximal in its production at 7 days (Fig. 9). Interferon-like activity could be detected after 3 days in culture providing that the lymphocytes were stimulated by PHA. Epstein and co-workers (1970) showed that the production of interferon by lymphocytes depends, to a certain extent, on the presence of macrophages.

Lymphocytes are cultured in the presence of 20–30% serum, as many investigators have found that the production of interferon by lymphocytes is usually serum dependent. This contrasts with production of other

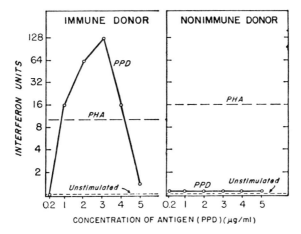

Fig. 9. Effect of antigen [tuberculin purified protein derivative (PPD)] concentration on the production of interferon by cultures of lymphocytes from immune and nonimmune donors. Interferon assays were done on culture supernatants collected on day 4. Copyright 1969 by the American Association for the Advancement of Science. (From Green *et al.*, 1969.)

lymphocyte mediators, such as MIF, chemotactic factor, lymphotoxin, where no serum is needed in the cultures. After various times in culture, the cell-free supernatants are harvested. To assay interferon activity, diluted fractions of the control- and interferon-containing supernatants then bathe confluent monolayers of neonatal foreskin fibroblasts for 18–24 hours at 37°C. The monolayers are washed and bovine vesicular stomatitis virus is absorbed. The monolayers are overlaid with agar for 48 hours to allow for plaque development. The interferon titer is defined as that dilution of supernatant which results in a 50% reduction of viral plaques.

The antigen- or mitogen-induced viral interferon inhibitors and virus-induced interferon behave somewhat similarly. They are stable at pH 4–10, stable at 4°C for 24 hours, nonsedimentable at 100,000 g for 2 hours, resistant to DNase and RNase (but destroyed by trypsin). Their effect is species specific for cells of human origin; i.e., it does not protect mouse L cells, chick embryo fibroblasts, or rabbit kidney cells against the viruses tested.

The cell types that synthesize lymphocyte-induced interferon have been investigated recently. Epstein et al. (1974) indicated that purified populations of human T and B lymphocytes are both capable of elaborating interferon-like material following stimulation by PHA and pokeweed. However, the kinetics of interferon production by these cell types are somewhat different. Human T cells stimulated by PHA or pokeweed produce significant amounts of interferon after 3, 5, or 7 days in culture. Human B cells, however, make interferon only after 5 or 7 days in culture following stimulation. Proliferative responses by B cells to PHA and pokeweed was delayed (thymidine incorporation was maximal after 5 or 7 days) and corresponded to the peak interferon activity in these cultures.

Interferon production following (or during) a specific immunological reaction is potentially very important to the host. Since persons who are unable to mount an adequate cellular immune response are plagued with viral infections, their lymphocytes may be unable to release interferon following stimulation by either antigens or mitogens. In fact, MacIntyre and co-workers have established that lymphocytes from patients with Hodgkin's disease were unable to produce normal amounts of interferon following stimulation by antigens. In more recent studies, Epstein and Ammann examined interferon production by lymphocytes obtained from patients with primary immunodeficiency diseases. They found a dissociation between lymphocyte-induced interferon production and proliferative responses to the same stimulant in some cases. Lymphocyte transformation to PHA and pokeweed was normal in 3 patients with selective IgA deficiency and in 1 patient with acquired hypogammaglobulinemia, but interferon levels were depressed. In another patient with selective IgA deficiency, lymphocyte transformation was depressed somewhat but interferon production was within normal limits. Epstein and Ammann also found that normal interferon responses could be obtained from 2 patients with thymic abnormalities following successful thymic transplants. By contrast, one patient with thymic hypoplasia, no serum IgA and low IgM, who had an unsuccessful thymic graft, had a markedly depressed inteferon response. In another study, Epstein *et al.* observed that interferon responses may be depressed in some patients with chronic lymphocytic leukemia.

VIII. Summary

An evaluation of lymphocyte function *in vitro* should include a measurement of the proliferative response to mitogens and antigens and one or more lymphocyte mediators. Because there is abundant evidence to indicate that these responses are functions of different subpopulations of cells, only a partial answer regarding cellular immune function will be obtained if either lymphocyte transformation or mediator production alone is employed. Furthermore, since there can be a dissociation between the different types of mediators that are produced, or between mediator production and the proliferative response, one may obtain a false impression if only one test is utilized. An example is given to illustrate this point. Some anergic sarcoid patients have intact lymphocyte transformation responses to mitogens and antigens as well as producing antigen-induced LMF. However, lymphocytes from these patients do not produce MIF. If only lymphocyte transformation had been measured, then one would have had the impression that lymphocyte function is normal. Moreover, if only LMF had been measured, then one would have had the impression that mediator production is likewise normal. The fact that lymphocytes from these patients do not produce MIF suggests that cutaneous anergy may stem from the absence of MIF production, not from a defect in the proliferative population. Thus, the use of multiple *in vitro* assays will furnish greater insight into the defects in lymphocyte function in patients having diseases associated with depressed immunity.

References

Altman, L. C., Chassy, B., and Mackler, B. F. (1975). *J. Immunol.* 115, 18.
Bennett, B., and Bloom, B. R. (1968). *Proc. Natl. Acad. Sci. U.S.* 59, 756.
Bloom, B. R. (1971). *Advan. Immunol.* 13, 102.
Bloom, B. R., and Glade, P. R., eds. (1971). "*In Vitro* Methods in Cell-Mediated Immunity." Academic Press, New York.

Chess, L., Rocklin, R. E., MacDermott, R. P., David, J. R., and Schlossman, S. F. (1975). *J. Immunol.* **115**, 315.

Coyne, J. A., Remold, H. G., Rosenberg, S. A., and David, J. R. (1973). *J. Immunol.* **110**, 1630.

David, J. R., and David, R. A. (1973). *Progr. Allergy* **16**, 300.

Epstein, L. B., Cline, M. J., and Merigan, T. C. (1970). *In* "Proceedings of the Fifth Leukocyte Culture Conference" (J. E. Harris, ed.), p. 506. Academic Press, New York.

Epstein, L. B., Kreth, H. W., and Herzenberg, L. A. (1974). *Cell. Immunol.* **12**, 407.

Gallin, J., Clark, R. A., and Kimball, H. R. (1973). *J. Immunol.* **110**, 233.

Geha, R. S., Schneeberger, E., Rosen, F. S., and Merler, E. (1973). *J. Exp. Med.* **138**, 1230.

George, M., and Vaughan, J. H. (1962). *Proc. Soc. Exp. Biol. Med.* **111**, 514.

Gordon, J., and MacLean, L. D. (1965). *Nature (London)* **208**, 795.

Granger, G. A., and Williams, T. W. (1968). *Nature (London)* **218**, 1253.

Green, J. A., Cooperband, S. R., and Kibrick, S. (1969). *Science* **164**, 3886.

Janis, M., and Bach, F. H. (1970). *Nature (London)* **225**, 238.

Jeffes, E. W. B., and Granger, G. A. (1975). *J. Immunol.* **114**, 64.

Kasakura, S., and Lowenstein, L. (1967). *Transplantation* **5**, 459.

Kolb, W. P., and Granger, G. A. (1968). *Proc. Natl. Acad. Sci. U.S.* **61**, 1250.

Mackaness, G. B. (1964). *J. Exp. Med.* **120**, 105.

Maini, R. N., Bryceson, A. D. M., Wolstencroft, R. A., and Dumonde, D. C. (1969). *Nature (London)* **224**, 43.

Mooney, J. J., and Waksman, B. H. (1970). *J. Immunol.* **105**, 1138.

Nathan, C. F., Karnovsky, M. L., and David, J. R. (1971). *J. Exp. Med.* **133**, 1356.

Nathan, C. F., Remold, H. G., and David, J. R. (1973). *J. Exp. Med.* **137**, 275.

Rich, A. R., and Lewis, M. R. (1932). *Bull. Johns Hopkins Hosp.* **50**, 115.

Rocklin, R. E. (1975). *J. Immunol.* **114**, 1161.

Rocklin, R. E., Lewis, E., and David, J. R. (1970a). *New Engl. J. Med.* **283**, 497.

Rocklin, R. E., Meyers, O. L., and David, J. R. (1970b). *J. Immunol.* **104**, 95.

Rocklin, R. E., Sheremata, W., Feldman, R., Kies, M. W., and David, J. R. (1971). *New Engl. J. Med.* **284**, 803.

Rocklin, R. E. (1974a). *J. Immunol.* **112**, 1461.

Rocklin, R. E. (1974b). *In* "Progress in Clinical Immunology" (R. Schwartz, ed.), Vol. 2, p. 21. Grune and Stratton, New York.

Rocklin, R. E., MacDermott, R. P., Chess, L., Schlossman, S. F., and David, J. R. (1974c). *J. Exp. Med.* **140**, 1303.

Rocklin, R. E., Winston, C. T., and David, J. R. (1974d). *J. Clin. Invest.* **53**, 559.

Ruddle, N. H., and Waksman, B. H. (1968). *J. Exp. Med.* **128**, 1237.

Snyderman, R., Altman, L. C., Hausman, M. S., *et al.* (1972). *J. Immunol.* **108**, 857.

Snyderman, R., Altman, L. C., Frankel, A., and Blaese, R. M. (1973). *Ann. Intern. Med.* **78**, 509.

Thor, D., Jureziz, R. E., Veach, S. R. Miller, E., and Dray, S. (1968). *Nature (London)* **219**, 755.

Valentinte, F. T., and Lawrence, H. S. (1969). *Science* **165**, 1014.

Ward, P. A., Remold, H. G., and David, J. R. (1969). *Science* **163**, 1079.

Ward, P. A., Remold, H. G., and David, J. R. (1970). *Cell. Immunol.* **1**, 162.

Ward, P. A., and Rocklin, R. E. (1975). *In* "The Immune System and Infectious Diseases. 4th International Convocation on Immunology," Buffalo, New York, 1974, p. 470. Karger, Basel.

Leukocyte Aggregation Test for Evaluating Cell-Mediated Immunity

BALDWIN H. TOM and BARRY D. KAHAN

Laboratory of Surgical Immunology, Departments of Surgery and Physiology,
Northwestern University Medical Center, and the Veterans Administration
Lakeside Hospital, Chicago, Illinois

I. Introduction

Cell-mediated immunity as demonstrated *in vitro* probably consists of
at least three steps—recognition, as evidenced by specific adhesion of
sensitized lymphocytes onto target cells; proliferation, as may be demonstrated by incorporation of ^{3}H-labeled thymidine in the presence of specific antigen; and performance, as shown by lysis of or by interference
with the function of target cells. Analysis of the recognition step of
cellular immunity offers advantages over the other two steps. Some investigators have observed increased numbers of spontaneously dividing

cells in the circulation of allotransplanted patients undergoing rejection. However, *in vitro* detection of immunospecific proliferation requires several days, which limits its usefulness as a routine tool. Indeed, it has not been possible to document a consistent relationship between rejection and the presence of circulating peripheral lymphocytes capable of proliferation upon contact with donor transplantation antigens as intact cells or subcellular extracts.

In vitro detection of immune performance, either target cell destruction or lymphokine release, tends to be erratic. The difficulties of precise analysis of performance include the obfuscation caused by the involvement of lymphokines and other soluble factors, as well as the activity of multiple rather than a single effector T-cell population, including immunologically specific and nonspecific cellular elements, such as B cells, macrophages, neutrophils, and subpopulations of T cells. Furthermore, the disparity between the poor results of cell-mediated cytotoxicity in the human setting compared to the excellent results in animal experimental models may be due to the use of immunosuppressive agents in man. Thus, Lundgren and colleagues (1970) could not detect killing of donor fibroblasts by immune lymphocytes from patients bearing renal allografts. Indeed, as described below, the authors have only been able to show chromium release from donor kidney cells during actual rejection crises in a few cases. However, Wolf and his colleagues (1971), using lymphocytes from patients who had undergone nephrectomy and were no longer on immunosuppressive drugs, showed radiochromium release from cultured donor kidney cells. The macrophage migration inhibition assay, which has been proposed as an indicator of cellular activity in renal transplant patients, rarely shows evidence of cellular reactivity long before rejection and also seems to be quite sensitive to immunosupportive therapy. Furthermore, these performance assays are somewhat nonspecific. Lundgren *et al.* (1970) showed that lymphocytes from patients immunized by allogeneic grafts produced plaques in monolayers of donor fibroblasts. However, the significance of these observations was unclear, since cytotoxicity both to allogeneic and to autochthonous cells could be obtained with nonimmune lymphocytes that were stimulated with phytohemagglutinin (PHA). Thus, after activation by any means, lymphocytes become indiscriminate aggressors.

On the other hand, recognition phenomena, which are by definition characterized by precise specificity, may afford more suitable tools for the *in vitro* assessment of cellular immunity. Algire and his collaborators (1954) demonstrated that intimate lymphocyte-target cell contact is required for immune destruction. Allografted cells survived in sensitized hosts, if they were enclosed within a cell-impermeable, Millipore chamber. Using an *in vitro* culture system in rats, Wilson (1965) showed that immune cells could not destroy monolayers, if they were separated by a Millipore membrane. Additional studies suggested that the destructive action of sensitized cells required not just transient contact, but also direct adherence to target cells. Immunological specificity of target recognition was demonstrated by the adsorption studies of Brondz and Snegirova (1971). They showed that lymphocytes immune to an H-2 antigen complex were only adsorbed by target cells possessing the proper specificities of the immunizing complex. More recently, in animal models studying *in vitro* induction of allograft immunity, Lonai and co-workers (1973) demonstrated that adherence was immunologically specific: preincubation of immune cells on target monolayers removed the reactive elements from the lymphocyte population. In the mouse model Rosenau and Moon (1962) found that although the immune performance of sensitized cells was blocked by corticosteroids, specific immune recognition, as exhibited by adherence to target cell surfaces, was unimpaired. Therefore, the recognition step offers an appropriate focus for the development of an assay which would be applicable as a routine test of cellular immunity.

The leukocyte aggregation test (LAT) was developed to evaluate the cellular immunity of patients undergoing renal transplantation. The LAT is based upon the adhesion of host leukocytes to target cells secondary to an immunospecific recognition of donor transplantation antigens by sensitized T lymphocytes. After this event, predominantly nonimmune leukocytes are captured at the reaction foci and appear as aggregates. The reaction requires the expenditure of metabolic energy; it is dependent upon physiological temperatures and is susceptible to inhibitors of protein and RNA synthesis. The LAT has several attributes that recommend it as a routine tool for assessing cell-mediated immunity in transplant patients: (1) completion within 5 hours; (2) requirement for only 10 ml of whole blood, permitting daily testing; (3) relative resistance to immunosuppressive agents; (4) immunological specificity; and (5) sensitivity to the modulating effects of serum factors on cellular immunity.

II. Method

A. PREPARATION OF TARGET CELLS

The LAT technique has been established as a routine procedure and can be briefly summarized as follows (Fig. 1): Cultured kidney or skin

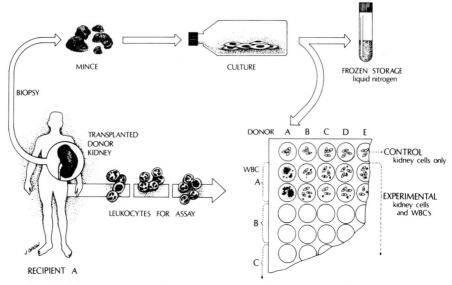

Fig. 1. Schematic protocol for assessment of cellular immunity toward allografted kidney.

fibroblast target cells are dispensed into 96 well flat-bottom microtiter plates (Falcon No. 3040) and allowed to adhere for 8–48 hours at 37°C in a humidified air–5% CO_2 incubator. Kidney and skin tissue are obtained as biopsies. Kidney cells are prepared by mincing, trypsinizing (0.25% for five 20–minute exposures), and plating the dissociated cells onto plastic tissue culture flasks (Falcon No. 3013 or 3024). Skin fibroblast cells are obtained from the outgrowth of minced skin pieces, which have been attached to the surface of culture flasks. Since reactions on kidney cells appear to be more vigorous, skin fibroblasts are utilized only when the kidney target is not available. In addition to maintaining cells in continuous culture, aliquots from tissue culture passages are frozen [1°C/minute with 10% dimethyl sulfoxide (DMSO) in minimum essential medium (MEM) plus 20% FCS] and stored under liquid nitrogen, in order to have early generations for future testing. Although the expression of histocompatibility antigens does not appear to decrease during the *in vitro* life-span of fibroblasts, it is probably preferable to avoid utilization of senescing cells. These cells can be recognized microscopically by their decreased viability, enlarged size, irregular margins, and cytoplasmic vacuolation, as compared to young cells, and by their reduced growth rate, as evidenced by the need for greater numbers of cells to establish desired monolayers.

Microbial infection of cultured cells should be avoided not only for practical but also for theoretical reasons. While bacterial and fungal contaminants are readily revealed, viral and mycoplasmal organisms may persist without detection. Cells "rescued" from infection by antibiotic or other therapy may well be unsatisfactory for subsequent use in the test, especially since they may now bear bacterial cell products, some of which are known to cross-react with HLA antigens to produce false test results.

In Fig. 1, the construction of an experimental plate is illustrated: Each vertical column is seeded with kidney cells of a single donor. Five cell donors are generally used. The first horizontal row is a series of control wells with only target cells plated, in order to ascertain the density of the monolayer. Each subsequent set of four rows are duplicate tests of a given leukocyte sample: two in the presence (A) and two in the absence (B) of serum.

A minimum of 8 hours are required for kidney cells to plate out in the wells. The length of the incubation period is determined by the initial number of cells seeded and the requisite density of the monolayer. Routinely, 8000 kidney or 3000 fibroblast cells suspended in 0.2-ml volume of MEM with antibiotics, glutamine, and 10% heat-inactivated fetal calf serum (FCS) are seeded into each well, and incubated for 24 hours. Contact-inhibited, confluent, cell monolayers have increased levels of cyclic AMP (cAMP), as contrasted to exponentially growing cultures. In parallel with the inhibiting effects of cAMP levels on migration inhibition factor activity, it is possible that similar local inhibitory effects could affect other cell-mediated immune parameters. As a precaution, 75% target cell monolayers are routinely used.

In order to determine the immunological specificity of the reactions, a variety of targets are used in each test, including kidney cells derived from (1) the donor; (2) patients with HLA antigens identical to those disparate between donor and recipient; (3) individuals bearing HLA antigens cross-reactive with the disparate factors; (4) persons with HLA phenotypes unrelated to these factors; and (5) the recipient himself.

B. Preparation of Leukocytes and Sera

Recipient cells and sera are collected by venipuncture into tubes with or without heparin (10 units/ml blood). Peripheral blood leukocytes from renal transplant patients have variable proportions of T lymphocytes, as defined by the nonimmune sheep erythrocyte rosette test. In unpublished studies the authors found that hemodialysis patients awaiting transplantation have an average of 40% (range 18–60%) T lympho-

cytes, while engrafted patients maintained on standard immunosuppressive drugs have 23% (range 1–51%) T lymphocytes. In contrast,
normal subjects exhibit 63% (range 57–70%) rosette-forming cells. Employing PHA stimulation as a measure of T-cell activity did not appear
to be particularly discriminative, since stimulation indices randomly
ranged from 3- to 253-fold in this entire group of patients.

Sera are heat-inactivated (56°C, 30 minutes) before use. Peripheral
blood leukocytes are prepared by plasmagel (15–20% v/v; Associated
Biomedic Systems, Buffalo) density sedimentation of erythrocytes. The
leukocytes in the enriched, upper layer are collected, washed, counted,
and added to wells from which the medium and unattached cells have
been drained. When sera are tested for the presence of humoral factors
affecting leukocyte reactivity, 0.05-ml aliquots are preincubated on target
monolayers (37°C/15 minutes). To perform the test, 400,000 leukocytes
in 0.2 ml of MEM with 10% FCS are added to the wells for a 5-hour reaction period. All test combinations are performed in duplicate. Leukocytes are also dispensed into an empty well to control for their spontaneous aggregation. At the end of the reaction period, the wells are
rinsed four times with MEM and refilled; the reactions observed under
150× magnification on an inverted microscope using bright-field optics
(Fig. 2). Figure 3 illustrates representative findings. The upper left panel
shows a kidney monolayer without added leukocytes. A negative reaction
with few aggregates and most of the leukocytes in a monodispersed pattern is seen in the upper right panel. Positive fields of leukocyte aggregation are shown in the lower panels.

C. Expression of Results

The tests are independently read by two or three individuals without
knowledge of the clinical condition of the patient. The scoring is based
on the number of 150× fields which contain at least 5 leukocyte-target
aggregates bearing more than 10 leukocytes per aggregate. A result of
25% aggregation indicates that one-quarter of the 150× fields had at
least 5 positive aggregates. Nonspecific reactions often occur along the
peripheral edges of the wells and should not be scored. Care should also
be taken to avoid scoring cell clusters formed in empty spaces between
target cells. If there is nonspecific aggregation of leukocytes alone or
when added to third-party, non-HLA cross-reactive targets, the test must
be repeated. In the latter case, one must include different targets, since
it is possible that the original target cells were abnormal, or that the re-

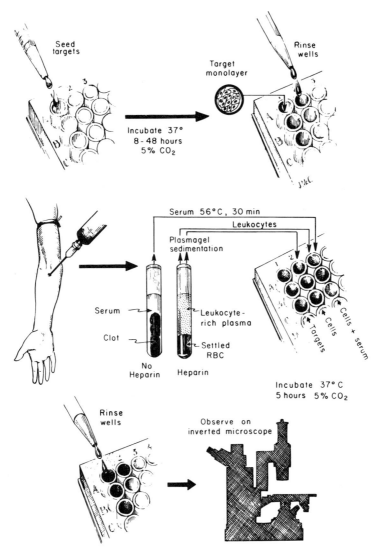

Fig. 2. Schematic protocol for actual performance of a leukocyte aggregation test.

actions on the third-party targets represented specific recognition of non-HLA, histocompatibility determinants. Individual values are corrected for the percentage of spontaneous aggregation by leukocytes incubated in the absence of target cells. All of the scores of duplicate wells by each observer are averaged to obtain the actual result.

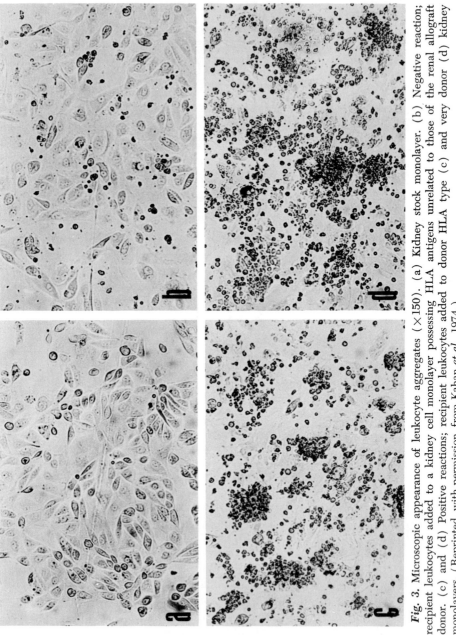

Fig. 3. Microscopic appearance of leukocyte aggregates (×150). (a) Kidney stock monolayer. (b) Negative reaction; recipient leukocytes added to a kidney cell monolayer possessing HLA antigens unrelated to those of the renal allograft donor. (c) and (d) Positive reactions; recipient leukocytes added to donor HLA type (c) and very donor (d) kidney monolayers. (Reprinted, with permission, from Kahan *et al.*, 1974.)

III. Results

A. CLINICAL APPLICATIONS

The leukocyte aggregation test has been employed in 52 patients on 275 occasions with 1180 target cells. It has proved to be useful in (1) detecting the onset of cellular immunity of engrafted patients toward donor transplantation antigens; (2) determining whether clinical deterioration of renal function was due to rejection, as opposed to other immunological, or pathological, causes; and (3) assessing the degree of cellular, immune presensitization.

There is a distinctive pattern of LAT reactivity correlating with the clinical course of graft rejection. As described in detail previously and summarized here in Table I, prior to rejection the nonpresensitized, transplant recipient does not exhibit cellular reactivity. Developing cellular activity is detected by leukocyte aggregation onto donor targets (AC), onto targets sharing the antigens disparate between donor and recipient (AD), and as sensitization proceeds, onto targets bearing antigens cross-reactive with the disparate antigens (FZ). During a rejection crisis, aggregation on donor targets is lost, while activity on shared (AD) and cross-reactive (FZ) targets persists and may increase. Furthermore, apparent nonspecific reactivity emerges: Aggregation is observed on nonspecific, HLA unrelated, target cells (UG). When the rejection episode is reversed, leukocyte aggregation is no longer visible. Following graft nephrectomy for irreversible rejection, aggregation activity shows a pattern reflecting HLA specificities disparate between donor and recipient.

TABLE I

SCHEMATIC REPRESENTATION OF LEUKOCYTE AGGREGATION RESULTS[a]

	Target cell antigens				
Clinical status	Donor AC	AD[b]	FZ[b]	UG[b]	Self XY
1. No rejection	0	0	0	0	0
2. Before clinical rejection	3.0	1.0	1.0	0	0
3. Rejection crisis	0	3.0	3.0	1.0	0
4. Between rejection crises	0	0	0	0	0
5. After graft nephrectomy	3.0	1.0	1.0	0	0

[a] Reprinted with permission from Kahan et al., 1974.

[b] Targets from individuals unrelated to the kidney donor: A is shared; F cross-reacts with A; and UG are noncross-reactive.

TABLE II

SUMMARY OF PATTERNS OF LEUKOCYTE AGGREGATION
TEST (LAT) REACTIONS IN 52 ALLOGRAFTED PATIENTS

Negative LAT, no rejection	12
Negative LAT, rejection phenomena	
Hyperacute rejection	2
Accelerated rejection	2
Chronic rejection	6
Negative LAT, decreased function from other causes	9
Positive LAT, no rejection	0
Positive LAT, prediagnosed rejection	14
Positive LAT, postgraft nephrectomy	14
Positive LAT enhanced by serum	8
Positive LAT blocked by serum	2

Patient 194, a 26-year-old woman (HLA, A2, A3, B12, and B13),[1] received an allograft bearing HLA, A1, A2, B8, and B18. Preoperatively she showed no evidence of aggregation on donor skin fibroblasts. There was no evident reactivity on postoperative days 5, 8, 11, 14, 19, 22, in spite of the fact that her serum creatinine rose on day 14 from 1.2 to 2.5. No antirejection therapy was administered, and the creatinine returned to 1.2. On day 26 when the creatinine was stable at 1.25, reactivity toward donor-type targets appeared, and increased by day 29. Overt clinical and chemical evidences of rejection were noted at day 32. Because of the information provided by the test, antirejection therapy was immediately administered, and the episode readily reversed. Of the nine patients showing negative reactivity in the face of deteriorating renal function (Table II), this patient is the only one who displayed rejection within 21 days of the negative test. In all other eight cases allograft biopsy confirmed the absence of rejection suggested by the LAT.

Patient 200 illustrates the parallel application of recognition and performance tests in clinical practice and the probable benefits of high-dose steroid therapy (Fig. 4). This 67-year-old man (HLA, A2, A9, B7, and B12) with polycystic kidney disease received a cadaveric allograft (HLA, A2, —, B12, and B27). Following a 7-day period of acute tubular necrosis, his renal function progressively improved as evidenced by a rising creatinine clearance and bladder/kidney ratio of excretion of ^{131}I-labeled hippuran. On day 26 there were clinical evidences of fever and oliguria

---

[1] According to the 1975 WHO Committee on leukocyte nomenclature (P. I. Terasaki, personal communication), the designation for the previous first locus LA antigens will be Locus A and written A1, A2 etc., while the second, or FOUR locus, will be Locus B, with antigen specificities B5, B7, etc. The third locus will now be called Locus C, and the former LD, MLC-1 locus, Locus D. HLA without the hyphen will now refer to the entire histocompatibility antigen complex.

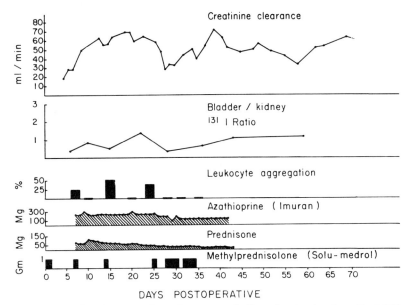

Fig. 4. Clinical and immunological patterns of allograft rejection in patient 200.

accompanied by chemical changes showing deterioration of allograft function. The leukocyte aggregation tests reflected developing cellular sensitization. On day 7 modest leukocyte aggregation was present, but was effectively diminished on the day 9 test by the routine 1-gm dose of methylprednisolone (Solu-Medrol). Similarly, the reactivity which was again evident at day 14 was presumably diminished on day 19 owing to the routine dose of Solu-Medrol. The reactivity at day 23 presaged a rejection episode which was clinically evident on day 26, and successfully treated with two courses of three, daily 1-gm intravenous boluses of Solu-Medrol. These findings suggest that high-dose, intravenous steroid, bolus therapy is effective in decreasing the cellular immunity of some patients in the LAT. At day 26, prelabeled donor kidney cells released 56% of their ^{51}Cr label after 24 hours in the presence of host lymphocytes, but only 1% in the presence of third-party lymphocytes, demonstrating the presence of cytotoxic effector cells. The patient released only 3% of the label which had been incorporated into third-party kidney target cells. This case represents one of the few in which it was possible to document cytotoxic performance by the chromium-release method. Whether a full course of antirejection therapy initiated at 7 days, that is, when there was the first evidence of cellular immunity, would have aborted the rejection episode, is uncertain. This becomes a matter of extreme importance since in 14 patients emerging cellular reactivity to donor antigens was detected 2–15 days before there were any clinical evidence of graft rejection.

The LAT test does not appear to discriminate allograft immunity in the settings of hyperacute, accelerated, and chronic rejection. In 11 such cases of 17, the test was negative and postnephrectomy specimens confirmed the clinical impression. While none of these 11 rejections were reversible by bolus therapy with methylprednisolone and local irradiation, the 6 rejections which elicited positive LAT results were reversed. In patients experiencing acute rejection, no cellular rejection was encountered when the LAT was negative. In 11 of 14 cases evaluated which exhibited a positive LAT, acute rejection was reversed by immunosuppressive therapy. Patients showing acute homograft rejection with negative LAT results were unresponsive to treatment and lost their grafts. Thus the LAT results appear to correlate with the response of the patient to bolus therapy, rather than with the timing of rejection.

The modulating effects of serum on cellular reactivity were of two types: (1) a suppression of reactivity seen immediately after transplantation, particularly in patients known to have produced lymphocytotoxic antibodies; and (2) a synergism of cellular activity, particularly at the time of overt transplant rejection. Suppressive effects of serum over 90 days after transplantation were not documented because none of the patients who were tested displayed cellular aggregation at that time.

B. Immunological Specificity

While an extensive analysis of specificity is now underway, it appears that the LAT reactivity conforms to the predictions of HLA cross-reactivity in 75–80% of the leukocyte–target combinations. The disparate reactions were of both possible types: apparently non-HLA-specific positive tests, and negative ones on targets with shared, or known cross-reactive, HLA factors. It is uncertain whether other systems, such as that defined by mixed lymphocyte culture reactions of Locus D, are reflected by these disparities, and whether the correlations with HLA merely reflect a marked linkage disequilibrium between serologically defined, HLA determinants and this other histocompatibility locus.

IV. Discussion

A. Utilization of the Test in Clinical Practice

Although the LAT has shown remarkable precision in the detection of cellular immunity toward allografts, it has been used only to clarify complex situations, not to dictate clinical practice. Routinely, intensified antirejection therapy, namely intravenous boluses of Solu-Medrol and local X-irradiation to the graft, are withheld until there are clinical or chemical evidences of rejection to support the immunological findings. However, the LAT represents a useful addition to the diagnostic armamentarium, since without this information one might frequently lose a precious 24–48 hours for the clinical situation to become clarified before initiating therapy. In the experience with 52 patients reported herein, a positive reaction has always signified incipient rejection. The cases of negative LAT reactions in the face of hyperacute, accelerated, or chronic graft rejection probably reflect the association of these processes with the reactions of humoral alloantibody.

It is important to perform reactions in the presence of host sera, particularly in cases where the patient is extensively presensitized. A positive synergism between serum and leukocytes always signified rejection. On the other hand, evident antagonism of serum on cellular activity was never associated with rejection, even when the leukocytes alone displayed marked reactions.

B. Possible Mechanism of the Phenomenon

The leukocyte aggregation test, which measures the adhesion of host leukocytes to cultured target cells, probably reflects a primary specific recognition to donor antigens by several populations of sensitized peripheral blood lymphocytes. Although the nature of the recognition process is unknown, it depends upon a trypsin-sensitive moiety on the immune cells. Further, aggregation requires the expenditure of metabolic energy, for it is dependent upon physiological temperatures and is susceptible to inhibitors of protein and RNA synthesis. On the other hand, inhibition of DNA synthesis by mitomycin C does not affect it. The immune lymphocyte responsible for initiating the reaction leading to aggregate formation appears to be thymus-derived, since treatment of the leukocyte population with antithymocyte globulin and complement totally ablated reactivity. It is possible that the recognizing cell can be distinguished from other T-cell subpopulations functioning as cytotoxic effectors against, or proliferating in response to, allogeneic antigens.

B lymphocytes also participate in the reaction. When immune leukocytes were treated with antiimmunoglobulin antisera and complement, the extent of the aggregates was reduced. The observation that reduction of the B-cell content of the leukocyte preparation produced a concomitant decrease, but did not ablate aggregate formation, is consistent with the possibilities: (1) that B cells participate as indifferent nonimmune elements responding to the lymphokines released by T cells; (2) that a portion of the reaction is mediated by a local release of specific antibodies; or (3) that the B cells produce nonantibody, amplifying substances which generate additional leukocyte aggregates.

The aggregates consist predominantly of nonimmune bystander cells. When 10,000 immune lymphocytes alone are reacted on a specific target cell monolayer, there are no visible aggregates. However, the admixture of 10,000 immune lymphocytes with 190,000 nonimmune leukocytes produces strong reactions. These results suggest that immune elements communicate with immunoincompetent cells to form the aggregates. As graphically depicted in Fig. 5 and described above, one possibility is that immune recognition by sensitized T cells activates the release of lymphokinetic mediators, such as chemotactic and migration inhibitory factors, to induce a reaction cascade yielding aggregate formation. Several alternative hypotheses are that the interaction of the immunocompetent lymphocyte with the target cell surface membrane initiates a nucle-

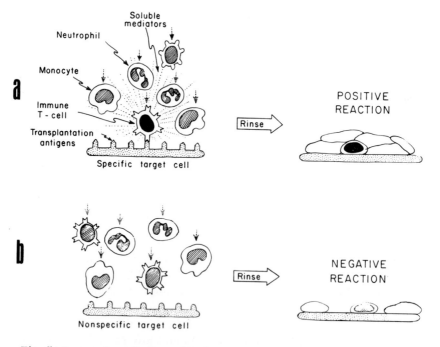

Fig. 5. Suggested mechanism of leukocyte aggregate formation. (a) Immune T cells direct the formation of specific aggregates by nonimmune cells after immunospecific adhesion. (b) Immune cells are unable to recognize surface markers on nonspecific target cells.

ation process, of the type described by Chipowsky and colleagues (Chipowsky *et al.*, 1973), leading to aggregate formation, or that the primary immune cell contact induces lymphocyte-lymphocyte aggregation by a transference phenomenon reported by Whitehead and Marcus (1975).

C. Actual and Potential Clinical and Experimental Applications

The LAT technique, which has been shown to be useful in human renal transplantation, has also detected allosensitization in a patient who displayed specific *in vivo* refractoriness following immunization by multiple platelet transfusions mismatched by the factor HLA-A8. Cellular immunity to HLA-A8 was detected by the reactivity of the patient's peripheral blood leukocytes on HLA-A8 specific kidney monolayers. Theoretically, this assay might be able to detect cell-mediated immunity toward the distinctive neoantigens on tumors. The test might also be useful for evaluating the biological activity of solubilized transplantation antigens, which during preincubation may specifically "defuse" immunoreactive cells either by an irreversible binding degradation as reported for insulin receptors, or by inactivation of responsive cells by contact with radioactively labeled antigen of high specific activity. Finally, the LAT may be applicable for studies identifying T-cell surface receptor molecules associated with cell-mediated reactions against determinants of the major histocompatibility complex.

Acknowledgments

Supported by Grants from the National Institutes of Health (RO-1-CA 14694 and R 26-CA-15434), from the Chicago and Illinois Heart Association (A-73-3), from the American Cancer Society (IC-84), and the Veterans Administration Lakeside Hospital, Chicago, Illinois. The HLA determinations were kindly provided by Dr. K. K. Mittal. We further thank Milda Jakstys, Li Huang, and AeZa Lee for excellent technical assistance.

References

Algire, G. H., Weaver, J. M., and Prehn, R. T. (1954). Growth of cells *in vivo* in diffusion chambers. I. Survival of homografts in immunized mice. *J. Nat. Cancer Inst.* **15,** 493.

Bloom, B. R. (1971). *In vitro* approaches to the mechanisms of cell-mediated immune reactions. *Advan. Immunol.* **13,** 101.

Brondz, B. D., and Snegiröva, A. E. (1971). Interaction of immune lymphocytes with the mixtures of target cells possessing selected specificities of the H-2 immunizing allele. *Immunology* **20,** 457.

Cerottini, J.-C., and Brunner, K. T. (1974). Cell-mediated cytotoxicity, allograft rejection, and tumor immunity. *Advan. Immunol.* **18,** 67.

Chipowsky, S., Lee, V., and Roseman, S. (1973). Adhesion of cultured fibroblasts to insoluble analogues of cell surface carbohydrates. *Proc. Nat. Acad. Sci. U.S.* **70,** 2309.

Kahan, B. D., Tom, B. H., Mittal, K. K., and Bergan, J. J. (1974). Immunodiagnostic test for transplant rejection. *Lancet* **1,** 37.

Kahan, B. D., Krumlovsky, F., Ivanovitch, P., Greenwald, J., Firlit, C., Bergan, J., and Tom, B. H. (1975). The leukocyte aggregation test. Immunodiagnostic applications and immunotherapeutic implications for clinical renal transplantation. *Arch. Surg.* **110,** 984.

Lonai, P., Eliraz, A., Wekerle, H., and Feldman, M. (1973). Specific depletion of GVH reactivity of mouse lymphocytes by adsorption on allogeneic fibroblast monolayers. *Transplant. Proc.* **5,** 857.

Lundgren, G., Möller, E., and Thorsby, E. (1970). *In vitro* cytotoxicity by human lymphocytes from individuals immunized against histocompatibility antigens. II. Relation to HL-A incompatibility between effector and target cells. *Clin. Exp. Immunol.* **6,** 671.

Rosenau, W., and Moon, H. D. (1962). The inhibitory effect of hydrocortisone on lysis of homologous cells by lymphocytes *in vitro. J. Immunol.* **89,** 422.

Tom, B. H., Jakstys, M. M., and Kahan, B. D. (1974). Leukocyte-aggregation: An *in vitro* assay for cell-mediated immunity. *J. Immunol.* **113,** 1288.

Tom, B. H., Huang, L. O., Jakstys, M. M., and Kahan, B. D. (1975). Characteristics of the leukocyte-aggregation assay for cell-mediated immunity. *Clin. Exp. Immunol.* **20,** 131.

Whitehead, J. S., and Marcus, F. S. (1975). Cell surface: Transfer of cellular adhesive properties from cell to cell by induced membrane alterations. *Proc. Soc. Exp. Biol. Med.* **148,** 160.

Wilson, D. B. (1965). Quantitative studies on the behavior of sensitized lymphocytes *in vitro. J. Exp. Med.* **122,** 143.

Wolf, J., Fawley, J., and Hume, D. (1971). *In vitro* quantitation of lymphocyte and serum cytotoxic activity following renal homograft rejection in man. *Transplant. Proc.* **3,** 449.

The HLA System:
Serologically Defined Antigens[1]

EKKEHARD D. ALBERT

Kinderpoliklinik der Universität München, Munich, Germany

I. The HLA System: Serologically Defined Antigens

A. Historical Introduction

Knowledge about the principal isoantigenic system of human leukocytes —now officially named Human Leukocyte System A, or HLA—begins in 1958 with Dausset's discovery of the antigen MAC (55). Soon thereafter van Rood (157) and Payne et al. (150), using statistical methods to measure the similarity or dissimilarity of reaction patterns, were able to recognize several more leukocyte groups and arranged these groups in diallelic (158) and multiallelic systems (31,150). The introduction by Terasaki and McClelland (185) of the microlymphocytotoxicity technique

[1] Supported by Sonderforschungsbereich 37, München, and by Deutsche Forschungsgemeinschaft, Bonn, Grant No. A2-92/7/9.

237

for leukocyte grouping provided the basis for the enormous numbers of tests that were necessary for the elucidation of the HLA system. When it became evident that the HLA antigens function as transplantation antigens (47,48,56,159), research in this field was strongly intensified. Dausset, in 1965 (57), postulated that all the antigens recognized by leukoagglutination and lymphocytotoxicity belong to a single genetic system, which he termed Hu-1 (later to be renamed HLA). The analysis of serological data obtained with HLA antisera was complicated by the fact that the vast majority of antisera is highly reactive and that inclusion phenomena are often observed. A new approach was introduced by Kissmeyer-Nielsen (101,103,104) who applied Hirschfeld's (93) serologic codes to the analysis of antisera, assuming that the antigen is simple and the antiserum is complex (i.e., multispecific). This principle was used by several investigators, who were able to define a large number of new HLA antigens in the years of 1969, 1970, and 1971 (2–4,51,52,59–61,63,64,99,105,106). The clear definition of so many antigens made it possible for the Fourth International Histocompatibility Workshop to prove the concept (99) of two closely linked loci within the HLA system, as it had been postulated by both Dausset (57,58) and Kissmeyer-Nielsen in 1967 (101). After the elucidation of the basic genetic organization of the HLA system the Fifth International Histocompatibility Workshop in 1972 undertook the task to test the distribution of HLA genes in the key human populations, thus providing the basis for the investigation of selection and mixture (35) of populations. The Sixth International Workshop in 1975 was mainly concerned with the definition of the genetic system determining the stimulation in mixed leukocyte culture. As is discussed in the next chapter, by Fritz H. Bach, this system is very closely linked and functionally related to the HLA system.

The rapid development of knowledge about this entire immunogenetic system, called Major Histocompatibility Complex, must be one of the striking success stories of international cooperation.

B. SEROLOGY AND GENETICS

1. Currently Used Methods

A detailed step-by-step description of most tissue typing procedures has been compiled in the "Manual of Tissue Typing Techniques" provided by the National Institute of Health (123).

a. The separation of lymphocytes. The most widely used method of separation of lymphocytes is that described by Boyum (37) and his co-workers in 1968 with more or less local variation. This method utilizes the separation of blood cells according to size and shape when passing through fluid of higher density (in this case Ficoll Isopaque of density 1.077). The lymphocytes are found in a faint white interphase layer after centrifugation of diluted whole blood (1:2 in saline) for 15 minutes at 1000 g. The lymphocytes are then washed twice, counted in a counting chamber, and adjusted to 1500–2000 cells per microliter.

b. *Lymphocytotoxicity test.* Two principally different methods of the cytotoxicity test are currently in use. In the following, these tests will be only briefly described with emphasis on the pecularities pertaining to the discussion of the problems of HLA serology. For details of the test, see the "Manual of Tissue Typing Techniques" (*123*).

1. Microlymphocytotoxicity test as introduced by Terasaki and McClelland in 1964 (*185*) (synonyms: NIH technique, two-stage technique, Terasaki technique). One microliter of antiserum is placed under a film of mineral oil into each of 60 wells of a plastic plate and mixed with $1\mu l$ of a lymphocyte suspension containing 1500 cells. This mixture is left at room temperature for 30 minutes. Then 5 μl of fresh frozen unabsorbed rabbit serum are added as complement. After an additional 60 minutes of incubation at room temperature, the test is terminated by staining with 2 μl of eosin and fixation is accomplished by adding 5 μl of formalin. Reading is performed in the plates using an inverted phase contrast microscope. The lymphocytes that were lysed by antigen-antibody reaction in the presence of complement are unable to exclude the dye and are therefore stained dark red. The unlysed cells appear as small bright spots in the phase contrast. Scoring is performed according to the proportion of stained cells in each well ($+$ = 10–25%; $++$ = 25–50%; $+++$ = 50–75%; and $++++$ = 75–100% stained cells). The important features of this test are its applicability to automated procedures, the long incubation period of 90 minutes, the excess amount of complement, and, by virtue of the latter two, a higher sensitivity.

2. Cytotoxicity test according to Kissmeyer–Nielsen (*102,123*) (synonym: one-stage test): In this test the reaction takes place on a glass plate under the protection of mineral oil. One microliter of antiserum is mixed with an equal volume of cells suspended in equal parts of fresh human AB serum and fresh rabbit serum. The incubation takes place at 37°C for 30 minutes, after which the staining of lysed cells is accomplished by incubation with Trypan blue. The typical features of this test are the short incubation of 37°C and the relatively small amount of complement used, both of which make this test clearly less sensitive than Terasaki's. This insensitivity, of course, may be advantageous, particularly in view of the

fact that most HLA sera are multispecific and can conceivably be reduced to a reasonably narrow specificity by lowering the test sensitivity.

In addition to these two principal techniques, there are many more tissue typing techniques such as Fluorchromasia assay and complement fixation, which, for the sake of simplicity will be omitted from this discussion.

2. Serology

There are a number of unusual features to the serology of the HLA system which are essential for the understanding and interpretation of serological results: The antisera for HLA typing come mainly from pregnant women and can therefore not be compared with the hyperimmune sera used for the classification of, for instance, the H-2 antigens of the mouse. The titers of antisera usually range between undiluted and 1:8. These in serologic terms very low titers severely limit the use of absorption procedures for the analysis of complex reaction patterns of sera with a broad reactivity. One of the most difficult problems in HLA serology is the large variation in reactivity of most sera when tests of only slightly different sensitivities are used. For example, a serum can react with 20% of the population when the Kissmeyer technique is used and with 40% in the Terasaki test. These results clearly indicate that even among the highly selected antisera used for typing, there are many sera that have one or more antibody populations at sublytic concentrations besides the one specificity they were selected for, and these populations could come into action with any minor accidental change in test sensitivity. Such changes may be a higher sensitivity of aged lymphocytes or of lymphocytes from patients, or an accidental 10-minute increase in incubation time. Antibodies present in sublytic concentrations need to be taken into account when "operationally" monospecific sera are used in blocking experiments or for typing of cultured lymphocytes and the like. These serological problems make it necessary to use at least two or three antisera for the definition of one HLA antigen (31), so that difficulties caused by occasional extra reactions are eliminated.

Cross-reactivity. This phenomenon is one of the typical features of the HLA serology. The term "cross-reactivity" has been used by workers in the field to describe the astonishing appearance in immunization experiments of antibody specificities that were not phenotypically present on the immunizing cells. For example, if an individual with the phenotype HLA-A1, A3; B7, B8 was immunized with the cells from a donor with HLA-A1, A3; B7, B12, the resulting antiserum could contain the specificities anti-HLA-B12, B13, and Bw21, although the latter two antigens cannot be found upon direct typing of the donor cells. As expected, however, in absorption experiments, the donor cell was able to completely remove the anti-12 as well as the anti-13 and anti-21 activity. The same situation was not only observed in planned immunizations (186–188), but also in pregnancy sera (5,176,178). It is important to note that all these cross-reactions occur only between antigens belonging to the same locus (5,51,52,135,136, 142). Within the two loci there are certain "families" of cross-reacting antigens such as HLA-A1, 3, and 11, or HLA-A2 and 28 in the first HLA series, and HLA-B5, Bw35, Bw15, 17, and B18 in one group as well as HLA-B7, Bw22, and B27, or Bw40 and HLA-B13 or HLA-B8 and B14, or Bw15 and HLA-Bw17, and many more in the second series (5,51,52,63, 135,136,142,176,179,189). The degree of cross-reactivity was assessed in a large series of absorption experiments by Mittal et al. (135,136) and in absorption elution techniques by Mueller-Eckhardt et al. (142). Similar results were obtained when the frequency of joint occurrence of antibody specificities in pregnancy sera was assessed (5). It was shown that certain antibody specificities tended to occur together in one serum while others were never found together and it was demonstrated that the frequency of joint occurrence of antibodies closely reflected the degree of cross-reactivity.

The explanation for these findings requires the following hypothesis: HLA antigens are composed of immunodominant and several less immunogenic features, the latter of which are common to more than one HLA antigen. The more common factors there are, the higher the degree of cross-reactivity between two antigens. Antibodies are produced primarily against the immunodominant factor. Other features also come into play, even though these antibodies are usually weaker than those elicited by immunodominant factor. The existence of such different antibody populations and therefore of the corresponding "antigenic" factors has been postulated on the basis of dilution and concentration experiments (5), and has been clearly demonstrated by the blocking of cytotoxicity with Fab fragments of the same antibody (114,154) and by absorption-elution experiments (142). The different antibody populations show a cumulative effect in the cytotoxicity test (4,94,177) so that it is possible that in an absorption experiment the removal of one antibody population might render a serum negative although another antibody population is left behind. For this reason, absorption experiments are unsafe in establishing monospecificity, at least as far as HLA serology is concerned.

The genetic interpretation of the existence of different highly associated antigenic factors is that the immunodominant group and all other factors of one HLA antigen must be coded by different but very closely linked genetic determinants that show strong linkage disequilibrium. From this interpretation the question arises of whether these determinants are different mutational sites of one gene or separate but closely linked genes. Studies of the molecular redistribution of HLA antigens (*24*) in capping-cocapping experiments (*109*) revealed that cross-reacting determinants (i.e., factors, such as the factor common to HLA-B5 and Bw35, to cite a typical example) are located on the same molecule as the immunodominant group (which is, in our example, HLA-B5). On the other hand, antigens belonging to different loci always reside on different molecules. These molecular findings therefore support the view that multiple mutational sites of one gene are responsible for the expression of these antigenic factors on the cell surface. The existence of a long-disputed third locus (*164,182*) may be proved by the demonstration that the AJ antigen is located on a different molecule than the specificity HLA-B27, with which AJ is highly associated (*126,192*).

3. Genetics of the HLA System: Current Status

a. The separation into two loci. Since the Fourth International Histocompatibility Workshop in Los Angeles in 1970, there is general agreement that the HLA system can be most economically described as consisting of two closely linked loci with a series of mutually exclusive specificities (i.e., alleles) belonging to each of these loci.

The subdivision of the HLA system into two loci is based on the following lines of evidence: 1. It is impossible to find individuals who possess more than two antigens belonging to the same series (in extremely rare cases, chimeric persons have been found with up to four antigens of each locus corresponding to the two cell populations they carried). As this "lack of triplets" is true for both loci, one can conclude that no individual carries more than a total of four antigens.

2. The alleles of each locus show among each other a negative correlation in an unrelated population. Antigens belonging to different loci generally have no correlation, or they are positively associated with each other. Occasionally, there are also negative correlations between antigens of different loci, as for example, between HLA-A2 and HLA-B8. This situation is explained by the fact that HLA-A8 is so highly positively associated with HLA-A1, which in turn is negatively correlated with HLA-A2, that a negative association between HLA-A2 and HLA-B8 results.

3. The relatively rare joint occurrence in a phenotype of two alleles, which is the basis for the negative correlation, can also be measured with the Hardy–Weinberg distribution. Two alleles, *a* and *b*, with the gene frequencies p and q are expected to occur together in a phenotype of one

person with a frequency of $2 \times p \times q$ and a will be homozygous with a frequency of p^2. These equations are valid for unrelated populations with random mating in the absence of selection.

Using these formulas, it is possible to calculate the expected frequencies of all possible homozygotes for each locus and to compare them with observed frequencies. It has been repeatedly shown that there is excellent agreement between expectation and observation if one assumes that HLA-A1, 2, 3, 9, 10, 11, 28; Aw29, 30/31, and 32 belong to the first HLA locus and HLA-B5, 7, 8, 12, 13, 14; Bw15, 16, 17; Bw18, 21, 22, 27; 35, and 40 belong to the second locus (2–4,6).

4. The segregation analysis of informative families has revealed that two antigens belonging to the same series were never coded for by genes in the cis position (i.e., on the same haplotype). For example, if the father of the family possesses HLA-A1 and A2 (both alleles of the first locus) and the mother is negative for these two antigens, the children will be either HLA-A1 positive, A2 negative, or HLA-A1 negative and A2 positive, but there will never be a A1-positive/A2-positive child, nor will there be a child who is negative for both antigens. Extensive family studies have established the allelism of the new antigens of the two loci beyond a reasonable doubt (6).

5. Final proof for the separation of both HLA loci is seen in the observation of crossing-over between the first and the second HLA locus (104). One example of crossover is shown in Table I. It can be seen that the children C_1, C_2, and C_5 have inherited the HLA 3–5 haplotype and C_4, the 9–13 haplotype from the mother. In child C_3 however, HLA-A3 was passed on together with HLA-B13, indicating a crossover between the two HLA loci. Thus it is demonstrated that the HLA loci are separable by recombination. In an attempt to estimate the frequency of crossover, Svejgaard et al. in 1971 (180) analyzed over 300 families and found a combined maternal and paternal frequency of 0.85%.

b. *The third HLA locus* (AJ) (164). Numerous attempts to show the existence of a third HLA locus proved unsuccessful because the serological data could be interpreted in various ways. The problem was that the sera defining the proposed third-locus antigens either included in their reaction patterns antigens of the established loci or they were highly associated with antigens of the second locus, so that cross-reactivity as described above might have served as an explanation for the observed reactions. More recently, however, Mayr et al. (126) and Solheim and Thorsby (172) demonstrated that the antigens of the proposed AJ locus move independently from second-locus antigens on the cell surface of lymphocytes, although there is a strongly positive association between

TABLE I
CROSSING-OVER BETWEEN FIRST AND SECOND HLA LOCUS[a]

	A2	A3	A9	B5	B7	B12	B13	Chromosome
Father	+	−	−	−	+	+	−	A/B
Mother	−	+	+	+	−	−	+	C/D
Child 1	+	+	−	+	−	+	−	A/C
Child 2	+	+	−	+	−	+	−	A/C
Child 3	+	+	−	−	+	−	+	B/C:D
Child 4	+	−	+	−	+	−	+	B/D
Child 5	+	+	−	+	−	+	−	A/C
Child 6	+	−	+	−	−	+	+	A/D

[a] Haplotypes: A:A2, B12; B:A2, B7; C:A3, B5; D:A9, B13. Schematic picture of crossing-over during the meiotic division:

Maternal chromosomes:

```
    C: HLA 3-⌃--HLA 5        HLA 3-⟍--HLA 5       HLA 3 - - - HLA 13
    D: HLA 9-⌄--HLA 13       HLA 9--⟍-HLA 13
       Chromosomal            Recombination         Recombinant
         break                                       chromosome
                                                        C:D
```

AJ and B27 in the random population. Thus, in contrast to the situation with the so-called cross-reacting antigens (or antigenic factors), the antigenic structures of AJ and B27 reside on different molecules and must therefore—by definition—be coded for by different genes. The association between AJ and second-locus antigens, however, suggests that the AJ locus and the second locus are very closely linked. The above given molecular experiments are further confirmed by the observation of a crossover between the third (AJ) and the second locus (120) which suggests that the order on the chromosome is First (HLA-A)-(HLA-C) (AJ)–Second (HLA-B) (Four). At present only a fairly limited number of specificities have been identified at this locus.

c. *Gene frequencies.* The HLA polymorphism can be described on the lowest level in terms of phenotype and gene frequencies in the random population. Several methods for the estimation of gene frequencies have been used (square root formula $g = 1 - \sqrt{1 - f}$ where f is the phenotype frequency; gene counting in families after deduction of genotypes; maximum likelihood gene counting method) and it may be shown that all methods yield virtually identical results. Gene frequencies of a representative Caucasian population are given in Table II. As can be observed in the "blank" gene frequency, there is still a considerable number of undetected genes at both loci. It is quite possible that the number of

TABLE II

HLA PHENOTYPE AND GENE FREQUENCIES
IN THE CAUCASIAN POPULATION ($N = 5046$)

Gene	Phenotype frequency	Gene frequency
I. HLA locus		
A1	0.28	0.152
A2	0.52	0.304
A3	0.30	0.165
A9	0.21	0.107
A10	0.11	0.057
A11	0.10	0.051
A28	0.07	0.036
A29	0.05	0.024
Aw30/31	0.04	0.021
Aw32	0.05	0.023
Blank	—	0.060
II. HLA locus		
B5	0.13	0.073
B7	0.27	0.145
B8	0.19	0.103
B12	0.23	0.119
B13	0.06	0.031
B14	0.05	0.026
Bw15	0.14	0.075
Bw16	0.05	0.023
Bw17	0.08	0.042
B18	0.09	0.044
Bw21	0.04	0.023
Bw22	0.03	0.015
B27	0.08	0.042
W5	0.17	0.091
W10	0.13	0.066
Blank	—	0.082

recognized antigens could increase since some "established" antigens could be subdivided into new specificities, as was the case for HLA-A10 (Aw25/Aw26) and HLA-A9 (Aw28 and Aw24).

C. HAPLOTYPE FREQUENCIES

Since the true unit of inheritance is the haplotype, it is important to determine the frequency of joint occurrence of two antigens from different loci in the cis position (presently for the AJ antigens not enough information is available). The estimation of haplotype frequencies can be done from families in which the genotypes have been deduced by the gene counting method. Ambiguous haplotypes must be tallied according to maximum likelihood criteria. Since families for deduction of genotypes are often not available, formulae have been developed by Mickey *et al.* (see Ref. *99*) and by Mattiuz *et al.* (*125*) for the estimation of haplotype frequencies from the phenotype data. It can be demonstrated in a large family that both methods, gene counting and calculation from phenotype data, yield almost identical results (*6*). Table III lists the haplotype frequencies in a large Caucasian sample. The frequencies are given in numbers per 1000. With 11 alleles of the first locus and 16 of the second, there are 176 different haplotypes that can be combined to over 18,000 possible genotypes. If the third locus is also taken into account, the number of theoretically possible genotypes reaches almost 1 million. This illustrates the extreme degree of polymorphism of the HLA system.

A wide variety of frequencies exists for different haplotypes: some are so rare that they have not been found in a sample of 4800 persons (i.e., 9600 haplotypes). On the other hand, there is a group of haplotypes that

TABLE III

HLA HAPLOTYPE FREQUENCIES OF THE CAUCASIAN POPULATION (N = 4306)[a]

	A1	A2	A3	A9	A10	A11	A28	A29	Aw 30/31	Aw 32	Blank	Total
B5	65	243	82	74	44	76	50	4	15	2	74	729
B7	112[b]	328[b]	638[c]	151	45	36	17	30	15	18	59	1449
B8	798[c]	110[b]	32[b]	31[b]	1	18	14	7	10	10	1[b]	1032
B12	15[b]	538[c]	82[b]	155	72	10[b]	65	124[c]	9	34	84	1188
B13	28	104	30	43	10	15	7	4	32	7	34	314
B14	24	60	9	30	2	7	22	8	10	11	73[c]	256
Bw15	47	422[c]	90	79	19	14	21	4	6	16	27	745
Bw16	30	17[b]	41	44	44	6	13	0	9	5	20	229
Bw17	122[c]	144	33	26	21	15	5	14	9	11	23	423
B18	5	121	41	45	124[c]	35	16	7	16	4	24	438
Bw21	22	67	30	46	18	8	3	3	7	8	14	226
Bw22	10	40	20	28	12	25	0	2	2	1	13	153
B27	35	177[c]	52	54	16	23	18	10	6	18	11	420
W5	40[b]	136[b]	333	93	26	138[c]	27	17	24	5	71	910
W10	32[b]	280[c]	89	75	17	19	30	4	20	36	59	661
Blank	133	252	51[b]	91	99[c]	60	48	0	23	44	26	827
Total	1518	3039	1653	1065	570	505	356	238	213	230	613	10,000

[a] Frequencies given as numbers per 10,000.
[b] Significant linkage disequilibrium at negative delta, p < 0.001.
[c] Significant linkage disequilibrium at positive delta, p < 0.001.

are relatively frequent in Caucasian populations such as HLA-A1, B8; A3, B7; A2, B12; A2, B7; A2, Bw15; A3-Bw35; and A2, B27, ranging in frequency from 25 to 80 per 1000 haplotypes. These haplotype frequencies provide the data basis for the calculation of the most probable genotype for any given phenotype, a procedure which is quite important for the assessment of incompatibility between unrelated persons, where one or both reveal 3 or fewer HLA antigens due to homozygosity or the presence of a serologically undetected antigen. For example, if a prospective donor has the phenotype HLA-A2, 3; B7, it would be important to know whether he is homozygous for B7 or whether he possesses an unknown antigen. The probability of the presence of an unknown antigen can be calculated as follows: The genotype can be either HLA-A2–7/3–7, or HLA 2-b1/3–7, or 3-b1/2–7. Thus

$$P \text{ (unknown)} = \frac{hf(2\text{–b1}) \times hf(3\text{–7}) + hf(2\text{–7}) \times hf(3\text{–b1})}{hf(2\text{–b1}) \times hf(3\text{–7}) + hf(2\text{–7}) \times hf(3\text{–b1}) + hf(2\text{–7}) \times hf(3\text{–7})}$$

P (unknown) = 0.46 (46% chance for the presence of an unknown antigen)

This shows that there is a fairly substantial chance that this donor could possess an unknown antigen. In contrast to this rather indecisive result in terms of which genotype is the most probable, a large proportion of the HLA phenotypes reaches a probability of 0.90 (a 90% chance) for one or the other possibility. The most common HLA phenotype, HLA-A1, 3; B7, 8, for example, has a greater than 98% chance for the genotype 1–8/3–7.

D. LINKAGE DISEQUILIBRIUM

It has been noted that some of the most frequent haplotypes consist of antigens that by themselves are uncommon. If crossing over can freely occur between two loci for a sufficiently large number of generations, then the alleles of one locus should be independent from the alleles of the other in the random population. In other words, there should be no gametic association between the alleles of two separate loci and the frequency of joint occurrence (i.e., haplotype frequency) should be equal to the product of the gene frequencies of both antigens involved. For instance, for HLA 1–8 the expected haplotype frequency = $g_{(1)} \times g_{(8)}$ which is a numerical value of 0.05.

If this expected frequency is compared to the observed frequency of 0.078, a large difference is observed (0.053). This differences is the so-called linkage disequilibrium parameter or delta. Since delta value is frequency-dependent use of the proportion of observed to expected haplo-type frequency instead of the difference (6) has been suggested. This linkage disequilibrium ratio (LDR) is then:

$$LDR_{(1-8)} = \frac{hf_{(1-8)} \text{ observed}}{g_{(8)} \times g_{(1)}}$$

Thus all positive deltas would have a ratio above 1.0, while negative deltas will be equivalent to ratios below 1.0. The use of a frequency-independent parameter for the linkage disequilibrium is particularly important when alleles of low gene frequencies are involved as is the case for the HLA disease associations.

In Table III the haplotypes with significant delta values are marked with an asterisk. The linkage disequilibrium parameters and ratios for some of the characteristic haplotypes are given in Table IV. If there are haplotypes which are more frequent than expected, then there must also be haplotypes less frequent than expected, for which a negative delta value can be found. It is an interesting phenomenon that the positive deltas generally have a higher numerical value than the negative deltas. Thus, the positive deviation from linkage equilibrium is based on rela-tively few haplotypes, while the negative deviation is distributed among a larger number of haplotypes and therefore reaches only lower numerical values.

TABLE IV

HLA HAPLOTYPES WITH POSITIVE AND NEGATIVE LINKAGE DISEQUILIBRIUM

Haplotype	Frequency	Delta[a]	Ratio[b]
HLA 1–8	0.0798	+0.0641	5.08
HLA 3–7	0.0638	+0.0398	2.66
HLA 2–12	0.0538	+0.0397	3.82
HLA 2–15	0.0422	+0.0196	1.87
HLA 3–W5	0.0333	+0.0183	2.22
HLA 10–18	0.0124	+0.0099	4.96
W29–12	0.0124	+0.0096	4.43
HLA 2–7	0.0328	−0.0112	0.75
HLA 1–12	0.0015	−0.0168	0.07
HLA 2–8	0.0110	−0.0204	0.35

[a] Delta: Linkage disequilibrium parameter is derived from observed haplotype frequency minus expected haplo-type frequency; see text.

[b] Ratio: Proportion of observed haplotype frequency over expected haplotype frequency; see text.

The reason for the linkage disequilibrium observed in the HLA system is not known. It has, however, been observed that the occurrence of linkage disequilibrium is a rather common feature of closely linked systems such as the immunoglobulins (45), the RH system, the MNS system, the HLA system, and the HLA–MLC system (8). This could be simply explained by the fact that whatever is causing the linkage disequilibrium it takes longer for cross-over to establish equilibrium again because with close linkage it will take more generations to permit the same number recombinations than it does with loose linkage. It is a favorite speculation of many immunogeneticists that selection could be the principal explanation for the observed linkage disequilibrium (35). It should be pointed out, however, that other mechanisms in population genetics will also influence the gametic association of linked genes such as genetic drift and migration and consecutive mixture of populations (71). It is conceivable, for example, that the observed linkage disequilibrium results from the recent mixture of a number of highly inbred populations (70,71) in which certain haplotypes become quite frequent, as has been observed for most of the isolated Indian populations with a restricted gene pool (113). After the mixture of two such populations the Hardy–Weinberg equilibrium is established within one generation of random breeding (44) but the linkage equilibrium will take a considerable number of generations to develop, depending on the distance between the loci under study (44). Thus the degree of linkage disequilibrium is in some way related to the recombination frequency as an indirect measure of chromosomal distance. The existence of nonrandom gametic association has been instrumental for the discovery of systems closely linked with the HLA loci such as the third HLA locus (164) and the MLC determinants (8,131,132). It can be expected that this will also be true for further HLA linked systems which hopefully will be found in the near future. In the outbred human population, the lack of inbred strains for experimentation is partially compensated by the existence of linkage disequilibrium and by the large number of recombinants that have taken place since the common origin of our haplotypes.

E. MAPPING OF THE HLA REGION

The chromosomal region in which the HLA system is located is known to include a number of other genetic systems: The system coding for structures which cause stimulation in mixed leukocyte culture (short: LD determinants, for lymphocyte-defined) is not only closely linked with the HLA loci (77), but it seems to have some functional interrelationship

(78). From studies in families with crossing-over (77–79,191) and from population data (131–133) there is evidence for the existence of two separate loci governing mixed leukocyte reactivity in man: one strong locus on the side of the second outside the immediate HLA region and possibly a second weak locus between the HLA loci (131,191). The special features of this extremely complex MLC polymorphism will be discussed elsewhere in this volume.

Classic linkage analyses by Lamm et al. (111,112) have demonstrated that the third locus of the phosphoglucomutase is linked with HLA at a distance of about 15% recombination units. With this rather high recombination frequency, linkage could be shown only in the male sex. The linkage between HLA and PGM_3 opened the way for hybridization experiments, which have resulted in the conclusion that PGM_3 and therefore HLA are located somewhere on chromosome 6 (80,173). More recently Allen (11) demonstrated linkage between the Bf polymorphism (formally known as glycinrich beta-globulin polymorphism, or GBG) and the HLA system without the observation of crossing-overs. In a somewhat larger material which also includes families with recombinants both between Bf and HLA and between HLA and MLC, the position of Bf could be located between the HLA-B and HLA-D loci. The addition of the Bf system into this linkage group may be of particular significance since the Bf protein acts as the proactivator of the C3 component in the complement system. It has been shown analogously in the mouse by Démant et al. (73) that the serum complement level is controlled by a gene linked with the major histocompatibility complex H-2. Interestingly enough, Fu et al. (88) observed a family in which a deficiency of the complement component C2 segregates with HLA in a family over three generations, strongly suggesting that C2 is controlled by an HLA linked gene. The rare blood group system Chido has also been shown to be linked with HLA (134). It should be stressed, however, that for the latter two genes the exact location within the MHC has not been established. The current knowledge about the mapping on chromosome 6 can be summarized in the following scheme:

$$\text{SDI–LD2}^?\text{–SDIII–SDII–AS}^?\text{–Bf–CD}^?\text{–MS}^?\text{–LD1–PGM}_3$$

SD = serologically defined, LD = lymphocyte defined (LD2 = minor, LD1 = major), $AS^?$, $CD^?$, and $MS^?$ are hypothetical disease susceptibility genes for ankylosing spondylitis (AS), coeliac disease (CD), and multiple sclerosis (MS), Bf = GBG polymorphism, and PGM_3 = phosphoglucomutase-3. The hypothetical disease susceptibility genes will be discussed in Section IV.

II. HLA and Transplantation

The HLA system owes the rapid discovery of at least some of its complexities to the fact that HLA antigens function as transplantation antigens (48,49,56,103). The hope, however, that matching for HLA antigens could circumvent the problems of graft rejection has not been fulfilled (133), particularly in the unrelated population. Nevertheless, there are unambiguous data indicating that HLA antigens play an important role in transplantation: (1) HLA antibodies are produced as the result of transplant rejection; (2) a positive crossmatch due to HLA antibodies will cause hyperacute rejection in over 80% of the cases (149); (3) HLA antigens (SD) form the major target in cell-mediated lymphocytolysis (12,78–80); and (4) HLA identical siblings have in all series of kidney grafts proved to have a significantly better graft prognosis than haploidentical siblings (65).

Observations (1–3) indicate that the HLA antigens themselves are somewhat involved in graft rejection, while observation (4) can be interpreted as also demonstrating that perhaps not only the HLA, but also a closely linked system may be important in rejection. The recently discovered MLC polymorphism is an obvious candidate for this role. Preliminary and retrospective data from Cochrum et al. (50) as well as experimental data from Koch et al. (108,109) seem to support this view: a lower stimulation ratio in MLC is associated with an improved graft prognosis. Clearly, the use of a simple stimulation ratio is a rather crude method, but it may be expected that MLC (LD) typing will provide a significantly improved matching scheme.

In spite of all these reservations, the matching for SD antigens in unrelated individuals has a benefit that is large enough to justify the existence of international organizations for the exchange of organs (159,160). In the Eurotransplant material of kidney grafts, matching for HLA seems to be of appreciable benefit only in preimmunized patients (165), while in the combined English–French data an overall correlation between HLA match and graft prognosis has been found. The presence of cytotoxic antibodies in recipients prior to transplantation indicates a poor prognosis as compared to those patients without antibodies (160). Since all the patients are transplanted only when the crossmatch is negative, one can assume that the presence of cytotoxic antibodies in a prospective kidney recipient indicates that this recipient is more prone to develop a strong immune response upon the allogenetic stimulus of a kidney graft.

In the Eurotransplant data it was shown that in the patients with antibodies matching was of particularly importance for the antigens of the second HLA locus. This would be in good agreement with the concept that the MLC determinants or other closely linked genes of this region perhaps play a major role in graft rejection. The matching for antigens of the second locus would to a certain degree also produce matching for MLC determinants by means of the linkage disequilibrium between HLA and MLC (8). Data from other transplantation organizations, however, did not confirm the importance of the antigens of the second HLA locus (69,147,148). In view of the often conflicting data about the importance of HLA matching, one must return to outbred experimental animals such as the dog, where some of the open questions may be investigated. For the time being, however, we can summarize the situation as follows: There is a discrepancy between the success of HLA matching in the family and the rather weak correlation between matching and graft survival among unrelateds. This suggests the importance of a rather closely linked system such as the MLC system. Indeed it seems that the MLC is a good *in vitro* model of antigen recognition during graft rejection (*17–20*). Experimental (*108,109*) and preliminary data about matching for MLC support this view (*50*). The HLA antigens (SD determinants), however, seem to play an important role as the target of cytotoxic cells in cell-mediated lysis (CML) (*12,36,78–80*), which is thought to represent the efferent limb of the transplantation reaction. Thus, the salomonic conclusion is that both systems are important for graft survival and should be matched. Furthermore, it must be expected that many more loci may be discovered in close proximity of HLA and MLC, all of which many participate in the role of the major histocompatibility complex, whatever its biological significance.

III. HLA and Disease

The era of HLA disease associations was introduced by Amiel in 1967, when he reported that patients with Hodgkin's disease had a higher than expected incidence of an antigen then called 4C (*14*). This report prompted a very large number of studies on HLA in Hodgkin's disease (*13,14,26,34,85,107,137,161,200*) and it is ironic to state that it is still undecided whether there is an association at all and, if so, with which antigen (*53,84,86,87,107,137,161,190,193,200*).

Nevertheless, in the wake of these Hodgkin's studies came investigations that resulted in clear and strong associations that could be reproduced in all subsequent studies. The first indication of a significant association came at the Fifth International Histocompatibility Workshop, when Terasaki presented a large family in which he had found that the

HLA haplotype 1-17 segregated together with the incidence of psoriasis over more than three generations. Soon thereafter a number of striking associations between HLA and disease were discovered, often independently at the same time by two or more investigators. Coeliac disease (*7,9,10,82,83,89,90,92,121,129,130,175,194*), psoriasis (*163,166,168,184, 197*), and ankylosing spondylitis (*9,10,38,43,74,169,174*) are the most outstanding examples of an ever-increasing list of diseases for which truly significant associations have been found (Table V).

The reports about associations between a blood group system and human diseases have been met with a great deal of skepticism, mainly for two good reasons (one remembers the reports about the ABO associations with a wide array of diseases). (1) The associations—although statistically significant—have not brought about any deeper insight into the genetic basis or the pathogenesis of the respective diseases, nor could they be used as diagnostic criteria. (2) It is quite difficult to assess the statistical significance of certain deviations in antigen frequencies when complex systems such as HLA are involved. Since one is looking at more than 20 variables (antigens) in the HLA system, one can expect that one of these antigens should show a deviation in frequency significant at the $p = 0.05$ level in any given population simply owing to chance. In order to overcome this problem, it was first suggested by Bodmer (33–35) to

TABLE V

LIST OF WELL-ESTABLISHED HLA DISEASE ASSOCIATIONS

Disease	HLA Association	References
Coeliac disease	B8	(*7,9,10,82,83,89,90,92,121,129,130, 141,170,175,194*)
Dermatitis herpetiformis	B8	(*195,196*)
Psoriasis	B8 and Bw 17	(*163,166,168,184,197*)
Ankylosing spondylitis	B27	(*9,10,38,43,74,169,174*)
Reiter's disease	B27	(*16,39,140,199*)
Acute anterior uveitis	B27	(*40,76,124*)
Juvenile rheumatoid arthritis	B27	(*153*, E. D. Albert *et al.*, unpublished)
Myasthenia gravis	B8	(*22,81,87*)
Addison's disease	B8	(*152*)
Chronic aggressive hepatitis	B8	(*122*)
Juvenile diabetes	B8 and Bw 15	(*54,144*)
Graves disease	B8	(*86*)
Psoriatic arthritis	Bw 16	(*41*)
Multiple sclerosis	HLA-A3, B7, B18, and HLA-Dw2	(*15,27–30,72,95,96,97,98,143*)
Paralytic poliomyelitis	HLA-A3 and B7	(*151*)

multiply the p values for each comparison between the disease group and the controls by the number of comparisons made. This is now a generally accepted procedure.

Despite the above-discussed reservations, the field of HLA and disease has become a topic for intensive research and scientific discussion. A list of presently well-established HLA disease associations is given in Table V. From this list it can be easily recognized that there are two groups of diseases: coeliac disease (CD) and dermatitis herpetiformis (DH), on one hand, and ankylosing spondylitis (AS), acute anterior uveitis, Reiter's disease, juvenile rheumatoid arthritis on the other, that show associations with the same HLA antigen, thus confirming the knowledge about the close relationship between, for example, AS and uveitis or Reiter's disease. Furthermore, there are a number of features common to most or all of these diseases:

(a) there is evidence for familial incidence for almost all these disorders; (b) immunological mechanisms are suspected (or proved) to play an important role in pathogenesis; and (c) almost without exception, the association is strongest with an antigen of the second HLA locus.

Since there are already a number of strongly HLA associated diseases, it seems fairly unlikely that this finding is merely coincidental. One is led rather to speculate that these associations should have a more general biological significance.

In trying to explain the observed associations between diseases and HLA antigens, it is necessary to discuss a number of possible situations that could lead to an association on the population level.

1. It could be that by chance two independent genes are both frequent in the tested subset of the population. In this situation of a spurious association, one would expect that in a family study the genes under consideration will show independent segregation. Therefore, all disease association studies should be followed by family investigations (7,9,10,25).

2. The antigen itself is involved in pathogenesis through its molecular configuration on the cell surface. One hypothesis is that there could be chance similarities between certain microorganisms and the HLA antigen, so that the individual would not be able to recognize the bacterium as foreign and therefore would be unable to mount an appropriate defense against it.

Another possibility is that the antigenetic structure itself would provide a fitting site for the binding of deleterious agents, such as viruses, bacteria, or food protein. The nature of the observed associations, however, makes these latter explanations rather unlikely, since not all patients with one particular disease are positive for the associated antigen, and conversely not all individuals positive for the respective antigen suffer from the disease. Furthermore, it is quite difficult to assume that the structure of one antigen, such as HLA-B8, could be directly involved in the pathogenesis of so many different diseases, such as coeliac disease, diabetes mellitus, hepatitis, myasthenia gravis, Addison's disease, and Graves disease.

3. The association observed between the disease and HLA antigens could be most economically explained by assumption of close linkage between the second HLA locus and a gene that is important in the pathogenesis of the disease.

If a disease is found in association with a certain dominant genetic marker, such as HLA, it is a logical consequence to investigate the inheritance of the diseases and of the genetic marker in families with more than one patient (9,10,25).

Such studies have been performed in CD and in AS, and have suggested joint segregation between HLA haplotypes and the disease (167,174). There is an incomplete penetrance for both AS and CD as is best demonstrated by the fact that discordance of monozygotic twins has been found for both diseases, clearly showing that environmental factors must be involved in the suppression or the expression of the disease (10,92). Thus it must be expected that a certain proportion of the carriers of the disease genes does not (yet) express the disease. That this is indeed the case was shown in family studies (174,194). Nevertheless the data also clearly demonstrate that the disease always follows one HLA haplotype in a family, except for one case of suspected crossover (74). Furthermore, it could be established for CD that the disease also segregates with haplotypes that do not carry the highly associated antigen HLA-B8 (92). This finding strongly supports the hypothesis that not B8, but a closely linked gene, separable from HLA by crossing-over, is involved in the pathogenesis of CD.

Family studies similar to those in AS and CD were also performed in psoriasis (166,184). With this disease, however, the situation seems much more complex: in some families there was strong indication for joint segregation of HLA-B13 or Bw17 with the disease. In numerous other families, however, HLA haplotypes and the disease segregated independently. These data may suggest that different disease entities might be comprised in the global diagnosis of psoriasis, a possibility which is strengthened by the wide variety of clinical "manifestations" of the disease and by the fact that certain forms, such as the acute exanthematous psoriasis, are more closely associated with Bw17 (166) than the total psoriasis group, whereas other forms of psoriasis do not show any significant association with HLA antigens (184).

In spite of these explanations it must be concluded that in the case of psoriasis a simple model accounting for the observed HLA association and the pattern of inheritance is not immediately available. In contrast, for AS and CD it can be proposed, on the basis of family and population data, that a HLA linked susceptibility gene is of paramount importance (9).

The assumption of a susceptibility gene would require the influence of environmental factors, such as infections, that are necessary for the development of the disease. The occasional observation of discordant monozygotic twins both in AS and CD demonstrates the importance of environmental factors. The predominance of males in AS and of females in CD could reflect the fact that for genetic, hormonal, or anatomical reasons one sex might have a greater tendency to be infected with certain microorganisms, which in genetically predisposed individuals (those possessing the susceptibility gene) will cause the disease. In such a disease susceptibility model, the epidemic distribution of the disease would depend on the frequency of the susceptibility gene, which follows a simple inheritance pattern, and on the occurrence of the causative environmental factor (e.g., bacteria or viruses), which would be expected to strike on a random basis. This combination of straightforward inheritance with the randomized attack of certain microorganisms creates a distribution compatible with the patterns observed for AS and CD. In this way, it can be easily explained why not all HLA-B27-positive first degree relatives of a B27-positive AS patient develop the disease.

Considering the mode of inheritance of the susceptibility gene, it seems quite obvious—as far as AS and CD are concerned—that susceptibility is dominant over resistance. The frequent occurrence of parent–child transmission, and more clearly the almost complete lack of B27 homozygotes in AS, as the scarcity of B8 homozygotes in CD (9,92) argue strongly in favor of a dominant inheritance for the HLA-linked susceptibility genes in these two diseases. In AS families with more than one patient there are approximately equal numbers of parent–child transmissions as there are cases with the disease occurring in two siblings. This finding suggests a dominant inheritance and demonstrates that only relatively few genes are involved in the genetic determination of AS (9,167).

Going back to the original finding of an association between the disease and an HLA antigen in the unrelated patient population, if one accepts the hypothesis of linkage of a disease gene with HLA, it is still necessary to explain why there is an association between the two linked markers. Such a gametic association or linkage disequilibrium (6,8,44,45) becomes detectable when—owing to close linkage, recent origin, mixture of the above-mentioned diseases suggests that disease susceptibility may been able to separate the two genes frequently enough to establish a linkage equilibrium, where the frequency of joint presence on one chromosome of the two markers equals the product of their respective gene frequencies. This equilibrium is quite regularly disturbed in closely linked systems such as Rh, MNS, HLA (33), and HLA-MLC (8).

This can be partly explained by the fact that linkage is too close to allow enough crossing-over after the origin of this gene combination. On the other hand, it is very well possible that selective advantage may have existed or may still exist for the carriers of certain gene complexes. It should be pointed out, however, that the gametic association of two linked genes is also subject to the influence of mixture of populations (71), inbreeding, and genetic drift, so that it is difficult to assess how much of the observed disequilibrium is due to selection. Such a selective influence would be all the more pronounced in a very closely linked system.

From all this it can be concluded that if two linked genes show a gametic association (e.g., the association between a disease and HLA-B8 antigen), it is likely that these genes are quite closely linked. In the case of two closely linked polymorphisms, it is, however, not possible to correlate the degree of linkage disequilibrium directly with the distance between two loci.

These more theoretical considerations can be summarized as follows: The observation of HLA disease associations can be most economically explained by the assumption of a disease susceptibility gene that is closely linked to the HLA locus and therefore exhibits strong linkage disequilibrium with one certain allele of the HLA system.

The above-mentioned concept is further strengthened by a wealth of data from experimental animals: disease susceptibility has been shown to be linked to the main histocompatibility complex (in the following short MHC) in inbred animals, where exact mapping has been possible. The first example was the observation by Lilly (116–119) that susceptibility to Gross leukemia virus was linked with H-2, the major histocompatibility complex in the mouse. Similarly, it has been shown in more recent experiments that susceptibility to LCM meningitis viruses (146), to experimental autoallergic encephalomyelitis (198), and to experimental autoimmune thyroiditis (162) is closely linked with the MHC of the respective species. The best example for this analogy between the situation in man with that in mice is autoimmune thyroiditis, which in man is associated with HLA and in the mouse with H-2 (92,162). These findings are particularly important in view of the fact that numerous immune response genes have been mapped in the same MHC-linked region (21, 23,127,128) as the disease susceptibility genes. The immunological nature of the above-mentioned diseases suggests that disease susceptibility may be determined by a defective immune response gene. From the recessive pattern of susceptibility for Gross leukemia it may be concluded that there might be a lack of immune responsiveness (this is in keeping with the immune surveillance theory), whereas there should be a pathogenic immune response in the disease where the susceptibility seems to be dominant as, for example, in AS (9,10). According to these considerations, it is advisable to investigate the relationship between homozygotes and heterozygotes (i.e., the Hardy–Weinberg law), as this might provide a hint about the pathophysiological nature of the disease.

Prompted by this highly suggestive evidence from experimental animals, there have been attempts to localize the hypothetical disease-susceptibility genes in man. It has been mentioned above that practically all significant disease associations involve antigens of the second HLA locus; this strongly suggests that the disease-susceptibility genes are located in close proximity to the second HLA locus. As there are now a number of genetic markers known to be located in this chromosomal region, it is obvious that they should be used for the precise mapping of the disease susceptibility genes within the major histocompatibility complex. One first step was taken in comparing the association of a disease with antigens of the second HLA locus. If the association of two closely linked genes is explained by linkage disequilibrium one would expect that the degree of association should decrease with increasing distance between both genes. Therefore one may conclude that the disease gene for CD is located closer to the second locus since the association of CD is greater with HLA-B8 of the second locus than with HLA-A1 which belongs to the first locus. There was, however, also a significant increase of A1 among CD patients so that the question arose whether this increase could be accounted for by the well-known linkage disequilibrium between A1 and B8 in the normal Caucasian population (6).

This question could be answered by analysis of haplotype frequencies in CD patients (7,92). If the CD gene were located between the first and the second HLA locus, one could expect that not only the HLA-A1, B8 haplotypes, but also the haplotypes carrying A1, but not B8, should show an increased frequency in CD patients. This, however, was clearly not the case. Conversely, the haplotypes carrying B8, but not A1, were significantly increased among CD patients. Although it cannot be excluded on the basis of these data that the CD gene could be located inside HLA and very close to the second locus, it is more likely that the CD locus lies outside of HLA (92). The same analysis showed analogous results with 250 patients suffering from AS (E. D. Albert et al., unpublished). It should be stressed that for this kind of orientation study it is absolutely necessary to use haplotype frequencies derived from a large patient population. To carry this orientation study even further, the newly devel-

oped principle of MLC-typing (7,8) has been applied to disease-associa-
tion studies (7,98). The system coding for major MLC determinants in
man has been shown to be located outside of HLA in the close proximity
of the second locus (77,78), which is the very region where one suspects
the disease-susceptibility and immune-response genes to occur in man.
Jersild et al. (98) were able to show that the MLC allele LD-7a (Pi) is
found in significantly increased frequency among patients with MS, a
disease known to have an association with HLA-A3 and HLA-B7 (16,
27–30,72,95,97,143). This finding of an association with alleles of another
locus of the MHC lends further support to the concept of close linkage as
an explanation for these associations. More recently, Jersild et al. (98)
provided data showing that MS has a significantly higher association with
LD7a (Pi) than with HLA-B7, indicating that the MS gene might be
located closer to the MLC locus than to the second HLA locus. From
this, the following tentative arrangement of genes can be constructed:
HLA–A--HLA–C--HLA–B--AS--Bf--CD–MS–HLA–D–PGM$_3$.

More intensive MLC typing of HLA-associated diseases will certainly
produce more results that can help in localizing the disease-susceptibility
genes within the major histocompatibility complex.

IV. Clinical Applications

After all these more or less theoretical considerations, the question
arises: What could be the clinical significance of these HLA disease
associations? The clinical importance can be seen in three fields: (1)
diagnosis, (2) prophylaxis, and, possibly, (3) therapy.

It must be stressed that the diagnostic value of HLA typing for certain
diseases is rather limited. Even the strongest association observed so
far—that of B27 and AS—does not provide any diagnostic certainty
that would be comparable to diagnostic laboratory tests, such as the
assays of enzyme activities or serum electrolyte levels. Nevertheless,
typing for B27 has become an important part of the diagnosis of AS. It
should always be borne in mind, however, that the presence of B27 is
only an indirect marker for the disease. Obviously, the diagnostic value
is given only in a highly selected group of patients who have rheumatic
manifestations and other symptoms highly suggestive of AS. In addition,
diagnostic information can be obtained from typing for B27 in acute
anterior uveitis, a disease known to be associated both with AS and B27
(40,76,124).

There are a number of different etiologies for acute anterior uveitis
besides the rheumatologic one, and it can be reasonably assumed that

the vast majority of the B27-positive cases of acute anterior uveitis belong
in the rheumatologic category. Similarly, in juvenile rheumatoid arthritis
(JRA), where an association has been found with B27 (*153*), one may
predict that most of the B27-positive cases will be early manifestations of
AS, as shown in a family where the father (B27 positive) suffered from
AS and his 10-year-old son (B27 positive) was treated for juvenile
rheumatoid arthritis. Close diagnostic scrutiny revealed the typical symptoms of AS (such as sacroileitis and lower back pain). It should be pointed
out that for most of the other HLA associated diseases, HLA typing is
of no diagnostic value in the unrelated patient population. There is important information, however, which can be obtained from testing the
families of patients. In CD, for example, it is possible by haplotype
analysis to point out the family members who might have an abortive form
and who are at risk to develop the disease. This is particularly important
in view of an increased frequency of malignant lymphoma in CD patients
(*92*).

From these clinical considerations it becomes clear that at present the
major importance of HLA-associated diseases lies in the field of theoretical immunogenetics. Nevertheless, one can reasonably expect this
situation to change as newly discovered marker systems make it possible
to further dissect the chromosomal region of the major histocompatibility
complex and to recognize the physiological functions of these probably
functionally related clusters of closely linked genes.

References

1. Aho, K., Ahvonen, P., Lassus, A., Sievers, K. and Tilikainen, A. (1973). HL-A antigen 27 and reactive arthritis. *Lancet* **2**, 157.
2. Albert, E. D., Mickey, M. R., McNicholas, A. C., and Terasaki, P. I. (1970). Seven new HL-A specificities and their distribution in three races. "Histo-compatibility Testing 1970" (P. J. Terasaki, ed.), pp. 221–230, Munksgaard, Copenhagen.
3. Albert, E. D., Mickey, M. R., and Terasaki, P. I. (1971). Genetics of four new HL-A specificities in the Caucasian and Negro populations. *Transplant. Proc.* **3**, 95–100.
4. Albert, E. D., Mickey, M. R., and Terasaki, P. I. (1972). Serology and ge-netics of Te58(W18) and other specificities included in the 4c complex. *Tissue Antigens* **2**, 47–56.
5. Albert, E. D., Mickey, M. R., and Terasaki, P. I. (1972). A new approach to crossreactivity in the HL-A system. *Int. Symp. Standardisation HL-A Reagents, 1972, Ser. Immunobiol. Standard.* **18**, 156–164.
6. Albert, E. D., Mickey, M. R., Ting, A., and Terasaki, P. I. (1973). Deduction of 2140 HL-A haplotypes and segregation analysis in 535 families. *Transplant. Proc.* **5**, No. 1, 215.
7. Albert, E. D., Harms, K., Wank, R., Steinbauer-Rosenthal, I., and Scholz, S.

(1973). Segregation analysis of HL-A antigens and haplotypes in 50 families of patients with coeliac disease. *Transplant. Proc.* **5**, No. 4, 1785–1789.

8. Albert, E. D., Mempel, W., and Grosse-Wilde, H. (1973). Linkage disequilibrium between HL-A7 and the MLC Specificity Pi. *Transplant. Proc.* **5**, No. 4, 1551.

9. Albert, E. D. (1975). The significance of HL-A disease associations. *Z. Immunitaetsforsch., Exp. Klin. Immunol.* **148**, 382–383.

10. Albert, E. D., Harms, K., Schattenkirchner, M., Scholz, S., Steinbauer-Rosenthal, I. and Wank, R. (1975). HL-A antigens—genetic markers for disease susceptibility genes? *Int. Congr. Internal Med., 12th, 1974.* In press.

11. Allen, F. H., Jr. (1974). Linkage of HL-A and GBG. *Vox Sang.* **27**, 382–384.

12. Alter, B. J., Schendel, D. J., Bach, M. L., Bach, F. H., Klein, J., and Stimpfling, J. H. (1973). Cell-mediated lympholysis. Importance of serologically defined H-2 regions. *J. Exp. Med.* **137**, 1303–1309.

13. Amiel, J. L. (1971). Hodgkin's disease and HL-A. *Transplant. Proc.* **3**, No. 3, 1277.

14. Amiel, J. L. (1967). Study of the leucocyte phenotypes in Hodgkin's disease. *In* "Histocompatibility Testing 1967" (E. S. Curtoni, P. L. Mattiuz, and M. R. Tosi, eds.), Munksgaard, Copenhagen, pp. 79–81.

15. Amor, B., Feldmann, J. L., Delbarre, F., Hors, J., Beaujan, M. M., and Dausset, J. (1973). *New Engl. J. Med.* **288**, 704.

16. Arnason, B. G., Fuller, T. C., Lehrich, J. R., and Winn, J. H. (1972). Leukocyte antigens (HL-A) in multiple sclerosis. *Proc. Transplant. Soc. Congr.*, p. 8 (abstr.).

17. Bach, F. H., and Hirschhorn, K. (1964). Lymphocyte interaction: A potential histocompatibility test *in vitro. Science* **142**, 813–814.

18. Bach, F. H., Albertini, R. J., Amos, D. B., Ceppellini, R., Mattiuz, P. L., and Miggiano, V. C. (1969). Mixed leukocyte culture studies in families with known HL-A genotypes. *Transplant. Proc.* **1**, 339–341.

19. Bach, F. H. (1973). The major histocompatibility complex in transplantation immunology. *Transplant. Proc.* **5**, 23–29.

20. Bach, F. H., Segall, M., Zier, K. S., Sondel, P. M., Alter, B., and Bach, M. L. (1973). Cell mediated immunity: Separation of cells involved in recognitive and destructive phases. *Science* **180**, 403–406.

21. Bach, F. H., and Klein, J. (1973). *In* "Genetic Control of Immune Responsiveness" (M. Landy and H. McDevitt eds.), Academic Press, New York.

22. Behan, P. O., Simpson, J. A., and Dick, H. (1973). Immune response genes in myasthenia gravis. *Lancet* **2**, 1033.

23. Benacerraf, B., and McDevitt, H. O. (1972). Histocompatibility-linked immune response genes. *Science* **175**, 273–279.

24. Bernoco, D., Cullen, S., Scudeller, G., Trinchieri, B., and Ceppellini, R. (1973). HL-A molecules at the cell surface. *In* "Histocompatibility Testing 1972" (J. Dausset and J. Colombani, eds.), pp. 527–537. Munksgaard, Copenhagen.

25. Bertrams, J., Schildberg, P., Hopping, P., Böhme, U., and Albert, E. (1973). HL-A antigens in retinoblastoma. *Tissue Antigens* **3**, 78.

26. Bertrams, J., Kuvert, E., Böhme, U., Reis, H. E., Gallmeier, W. M., Wetter, O., and Schmidt, C. G. (1972). HL-A antigens in Hodgkin's disease and multiple myeloma. *Tissue Antigens* **2**, 41.

27. Bertrams, J., Kuwert, E., and Liedtke, U. (1972). HL-A antigens and multiple sclerosis. *Tissue Antigens* **2**, 405.

28. Bertrams, J., and Kuwert, E. (1972). HL-A-antigen frequencies in multiple

sclerosis: significant increase of HL-A 3, HL-A 10 and W 5 and decrease of HL-A 12. *Eur. Neurol.* **7**, 74.

29. Bertrams, J., and Kuwert, E. (1974). HL-A antigen segregation analysis in multiple sclerosis. *Lancet* **II**, 43–44.

30. Bertrams, J., Kuwert, E., von Fisenne, E., and Höher, P. G. (1974). Measles antibodies and HL-A antigens in multiple sclerosis. *Z. Immunitaetsforsch., Exp. Klin. Immunol.* **147**, 4.

31. Bodmer, W. F., and Payne, R. (1965). Theoretical consideration of leukocyte grouping using multispecific sera. "Histocompatibility Testing 1965," p. 141. Munksgaard, Copenhagen.

32. Bodmer, W. F., Bodmer, J., Adler, S., Payne, R., and Bialek, J. (1966). Genetics of 4 and LA human leukocyte groups. *Ann. N.Y. Acad. Sci.* **129**, 673.

33. Bodmer, W. F. (1972). Evolutionary significance of the HL-A system. *Nature (London)* **237**, 139–145.

34. Bodmer, W. F. (1973). Genetic factors in Hodgkin's disease: Association with a disease-susceptibility locus (DS-A) in the HL-A region. International Symposium on Hodgkin's Disease. *Nat. Cancer Inst. Monog.*

35. Bodmer, W. F. (1973). Population genetics of the HL-A system retrospect and prospect. *In* "Histocompatibility Testing 1972" (J. Dausset and J. Colobani, eds.), pp. 611–617. Munksgaard, Copenhagen.

36. Bonnard, G. D., Chappnis, M., Clauser, A., Mempel, W., Baumann, P., Grosse-Wilde, H., and Albert, E. D. (1973). SD versus LD antigens as target for lymphocyte mediated cytotoxicity. Study of a family presenting a recombination event within the MHR. *Transplant. Proc.* **5**, 1679–1682.

37. Boyum, A. (1968). Separation of leukocytes from blood and bone marrow. *Scand. J. Clin. Lab. Invest. Suppl.* **97**, 21.

38. Brewerton, D. A., Caffrey, M., Hart, F. D., James, D. C. O., Nicholls, A., and Sturrock, R. D. (1973). Ankylosing spondylitis and HL-A27. *Lancet* **2**, 904–907.

39. Brewerton, D. A., Caffrey, M., Nicholls, A., Walters, D., Oates, J. K., and James, D. C. O. (1973). Reiters disease and HL-A27. *Lancet* **2**, 996–999.

40. Brewerton, D. A., Caffrey, M., Nicholls, A., Walters, D., Oates, J. K., and James, D. C. O. (1973). Acute anterior uveitis and HL-A27. *Lancet* **2**, 994–996.

41. Brewerton, D. A., Nicholls, A., Caffrey, M., and Walters, D. (1974). HL-A27 and arthopathies associated with ulcerative colitis and psoriasis. *Lancet* **1**, 956–957.

42. Brown, J. L., Ferguson, A., Carswell, F., Horne, C. H. W., and Macsween, R. N. M. (1973). Autoantibodies in children with coeliac disease. *Clin. Exp. Immunol.* **13**, 373–382.

43. Caffrey, M. F. P., and James, D. C. O. (1973). Human lymphocyte antigen association in ankylosing spondylitis. *Nature* (London) **242**, 121.

44. Cavalli Sforza, L. L., and Bodmer, W. F. (1971). "The Genetics of Human Populations." Freeman, San Francisco.

45. Ceppellini, R. (1967). Genetica delle Immunoglobuline. *Ann. Meet. Assoz. Genet. Ital., 1967* Vol. 12, p. 3.

46. Ceppellini, R., Curtoni, E. S., Mattiuz, P. L., Miggiano, V., Scudeller, G., and Serra, A. (1967). Genetics of leukocyte antigens. A family study of segregation and linkage. *In* "Histocompatibility Testing 1967" (E. S. Curtoni, P. L. Mattiuz and M. R. Tosi, eds.), p. 169. Munksgaard, Copenhagen.

47. Ceppellini, R. (1968). The genetic basis of transplantation. *In* "Human Trans-

plantation" (F. T. Rapaport and J. Dausset, eds.), pp. 21–34. Grune & Stratton, New York.

48. Ceppellini, R., Mattiuz, P. L., Scudeller, G., and Visetti, M. (1969a). Experimental allotransplantation in man: I. The role of the HL-A system in different genetic combinations. *Transplant. Proc.* 1, 385–389.

49. Ceppellini, R. (1971). Old and new facts and speculations about transplantation antigens of man. *In* "Progress in Immunology" (B. Amos, ed.), pp. 973–1025. Academic Press, New York.

50. Cochrum, K., Salvatierra, O., Jr., Perkins, H. A., and Belzer, F. O. (1975). MLC-Testing in renal transplantation. *Transplant. Proc.* 7, No. 1, 659–662.

51. Colombani, M., Colombani, J., Dastot, H., Meyer, S., Tongio, M. M., and Dausset, J. (1969). Définition de deux nonveaux antigènes du système HL-A: Da19 et Da20. Réaction croisée entre les antigènes Da19, Da20, HL-A5 et Da6. *Rev. Franc. Etud. Clin. Biol.* 14, 995.

52. Colombani, J., Colombani, M., and Dausset, J. (1970). Cross-reactions in the HL-A system with special reference to the Da6 cross-reacting group. Description of HL-A antigens Da22, Da23, Da24 defined by platelet complement fixation: "Histocompatibility Testing 1970" (P. I. Terasaki, ed.), pp. 79–92. Munksgaard, Copenhagen.

53. Coukell, A., Bodmer, J. G., and Bodmer, W. F., (1971). HL-A types of fortyfour Hodgkin's patients. *Transplant. Proc.* 3, No. 3, 1291.

54. Cudworth, A. G., and Woodrow, J. C. (1974). HL-A antigens and diabetes mellitus. *Lancet* 2, 1153.

55. Dausset, J. (1958). Iso-leuco-anticorps. *Acta Haematol.* (*Basel*) 20, 156–166.

56. Dausset, J., Rapaport, F. T., Ivanyi, P., and Colombani, J. (1965). Tissue alloantigens and transplantation. *In* "Histocompatibility Testing 1965," pp. 63–69. Munksgaard, Copenhagen.

57. Dausset, J., Ivanyi, P., and Ivanyi, D. (1965). Tissue alloantigens in human. Identification of a complex system (Hu-1). *In* "Histocompatibility Testing 1965," p. 51. Munksgaard, Copenhagen.

58. Dausset, J., Ivanyi, P., Colombani, J., Feingold, N., and Legrand, L. (1967). The Hu-1 system. "Histocompatibility Testing 1967," p. 189. Munksgaard, Copenhagen.

59. Dausset, J., Colombani, J., Colombani, M., Legrand, L., and Feingold, N. (1968). Un nouvel antigène du système HL-A (Hu-1), l'antigène 15 allèle possible des antigènes 1, 11, 12. *Nouv. Rev. Franc. Hematol.* 8, 398.

60. Dausset, J., Colombani, J., Legrand, L., and Feingold, N. (1968). Le deuxième sub-locus du système HL-A. *Nouv. Rev. Franc. Hematol.* 8, 861.

61. Dausset, J., Colombani, J., Colombani, M., Legrand, L., and Feingold, N. (1969). Génétique du système HL-A. Fréquences génique, haplotypique et génotypique observées dans 113 familles. *Nouv. Rev. Franc. Hematol.* 9, 749.

62. Dausset, J., Colombani, J., Legrand, L., and Feingold, N. (1969). Les sub-loci du système HL-A. Le système principal d'histocompatibilité de l'homme. *Presse Med.* 77, 849–853.

63. Dausset, J., Colombani, J., Legrand, L., and Feingold, N. (1969). Relation of antigens Da6 and 6ᵇ (Da9) with the antigens of the second sub-locus of the HL-A system. *Transplantation* 8, 739.

64. Dausset, J., and Legrand, L. (1969). Antigène Da17: Un nouvel allèle du premier sub-locus du système HL-A. *Nouv. Rev. Franc. Hematol.* 9, 655.

65. Dausset, J., Walford, R. L., Colombani, J., Legrand, L., Feingold, N., and

Rapaport, F. T. (1969). The HL-A sub-loci and their importance in transplantation. *Transplant. Proc.* 1, 331.

66. Dausset, J. (1971). The polymorphism of the HL-A system. *Transplant. Proc.* 3, 1139–1146.

67. Dausset, J. (1971). Correlation between histocompatibility antigens and susceptibility to illness. *In* "Progress in Clinical Immunology" (R. Schwartz, ed.), pp. 183–210. Grune & Stratton, New York.

68. Dausset, J., Florman, A. L., Bachvaroff, R., Kanra, G. Y., Sasportes, M., and Rapaport, F. T. (1972). *In vitro* approach to a correlation of cell susceptibility to viral infection with HL-A genotypes and other biological markers. *Proc. Soc. Exp. Biol. Med.* 140, 1344.

69. Dausset, J. (1973). Some remarks about the preceding paper by Prof. J. J. van Rood with regard to the interpretation of the results of kidney and skin allograft studies in man. *Transplant. Proc.* 5, No. 4, 1751–1753.

70. Degos, L., and Bodmer, W. F. (1973). The effects of inbreeding on a two locus system. *In* "Histocompatibility Testing 1972" (J. Dausset and J. Colombani, eds.), pp. 545–547. Munksgaard, Copenhagen.

71. Degos, L., and Dausset, J. (1974). Human migrations and linkage disequilibrium of HL-A system. *Immunogenetics* 3, 195–210.

72. Degos, L., and Dausset, J. (1974). Histocompatibility determinants in multiple sclerosis. *Lancet* 1, 307–308.

73. Démant, P., Capková, J., Hinzová, E., and Vorácová, B. (1973). The role of the histocompatibility-2-linked Ss-Slp region in the control of mouse complement. *Proc. Nat. Acad. Sci. U.S.A.* 70, 863–864.

74. Dick, H. M., Dick, W. C., Sturrock, R. D., and Buchanan, W. W. (1974). Inheritance of ankylosing spondylitis and HL-A antigen W27. *Lancet* 2, 24–25.

75. Doe, W. F., Booth, C. C., and Brown, D. L. (1973). Evidence for complement-binding immune complexes in adult coeliac disease, Crohn's disease, and ulcerative colitis. *Lancet* 1, 402–403.

76. Ehlers, N., Kissmeyer-Nielsen, F., Kjerbye, K. E., and Lamm, L. (1974). HL-A27 in acute and chronic uveitis. *Lancet* 1, 99.

77. Eijsvoogel, V. P., Rood, J. J. van, Toit, E. D., and Schellekens, P. T. A. (1972). Position of a locus determining mixed lymphocyte reaction distinct from the known HL-A loci. *Eur. J. Immunol.* 2, 413–418.

78. Eijsvoogel, V. P., Bois, M. J. G. J. du, Melief, C. J. M., Groot-Kooy, M. L. de, Koning, C., Rood, J. J. van, Leeuwen, A. van, Toit, E. D., and Schellekens, P. T. A. (1973). Position of a locus determining mixed lymphocyte reaction (MLR), distinct from the known HL-A loci, and its relation to cell-mediated lympholysis (CML). *In* "Histocompatibility Testing 1972" (J. Dausset and J. Colombani, eds.), pp. 501–508. Munksgaard, Copenhagen.

79. Eijsvoogel, V. P., Bois, R. du, Melief, C. J. M., Zeylemaker, W. P., Koning, L., and Groot-Kooy, L. de (1973). Lymphocyte activation and destruction *in vitro* in relation to MLC and HL-A. *Transplant. Proc.* 5, 415–420.

80. Eijsvoogel, V. P., du Bois, M. J. G. J., Meinesz, A., Bierhorst-Eijlander, A., Zeylemaker, W. P., and Schellekens, P. Th. A. (1973). The specificity and the activation mechanism of cell-mediated lympholysis (CML) in man. *Transplant. Proc.* 5, 1675–1678.

81. Engelfriet, C. P., Feltkamp, Th. E. W., Nijenhuis, L. E., Galama, S. M. D., Rijn, A. van, Loghem, E. van, Berg-Loonen, E. van den, Possum, A. van, and Loghem, J. van. HL-A phenotype and haplotype frequencies in patients with myasthenia gravis. Personal communication.

82. Evans, D. A. P. (1973). Coeliac disease and HL-A 8. *Lancet* **2**, 1096.
83. Falchuk, J. M., Rogentine, G. N., and Strober, W. (1972). Predominance of histocompatibility antigen HL-A 8 in patients with gluten-sensitive enteropathy. *J. Clin. Invest.* **51**, 1602.
84. Falk, J., and Osoba, D. (1971). HL-A antigens and survival in Hodgkin's disease. *Lancet* **2**, 1118.
85. Forbes, J. K., and Morris, P. J. (1972). Analysis of HL-A antigens in patients with Hodgkin's disease and their families. *J. Clin. Invest.* **51**, 1156.
86. Forbes, J. F., and Morris, P. J. (1970). Leucocyte antigens in Hodgkin's disease. *Lancet* **2**, 849.
87. Fritze, D., Herrman, Ch., Naeim, F., Smith, G. G., and Walford, R. L. (1974). HL-A antigens in myasthenia gravis. *Lancet* **1**, 240–243.
88. Fu, S. M., Kunkel, H. C., Brusman, H. P., Allen, F. H., and Fotino, M. (1974). Evidence for linkage between HL-A histocompatibility genes and those involved in the synthesis of the second component of complement. *J. Exp. Med.* **140**, 1108.
89. Gebhard, R. L., Katz, S. J., Marks, J., Shuster, S., Trapani, R. J., Rogentine, G. N., and Strober, W. (1973). HL-A antigen type and small intestinal disease in dermatitis herpetiformis. *Lancet* **2**, 760–763.
90. Granditsch, G., Ludwig, H., Polymenidis, Z., and Wick, G. (1973). Coeliac disease and HL-A 8. *Lancet* **2**, 908.
91. Grumet, F. C., Payne, R. O., Konishi, J., and Kriss, J. (1974). HL-A antigens as markers for disease susceptibility and autoimmunity in Graves' disease. *J. Clin. Endocrinol. Metab.* **39**, 1115–1119.
92. Harms, K., Granditsch, G., Rossipal, E., Ludwig, H., Polymenidis, Z., Scholz, S., Wank, R., and Albert, E. D. (1974). *In* "Coeliac Disease" (W. Th. J. M. Hekkens, and A. S. Pena, eds.), pp. 215–228. H. E. Stenfert Kroese, Leiden.
93. Hirschfeld, J. (1965). Serologic codes: interpretation of immunogenetic systems. *Science* **148**, 968–971.
94. Ivasková, E., Vybiralová, H., Raue, I., Démant, P., and Ivanyi, P. (1969). Synergic action of HL-A antibodies. *Folia Biol. (Prague)* **15**, 26–34.
95. Jersild, C., Ammitzbøll, T., Clausen, J., and Fog, T. (1973). Association between HL-A antigens and measles antibody in multiple sclerosis. *Lancet* **1**, 151.
96. Jersild, C., Fog, T., Hansen, G. S., Thomsen, M., Svejgaard, A., and Dupont, B. (1973). Histocompatibility determinants in multiple sclerosis, with special reference to clinical course. *Lancet* **2**, 1221–1225.
97. Jersild, C., Svejgaard, A., and Fog, T. (1972). HL-A antigens and multiple sclerosis. *Lancet* **1**, 1240.
98. Jersild, C., Dupont, B., Fog, T., Hansen, G. S., Nielsen, L. S., Thomsen, M., and Svejgaard, A. (1973). Histocompatibility-linked immune response determinants in multiple sclerosis. *Transplant. Proc.* **5**, No. 4, 1791–1796.
99. "Joint Report of the Fourth International Histocompatibility Workshop." *In* "Histocompatibility Testing 1970" (P. I. Terasaki, ed.), pp. 2–47. Munksgaard, Copenhagen.
100. Jongsma, A., van Someren, H., Westerveld, A., Hagemeijor, A., and Pearson, P. (1973). Localization of genes on human chromosomes using human-Chinese hamster somatic cell hybrids. Assignment of PGM₃ to chromosome C6 and regional mapping of the PGD, PGM₁ and Pep-C genes on chromosome A1. *Humangenetik* **20**, 195.
101. Kissmeyer-Nielsen, F., and Kjerbye, K. E. (1967). The human HL-A locus. Antibodies and antigens belonging to the LA- and 4-series. *Bull. Eur. Soc. Hum. Genet.* **1**, 58–63.

102. Kissmeyer-Nielsen, F., and Kjerbye, K. E. (1967). Lymphocytotoxic micro-
     technique. Purification of lymphocytes by flotation. In "Histocompatibility Test-
     ing, 1967" (E. S. Curtoni, P. L. Mattiuz, and R. M. Tosi, eds.), pp. 381–383.
     Munksgaard, Copenhagen.
103. Kissmeyer-Nielsen, F., Svejgaard, A., and Hauge, M. (1968). Genetics of the
     human HL-A transplantation system. Nature (London) 219, 1116.
104. Kissmeyer-Nielsen, F., Svejgaard, A., Ahrons, S., and Nielsen, L. S. (1969).
     Crossing-over within the HL-A system. Nature (London) 224, 75.
105. Kissmeyer-Nielsen, F., Kjerbye, K. E., Mayr, W., and Thulstrup, H. (1970). The
     HL-A antigen KN-HN Vox Sang. In press.
106. Kissmeyer-Nielsen, F., Staub-Nielsen, L., Sandiberg, L., Svejgaard, A., and
     Thorsby, E. (1970). The HL-A system in relation to human transplantations.
     In "Histocompatibility Testing, 1970" (P. I. Terasaki, ed.), pp. 105–135. Munks-
     gaard, Copenhagen.
107. Kissmeyer-Nielsen, F., Jensen, K. B., Ferrara, G. B., Kjerbye, K. E., and Svej-
     gaard, A. (1971). HL-A phenotypes in Hodgkin's disease. Preliminary report.
     Transplant. Proc. 3, 1287.
108. Koch, C. R., Frederiks, E., Eijsvoogel, V. P., and Rood, J. J. van (1971). Mixed-
     lymphocyte-culture and skin-graft data in unrelated HL-A identical individuals.
     Lancet II, 1334–1336.
109. Koch, C., Hooff, J. P. van, Leeuwen, A. van, Tweel, J. van den, Frederiks, E.,
     Steen, G. van den, Schippers, H. M. A., and Rood J. J. van (1973). The relative
     importance of matching for the MLC versus the HL-A loci in organ transplanta-
     tion. In "Histocompatibility Testing 1972" (J. Dausset and J. Colombani, eds.),
     pp. 521–524. Munksgaard, Copenhagen.
110. Kourilsky, F. M., Silvestre, D., Neaport-Sautes, C., Loosfelt, Y., and Dausset, J.
     (1972). Antibody-induced redistribution of HL-A antigens at the cell surface.
     Eur. J. Immunol. 2, 249–257.
111. Lamm, L. U., Svejgaard, E., and Kissmeyer-Nielsen, F. (1971). PGM₃: HL-A
     is another linkage in man. Nature (London) 231, 109–111.
112. Lamm, L. U., Kissmeyer-Nielsen, F., Svejgaard, A., Brunn Petersen, G., Thorsby,
     E., Mayr, W., and Høgman, C. (1972). On the orientation of the HL-A region
     and the PGM₃ locus in the chromosome. Tissue Antigens 2, 205–214.
113. Layrisse, Z., Terasaki, P., Wilbert, J., Seinen, H. D., Arredondo, B., Soyano, A.,
     Mittal, K., and Layrisse, M. (1973). Study of the HL-A system in the warao
     population. In "Histocompatibility Testing 1972" (J. Dausset and J. Colombani,
     eds.), pp. 377–386. Munksgaard, Copenhagen.
114. Legrand, L., and Dausset, J. (1973). Serological evidence of the existence of
     several antigenic determinants (or factors) on the HL-A gene products. In "His-
     tocompatibility Testing 1972" (J. Dausset and J. Colombani, eds.), pp. 441–
     453. Munksgaard, Copenhagen.
115. Levine, B. B., Stember, R. H., and Fotino, M. (1972). Science 178, 1201.
116. Lilly, F. (1973). In "Genetic Control of Immune Responsiveness" (M. Landy
     and H. McDevitt, eds.), pp. 279–288. Academic Press, New York.
117. Lilly, F. (1971). The influence of H-2 type on gross virus leukemogenesis in
     mice. Transplant. Proc. 3, 1239.
118. Lilly, F. (1966). The histocompatibility-2 locus and susceptibility to tumor in-
     duction. In "Murine Leukemia," Nat. Cancer Inst. Monogr. 22, 631–641.
119. Lilly, F., Boyse, E. A., and Old, L. J. (1964). Genetic basis of susceptibility to
     viral leukemogenesis. Lancet 2, 1207.

120. Löw, B., Messeter, S., Mansson, S., and Lindholm, T. (1974). Crossing-over between the SD-2 (FOUR) and SD-3 (AJ) loci of the human major histocompatibility chromosomal region. *Tissue Antigens* 4, 405.

121. Ludwig, H., Polymenidis, Z., Granditsch, G., and Wick, G. (1973). HL-A1 and HL-A8 bei kindlicher Coeliakie. *Z. Immunitaetsforsch., Exp. Klin. Immunol.* 146, 158.

122. Mackay, I. R., and Morris, P. J. (1972). Association of autoimmune active chronic hepatitis with HL-A1, 8. *Lancet* 2, 793.

123. "Manual of Tissue Typing Techniques" (1974). (J. G. Ray, D. B. Hare, P. D. Pederson, and D. A. Kayhoe, eds.), NIAID Transplant. Immunol. Branch DHEW Publ. No. (NIH) 75–545.

124. Mapstone, R., and Woodrow, J. C. (1974). Acute anterior uveitis and HL-A27. *Lancet* 1, 681–682.

125. Mattiuz, P. L., Ihde, D., Piazza, A., Ceppellini, R., and Bodmer, W. F. (1970). New approaches to population genetic and segregation analysis of the HL-A System. *In* "Histocompatibility Testing 1970" (P. I. Terasaki, ed.), 193. Munksgaard, Copenhagen.

126. Mayr, W., Bernoco, D., De Marchi, M., and Ceppellini, R. (1973). Genetic analysis and biological properties of products of the third SD (AJ) locus of the HL-A region. *Transplant. Proc.* 5, 1581–1593.

127. McDevitt, H. O., and Benacerraf, B. (1969). Genetic control of specific immune responses. *Advan. Immunol.* 11, 31–74.

128. McDevitt, H. O., and Bodmer, W. F. (1972). Histocompatibility antigens, immune responsiveness and susceptibility to disease. *Amer. J. Med.* 52, 1–8.

129. McDonald, W. C., Dobbins, W. O., and Rubin, C. E. (1965). Studies of the familial nature of celiac sprue using biopsy of the small intestine. *New Engl. J. Med.* 272, 448–456.

130. McNeish, A. S., Nelson, R., and Mackintosh, P. (1973). HL-A 1 and 8 in childhood coeliac disease. *Lancet* 1, 668.

131. Mempel, W., Grosse-Wilde, H., Albert, E., and Thierfelder, S. (1973). Atypical MLC reactions in HL-A typed related and unrelated pairs. *Transplant. Proc.* 5, 401–408.

132. Mempel, W., Grosse-Wilde, H., Baumann, P., Netzel, B., Steinbauer-Rosenthal, I., Scholz, S., Bertrams, J., and Albert, E. D. (1973). Population genetics of the MLC response: Typing for MLC determinants using homozygous and heterozygous reference cells. *Transplant. Proc.* 5, 1529–1534.

133. Mickey, M. R., Terasaki, P. I., Kreisler, M., Albert, E. D., and Sengar, D. P. S. (1971). Analysis of histocompatibility data from 1000 kidney transplants. *Tissue Antigens* 1, 57–67.

134. Middleton, J., Crookston, M. C., Falk, J. A., Robson, E. M., Cook, P. J. L., Batchelor, J. R., Bodmer, J., Ferrara, G. B., Festenstein, H., Harris, R., Kissmeyer-Nielsen, F., Lawler, S. D., Sachs, J. A., and Wolf, E. (1974). Linkage of Chido and HL-A. *Tissue Antigens* 4, 366–373.

135. Mittal, K. K., Mickey, M. R., and Terasaki, P. I. (1972). Crossreactive antibodies in "duospecific" anti-HL-A antisera. *Int. Symp. Standardisation HL-A Reagents, Copenhagen, Symp. Ser. Immunobiol. Standard* 18, 165–170.

136. Mittal, K. K., and Terasaki, P. I. (1972). Cross-reactivity in the HL-A system. *Tissue Antigens* 2, 94–104.

137. Morris, P. J., and Forbes, J. F. (1971). HL-A and Hodgkin's disease. *Transplant. Proc.* Vol. III, 1275.

138. Morris, P. J., Lawler, S., and Oliver, R. T. (1973). HL-A and Hodgkin's disease. *In* "Histocompatibility Testing 1972" (J. Dausset and J. Colombani, eds.), pp. 669–677. Munksgaard, Copenhagen.

139. Morris, P. J. (1973). Histocompatibility systems, immune response and disease in man. *Contemp. Top. Immunobiol.* 3, 141–169.

140. Morris, R., Metzger, A. L., Bluestone, R., and Terasaki, P. I. (1974). HL-A-W27—A clue to the diagnosis and pathogenesis of Reiter's syndrome. *New Engl. J. Med.* 290, 554.

141. Mowbray, J. F., Hoffbrand, A. V., Holborow, E. J., Seah, P. P., and Fry, L. (1973). Circulating immune complexes in dermatitis herpetiformis. *Lancet* 1, 400–401.

142. Mueller-Eckhardt, C., Heinrich, D., and Rothenberg, V. (1972). Frequency and complexity of crossreactive HL-A antibodies. Elution studies with platelets. *Int. Symp. Standardisation HL-A Reagents, Ser. Immunobiol. Standard* 18, 171–178.

143. Naito, S., Namerow, N., Mickey, M. R., and Terasaki, P. I. (1972). Multiple sclerosis: association with HL-A3. *Tissue Antigens* 2, 1–4.

144. Neauport-Sautes, C., Silvestre, D., Kourilsky, F. M., and Dausset, J. (1973). Independence of HL-A antigens from the first and second locus at the cell surface. *In* "Histocompatibility Testing 1972" (J. Dausset and J. Colombani, eds.), pp. 539–544. Munksgaard, Copenhagen.

145. Nerup, J., Platz, P., Andersen, O. O., Christy, M., Lyngsøe, J., Poulsen, J. E., Ryder, L. P., Nielsen, L. S., Thomsen, W., and Svejgaard, A. (1974). HL-A antigens and diabetes mellitus. *Lancet* 2, 864–866.

146. Oldstone, M. B., Dixon, F. J., Mitchell, G. F., and McDevitt, H. O. (1973). Histocompatibility-linked genetic control of disease susceptibility Murine lymphocytic choriomeningitis virus infection. *J. Exp. Med.* 137, 1201–1212.

147. Opelz, G., and Terasaki, P. I. (1972). The role of the HL-A system in kidney transplants. *Transplant. Proc.* 4, 433–438.

148. Opelz, G., Mickey, M. R., and Terasaki, P. I. (1972). Identification of unresponsive kidney transplant recipients. *Lancet* 1, 868–871.

149. Patel, R., and Terasaki, P. I. (1969). Significance of the positive cross match test in kidney transplantation. *New Engl. J. Med.* 280, 735.

150. Payne, R., Tripp, M., Weigle, M., Bodmer, W., and Bodmer, J. (1964). A new leukocyte isoantigen system in man. *Cold Spring Harbor Symp. Quant. Biol.* 29, 285.

151. Pietsch, M., and Morris, P. J. (1974). An association of HL-A3 and HL-A7 with paralytic poliomyelitis. *Tissue Antigens* 4, 50–55.

152. Platz, P., Ryder, L., Staub Nielsen, L., Svejgaard, A., Thomsen, M., Nerup, J., and Christy, M. (1974). HL-A and idiopathic Addison's disease. *Lancet* 2, 289.

153. Rachelewski, G. S., Terasaki, P. I., Katz, R., and Stiehm, E. R. (1974). Increased prevalence of W27 in juvenile rheumatoid arthritis. *New Engl. J. Med.* 290, 892–893.

154. Richiardi, P., Carbonara, A. O., Mattiuz, P. L., and Ceppellini, R. (1973). Inhibition of cytotoxic anti HL-A sera by their F(ab)₂. *In* Histocompatibility Testing 1972" (J. Dausset and J. Colombani, eds.), pp. 455–464. Munksgaard, Copenhagen.

155. Rittner, Ch., Rittner, B., Scholz, S., Lorenz, H., and Albert, E. D. (1974). Data on a new linkage group: HL-A-Bf (Factor B of the properdin system). *Z. Immunitaetsforsch., Exp. Klin. Immunol.* In press.

156. Rittner, Ch., Grosse-Wilde, H., Rittner, B., Netzel, B., Scholz, S., Lorenz, H.,

and Albert, E. D. (1975). Linkage group HL-A-MLC-Bf (properdin Factor B). The site of the Bf locus at the immunogenetic linkage group on chromosome No. 6. *Humangenetik* **27**, 173–183.

157. Rood, J. J. van (1962). "Leukocyte Grouping. A Method and Its Application." Thesis, Leyden. Drukkeris Pasmans, Dan Haag.

158. Rood, J. J. van, and Leeuwen, A. van (1965). Defined leukocyte antigenic groups in man. *In* "Histocompatibility Testing" Nat. Acad. Sci. Publ. 1229, p. 21. Washington, D.C.

159. Rood, J. J. van (1967). A proposal for international cooperation in organ transplantation: Eurotransplant. *In* "Histocompatibility Testing 1967" (E. S. Curtoni, P. L. Mattiuz, and M. R. Tosi, eds.), pp. 451–452. Munksgaard, Copenhagen.

160. Rood, J. J. van (1973). LD-SD interaction *in vivo* and the allograft reaction. *Transplant. Proc.* **5**, 1747–1750.

161. Rood, J. J. van and Leeuwen, A. van (1973). HL-A and the group five system in Hodgkin's disease. *Transplant. Proc.* 3, 1283.

162. Rose, N. R., Twarog, F. J., and Crowle, A. J. (1970). *J. Immunol.* **106**, 698.

163. Russell, Th. J., Schultes, L. M., and Kuban, D. J. (1973). Histocompatibility (HL-A) antigens associated with psoriasis. *New Engl. J. Med.* **287**, 738–740.

164. Sandberg, L., Thorsby, E., Kissmeyer-Nielsen, F., and Lindholm, A. (1970). Evidence of a third sublocus within the HL-A chromosomal region. *In* "Histocompatibility Testing 1970" (P. I. Terasaki, ed.), pp. 165–170. Munksgaard, Copenhagen.

165. Schippers, H. M. A. (1973). Annual Report. Eurotransplant Foundation, Leiden, The Netherlands.

166. Schoefinius, H. H., Braun-Falco, O., Scholz, S., Steinbauer-Rosenthal, I., Wank, R., and Albert, E. D. (1974). Histokompatibilitätsantigene (HL-A) bei Psoriasis. *Deut. Med. Wochschr.* **99**, 440–444.

167. Scholz, S., Schattenkirchner, M., Harms, K., Steinbauer-Rosenthal, I., and Albert, E. D. Family studies in HL-A associated diseases. *Z. Immunitaetsforsch., Exp. Klin. Immunol.* **148**, 387–388.

168. Scholz, S., Schoefinius, H., Steinbauer-Rosenthal, I., Wank, R., Albert, E. and Braun-Falco, O. (1974). Association between HL-A antigen and psoriasis vulgaris. *Z. Immunitaetsforsch.* 147, 4 (abstr.).

169. Schlosstein, I., Terasaki, P. J., Bluestone, R., and Pearson, C. M. (1973). High association of an HL-A antigen, W27, with ankylosing spondylitis. *New Engl. J. Med.* **288**, 704–706.

170. Shiner, M., and Shmerling, D. H. (1972). The immunopathology of coeliac disease. *Digestion* **5**, 77.

171. Snell, G. D. (1968). The H-2 locus of the mouse: observations and speculations concerning its comparative genetics and its polymorphism. *Folia Biol.* 14, 335.

172. Solheim, B. G., and Thorsby, E. (1973). Evidence of a third HL-A locus. *Transplant. Proc.* **5**, No. 4, 1579–1580.

173. Someren, H. von, Westerveld, A., Hagemeijer, A., Mees, J. R., and Meera Khan, P. Human antigen and enzyme markers in man-Chinese hamster somatic cell hybrids. Evidence for synteny between the HL-A, PGM_3, ME_1, and IPO-B loci. *Proc. Nat. Acad. Sci. U.S.A.* **71**, 962(1974).

174. Steinbauer-Rosenthal, I., Schattenkirchner, M., Schürer, W., Wank, R., Scholz, S., Schiessl, B., Brandenburg, H., and Albert, E. D. (1974). HL-A 27 in patients with ankylosing spondylitis (AS). *Z. Immunitaetsforsch., Exp. Klin. Immunol.* **147**, 6 (abstr.).

175. Stokes, P. L., Asquith, P., Holmes, G. K. T., Mackintosh, P., and Cooke, W. T. (1972). Histocompatibility antigens associated with adult coeliac disease. *Lancet* 2, 162.

176. Svejgaard, A., and Kissmeyer-Nielsen, F. (1968). Cross-reactive human HL-A isoantibodies. *Nature (London)* 219, 868–869.

177. Svejgaard, A. (1969). Synergistic action of HL-A isoantibodies. *Nature (London)* 222, 94–95.

178. Svejgaard, A., Kissmeyer-Nielsen, F., and Thorsby, E. (1970). HL-A typing of platelets. *In* "Histocompatibility Testing 1970" (P. I. Terasaki, ed.), pp. 153–164. Munksgaard, Copenhagen.

179. Svejgaard, A., Thorsby, E., Hauge, M., and Kissmeyer-Nielsen, F. (1970). Genetics of the HL-A system. A population and family study. *Vox Sang.* 18, 97–133.

180. Svejgaard, A., Bratlie, A., Hedin, P. J., Høgman, C., Jersild, C., Kissmeyer-Nielsen, F., Lindblom, B., Lindholm, A., Løw, B., Messeter, L., Møller, E., Sandberg, L., Staub-Nielsen, L., and Thorsby, E. (1971). The recombination fraction of the HL-A system. *Tissue Antigens* 1, 81–88.

181. Svejgaard, A., Hauge, M., Kissmeyer-Nielsen, F., and Thorsby, E. (1971). HL-A haplotype frequencies in Denmark and Norway. *Tissue Antigens* 1, 184–195.

182. Svejgaard, A., Staub-Nielsen, L., Ryder, L., Kissmeyer-Nielsen, F., Sandberg, L., Lindholm, A., and Thorsby, E. (1973). Subdivisions of HL-A antigens. Evidence of a 'new' segregant series. *In* "Histocompatibility Testing 1972" (J. Dausset and J. Colombani, eds.), pp. 465–473. Munksgaard, Copenhagen.

183. Svejgaard, A., Jersild, C., Staub Nielsen, L., and Bødmer, W. F. (1974). HL-A antigens and disease statistical and genetical consideration. *Tissue Antigens* 4, No. 2, 95–105.

184. Svejgaard, A., Staub Nielsen, L., Svejgaard, E., Kissmeyer-Nielsen, F., Hjortshøj, A., and Zachariae, H. (1974). HL-A in psoriasis vulgaris and in pustular psoriasis—population and family studies. *Brit. J. Dermatol.* 91, 145.

185. Terasaki, P. I., and McClelland, J. D. (1964). Microdroplet assay of human serum cytotoxins. *Nature (London)* 206, 998.

186. Thorsby, E., and Kissmeyer-Nielsen, F. (1968). Lymphocytotoxic antisera of limited isospecificity after skin grafting in man. *Vox Sang.* 14, 417.

187. Thorsby, E., and Kissmeyer-Nielsen, F. (1969). HL-A antigens and genes. III. Production of HL-A typing antisera and desired specificity. *Vox Sang.* 17, 102.

188. Thorsby, E., and Kissmeyer-Nielsen, F. (1970). New alleles of the HL-A system. Identification by planned immunization. *Vox Sang.* 18, 134–147.

189. Thorsby, E., Kjerbye, K. E., and Bratlie, A. (1970). Cross-reactive HL-A antibodies. Absorption and immunization studies. *Vox Sang.* 18, 373–378.

190. Thorsby, E., Falk, J., Engeset, A., and Osoba, E. (1971). HL-A antigens in Hodgkin's disease. *Transplant. Proc.* 3, 1279.

191. Thorsby, E., Hirschberg, H., and Helgesen, A. (1973). A second locus determining Human MLC response: Separate lymphocyte populations recognise the products of each different MLC locus allele in allogeneic combinations. *Transplant. Proc.* 5, No. 4, 1523–1528.

192. Thorsby, E. (1974). The human major histocompatibility system. *Transplant. Rev.* 18, 51–129.

193. Walford, R. L. (1972). Histocompatibility systems and disease states with particular reference to cancer. *Transplant. Rev.* 8, 1.

194. Wank, R., Harms, K., Scholz, S., Steinbauer-Rosenthal, I., Brandenburg, H.,

Schiessl, B., and Albert, E. (1974). A study of HL-A antigens in 50 families of patients with coeliac disease. *Z. Immunitaetsforsch., Exp. Klin. Immunol.* **147**, 147 (abstr.).

195. White, A. G., Barnetson, R. St. C., Da Costa, J. A., and McClelland, D. B. L. (1973). HL-A and disordered immunity. *Lancet* **1**, 108.

196. White, A. G., Barnetson, R. St. C., Da Costa, J. A. G., and McClelland, D. B. L. (1973). The incidence of HL-A antigens in dermatitis herpetiformis. *Brit. J. Dermatol.* **89**, 133–136.

197. White, S. H., Newcomer, V. D., Mickey, M. R., and Terasaki, P. I. (1972). Disturbance of HL-A antigen frequency in psoriasis. *New Engl. J. Med.* **287**, 740.

198. Williams, R. M., and Moore, M. J. (1973). Linkage of susceptibility to experimental allergic encephalomyelitis to the major histocompatibility locus in the rat. *J. Exp. Med.* **138**, 775–783.

199. Zachariae, H., Hjortshøj, A., and Kissmeyer-Nielsen, F. (1973). Reiter's disease and HL-A27. *Lancet* **2**, 565–566.

200. Zervas, J. D., Delamore, L. W., and Israels, M. C. O. (1970). Leucocyte phenotypes in Hodgkin's disease. *Lancet* **2**, 634.

Mixed Leukocyte Cultures: A Cellular Approach to Histocompatibility Testing[1]

FRITZ H. BACH

Immunobiology Research Center and Departments of Medical Genetics and Surgery, The University of Wisconsin, Madison, Wisconsin

I. Introduction

The mixed leukocyte culture (MLC) test represents an *in vitro* model of the recognitive phase of the allograft reaction. Lymphocytes of a potential recipient are mixed with lymphocytes of a potential donor to assay the response of lymphocytes of the recipient as they recognize foreign histocompatibility antigens on the cells of the donor. If incompatibility for the major histocompatibility complex, human leukocyte system A (HLA), in humans exists between the two individuals, cells

[1] This work is supported by NIH grants AI-08439, AI-11576, CA-14520, and CA-16836 and National Foundation March of Dimes grant CRBS 246. This is paper No. 67 from Immunobiology Research Center and paper No. 1933 from Laboratory of Genetics, The University of Wisconsin, Madison, Wisconsin 53706.

of the recipient will respond to these foreign antigens on the cells of the donor by differentiating to blastlike cells, incorporating thymidine during DNA synthesis, and cell division. This response is thought to represent, at least in part, the similar morphological changes that are observed at the site of allograft rejection *in vivo*.

Lymphocytes are used both as the *responding* cells (of the potential recipient) and as the *stimulating* cells (of the potential donor) based on the following considerations. It has been shown by many workers that lymphocytes are the cells of prime import in the recognition of foreign histocompatibility antigens and that these cells can react to such antigens by the sequence described above. Further it has been demonstrated that lymphocytes carry the cell surface antigens that are associated with the major histocompatibility complex (MHC); they are thus used as the test cells reflecting the histocompatibility antigens which are carried by tissues to be transplanted. It should be noted that, whereas the lymphocytes thus represent a useful cell population for interaction, macrophages (or adherent cells) must be present in the MLC to allow the lymphocytes to interact.

Under many circumstances, such as kidney transplantation, we are interested in the response of the recipient as that recipient's immune system recognizes foreign antigens on the transplanted kidney; one would not consider the potential immunological response of the kidney donor as playing an important role in the potential rejection of that graft. As such, the one-way MLC test was developed in which the proliferative response of recipient lymphocytes as they recognize foreign histocompatibility antigens on the lymphocytes of the donor could be measured independently of the potential response of donor lymphocytes to recipient foreign histocompatibility antigens. This was achieved in the following manner. Since the assay of the MLC test, which has been used in the vast majority of laboratories, is to study the incorporation of radioactive thymidine into the responding cells, donor lymphocytes were treated with agents, such as mitomycin C or X-irradiation, which would prevent the replication of DNA in those cells yet allow them to express their antigens. Thus in an MLC, recipient cells, e.g., A (a mixture of lymphocytes and monocytes), were mixed with cells of the potential donor, e.g., B, treated with either mitomycin C or X-irradiation. In such a mixture, designated AB_m or AB_x, the only cells that could incorporate radioactive thymidine were cells of the recipient. The mitomycin C-treated or X-irradiated cells are referred to as the stimulating cells.

Data accumulated in family studies suggested very strongly that the only genetic region in humans that could lead to stimulation in the MLC test, if different in two individuals, was the HLA complex. As detailed previously in *Clinical Immunobiology*, Volume 1, and in a chapter by Albert in this volume, one assay of this region is to measure the serologically defined (SD) antigens of HLA. Whereas many workers initially assumed that stimulation in the MLC test was a reflection of disparity for these SD antigens, evidence accumulating during the last few years in humans, as well as studies in mouse, suggest that the SD system determines cell surface antigens which can be recognized by serological methods and that the antigens are present on essentially all tissues of the body; stimulation in the MLC test is primarily determined by genetic differences of a lymphocyte-defined (LD) locus (loci), which is genetically separable from the SD loci. A map of the HLA region indicating these different loci is presented in Fig. 1. Whereas it is not clear that the SD antigens (HLA-A, -B, and -C) cannot lead to low-level proliferation in MLC tests, and it may well be that the LD differences (HLA-D) can be recognized serologically, we will for purposes of this discussion separate the HLA complex into the LD and SD systems.

The recognition that the MLC test is under control of the same genetic region as the SD antigens and yet depends on differences at loci that are separable from those determining the SD antigens, made the test

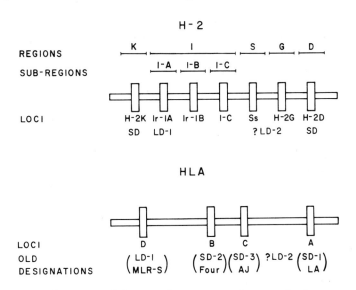

Fig. 1. Major histocompatibility complex: mouse and man. The four mapped loci of human leukocyte system A (HLA) are given with the new terminology (HLA-A, -B, -C, and -D) and the old designations. The A, B, and C loci and their phenotypic product are referred to as the serologically defined (SD) system; the HLA-D locus is the LD locus. The loci determining the Ia-like (or B cell) antigens have not been formally mapped.

potentially complementary to the information obtained by studies defining the SD antigens.

In this context the MLC test, representing the LD approach to histocompatibility testing, attempts to define compatibility between two individuals based on the degree of difference at the HLA-D locus (loci). Ideally, a donor should be identical for the HLA LD loci; less ideally a donor should be chosen whose cells stimulate the lymphocytes of the recipient to a lesser extent than those of another donor.

II. Methods

The methods most commonly used for the MLC test at the present time attempt to conserve on the number of cells needed to obtain results. In addition, a number of technical modifications have been introduced to save time needed to perform the assay. Although several different assays are in use, we will limit our description in this article to one method which involves the use of microtiter plates in each well of which a total of 0.2 ml of culture medium and cells are employed. The cultures are labeled at the end of the incubation period with radioactive thymidine, and the counts per minute incorporated into the responding cells are assessed by use of a multiple automated sample harvester (Otto Hiller, Madison, Wisconsin).

Either defibrinated or heparizined peripheral blood is drawn from the subjects to be studied, and the lymphocyte–monocyte preparation is obtained in one of several ways, most commonly by spinning the cells on a Ficoll-Hypaque gradient, which allows the red blood cells and polymorphonuclear leukocytes to sediment to the bottom of the gradient and retains the lymphocytes and monocytes at the interface. Responding cells (from the potential recipient) are suspended in tissue culture medium TC 199 (a number of different media can be used) containing human plasma or serum. The stimulating cells are treated either with mitomycin C or X-irradiation and then mixed with the responding cells.

In the microtiter plates in which each well contains a total of 0.2 ml, the usual number of responding lymphocytes per well is 1×10^5 with an equal number of stimulating cells. Several points are of importance here. First, although this number of responding and stimulating cells is adequate to give a response if the responding cell donor and the stimulating cell donor differ for HLA, there are some cases where minimal disparity exists which may not be seen using these numbers of cells. Thus, to assure MLC identity it is wise, in cases where no stimulation is seen at the numbers of cells mentioned above, to test the same individuals using 2×10^5 and 4×10^5 stimulating cells. Second, to test whether a case of nonresponse is a reflection of true HLA identity or may be due to technical problems, it is important to do the following controls. If a mixture AB_m does not show any stimulation, one must, in the same experiment using the same experimental conditions, show that the cells of individual A can respond to the cells of an unrelated individual X in the MLC, AX_m, and that the mitomycin C-treated cells of B can stimulate in a mixture XB_m.

The usual MLC tests are assayed on day 4 or day 5 by studying the incorporation of radioactive thymidine into the mixture. In some sensitive systems it is possible to show differences in thymidine incorporation as early as day 3 between an allogeneic mixture (AB_m) and the control isogeneic one (e.g., AA_m). This is still a very long period of time when considering the time available for, let us say, renal allografting from a cadaver donor. Some investigators have thus attempted to develop more rapid assays of the MLC reaction; most of these have used the incorporation of radioactive amino acids into the culture. Although these methods have not been extensively tested, it appears that one can obtain significant stimulation as early as 24 hours after the initiation of culture, although it is not clear whether under these conditions significant stimulation is seen with mixtures which are, by thymidine incorporation on day 5, only minimally (although significantly) MLC disparate.

One of the major uses for the MLC test has been to assess HLA LD identity. As such the question has frequently been raised in the past how to define nonstimulation in MLC. Given the present technology, it would seem to us that this will rarely be a problem (as will be illustrated in some of the family data to be presented in the next section). If multiple doses of stimulating cells are used in a sensitive microculture system, zero stimulation is easily distinguished from low levels of stimulation in the vast majority of cases. Two statistical approaches are sound: first, to test the mixture in question several times and ask, using nonparametric statistics, whether the counts per minute of tritiated thymidine incorporated into the allogeneic mixture are greater than those in the isogeneic control a significant percentage of the times tested; second, to convert the raw counts per minute incorporated to log values and then test whether a significant difference exists by a t test.

The second, and probably much more widely used, aspect of MLC testing is the attempt to quantify the amount of stimulation found between two individuals. Most important in performing such tests are (1) to use numbers of test cells that are not inhibitory (i.e., not too many stimulating or responding cells), (2) to assay the MLC on a day when there is still a log-linear increase in the number of counts per minute incorporated when plotting the counts per minute against the day of assay, and (3) to have some standard against which to measure the response.

The first two of the requirements listed have been discussed in extenso in some of the references given at the end of this chapter; the standard against which to compare the counts per minute incorporated into a given allogeneic mixture on a given day has only more recently become available, and needs extensive further testing; its potential usefulness encourages us to include it in this chapter despite the preliminary nature of some of the findings.

III. Results

A. FAMILY STUDIES

The data from an MLC experiment testing a large family is given in Table I. Two major points are apparent. First, siblings within the family who have inherited the same HLA chromosomes from their parents as determined by HLA SD typing (see *Clinical Immunobiology*, Volume 1 and chapter by Albert in this volume) do not stimulate each other in MLC. These are the classical HLA identical, MLC identical siblings. We now recognize that this is a reflection of HLA LD identity and tells us relatively little about HLA SD, except that in the case of siblings we would expect that in approximately 99/100 cases, HLA LD identity will also mean HLA SD identity. Second, it has been extensively documented

TABLE I

RESULTS OF MIXED LEUKOCYTE CULTURE (MLC) TESTS ON SIBLINGS
TESTED IN ONE-WAY CULTURE IN ALL COMBINATIONS

Responding cells	Stimulating cells						
	Am	Bm	Cm	Dm	Em	Fm	Gm
A	(43)	35	−9	2426	1737	11340	1685
B	57	(95)	14	2846	1623	4695	1165
C	22	23	(17)	1672	1763	1193	1284
D	2055	2365	1970	(25)	13	392	746
E	8663	5743	12815	56	(52)	2431	515
F	4251	5030	6989	1554	1138	(89)	1325
G	1505	1253	1649	472	432	263	(33)

that siblings who differ by only one HLA haplotype stimulate each other less in MLC than those siblings who differ by two HLA haplotypes. This is still the most direct and strongest evidence that the MLC test can be meaningfully quantitated, since one would expect that siblings differing by two haplotypes will have a greater immunogenetic disparity than those differing by only one haplotype, or parent–child combinations which in the great majority of cases will also differ by only one haplotype.

Thus, from family studies two findings emerge that are of prime importance in MLC studies and have direct usefulness in clinical testing using the MLC test. MLC identity is most clearly defined in siblings inheriting the same HLA haplotypes from their parents; these siblings, as will be discussed later, are the ideal donors for kidney transplantation and the only donors presently used in any numbers for bone marrow transplantation. Further, it is possible to define different degrees of HLA LD disparity using the MLC test.

It is within-family studies that the strongest evidence for the existence of an HLA LD locus separable for the HLA SD loci has been obtained.

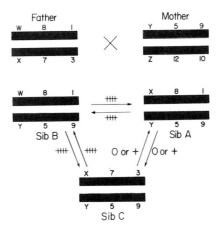

Fig. 2. Schema of the human leukocyte system A (HLA) including the HLA-D locus. Presumed major histocompatibility complex (MHC) chromosomes in a human family. The numbers refer to the HLA SD antigens of the A and B loci; the letters, to presumed alleles of the D locus. The one parent carries a 1, 8 W and a 3, 7 X haplotype; the other parent carries a 9, 5 Y and 10, 12 Z haplotype. Two siblings who inherit the same HLA SD loci alleles—and thus the same HLA SD antigens—can differ for the D locus secondary to a recombinational event in one of the parents. In this particular case, a recombinational event in the first parent resulted in a 1, 8, X haplotype. These two siblings thus stimulate in MLC. The + signs refer to MLC stimulation in a quantitative sense.

Hypothetical results that reflect the findings in a large number of families now studied and demonstrating the separation of the HLA LD locus from the SD loci is shown in Fig. 2. It should be noted that child A carries a recombinant chromosome from the father. The child has inherited that portion of the HLA chromosome which determines the SD antigens, which has also been inherited by child B. However, owing to a recombinational event in the father, child A has inherited the HLA LD locus from the other chromosome in the father. Thus children A and B are HLA SD identical but differ for the HLA LD locus. The resulting strong MLC activation demonstrates the importance of the LD locus in this regard. Most critical for this model are the MLC test results between child A and child C. These two children have inherited different SD haplotypes but, on the basis of the recombinant chromosome carried by child A, are HLA LD identical. In these instances there is little or no MLC stimulation between such siblings, providing strong support for the differential role of LD antigens and SD antigens in activating the MLC proliferative response.

B. Studies in the Unrelated Population

Most unrelated individuals differ for their HLA LD antigens as evidenced by reciprocal stimulation in one-way MLC tests between such individuals. Unrelated individuals who carry the same HLA SD antigens are in certain instances also HLA LD identical. This is true, however, only in a small percentage of individuals identical for their SD antigens. An occasionally unrelated pair have been found who are identical for their LD antigens while differing for the SD antigens.

If a single responder is tested against a large panel of stimulating cell donors (in analogy with a recipient being tested for response to a large panel of potential donors), large differences in the amount of response can be seen. This finding is demonstrated in Table II, in which certain values are chosen from 20 different mixtures that were tested with cells of individual A used as the responding cell donor. To the extent that the amount of stimulation in the MLC test reflects immunogenetic disparity for the HLA LD locus, these findings would suggest that great variability exists. This will be an important point in our discussion below of the role of MLC testing in clinical transplantation. Clearly the objective for clinical testing is to choose a donor who is either HLA LD identical or only minimally disparate with the recipient.

TABLE II
RANGE OF MIXED LEUKOCYTE
CULTURE (MLC)
INCOMPATIBILITY IN THE
UNRELATED POPULATION

$AA_m{}^a$	386^b
AB_m	491
AC_m	7312
AD_m	28401
AE_m	86922

^{a} AA_m is the control MLC; individuals B through E are unrelated to individual A. Individual B is obviously either identical for the MLC antigens or very similar.

^{b} Counts per minute.

C. A Standard Stimulating Cell

One of the major problems that has existed in applying the MLC test to clinical problems has concerned the evaluation of the amount of stimulation found in a given culture. The same two individuals tested on different days in MLC may stimulate each other to apparently different extents as assayed by the counts per minute of radioactive thymidine incorporated into the cultures. An attempt to circumvent this problem has been the use of "standard stimulating cells" that provide a "standard" with which to compare the counts per minute found in a given allogeneic mixture.

The standard stimulating cell used in our laboratory consists of a pool of twenty different stimulating cells chosen at random. The rationale for adopting this approach is that the twenty stimulating cells will represent most of the different HLA LD specificities found in the population and will thus, for any given responding cell, provide a maximal or near-maximal response for that cell on a given day. Whereas the response of cells of a given individual to the stimulus provided by the standard stimulating cell may once again vary from day to day in terms of the counts per minute of radioactive thymidine incorporated into the cultures, the relationship between the counts per minute incorporated on a given day in response to the standard stimulating cell and those incorporated in response to a given allogeneic cell may remain a constant from day to day. That this is in fact the case is illustrated in Fig. 3.

Cells from a single responder were tested against a number of different allogeneic stimulating cells as well as a pooled standard stimulating cell

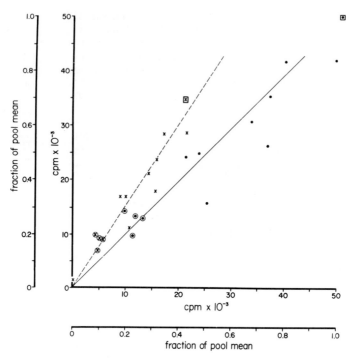

Fig. 3. The data presented in this figure represent results of mixed leukcoyte culture (MLC) experiments plotted in two different ways. In each experiment the response of cells of one individual are tested against 12 different allogeneic stimulating cells as well as a "standard stimulating cell." These same cell combinations are tested on the two different days. The results, in counts per minute of tritiated thymidine incorporated, on the two different days are plotted on the abscissa and ordinate, respectively. Each cross gives the values for a given allogeneic mixture for the 2 days of testing. The four crosses with a circle around them represent mixtures in which the two individuals are identical for the human leukocyte system A serologically defined (HLA SD) antigens (Bach and van Rood, 1975; HLA-LD Workshop, 1975; Segall and Bach, 1976; Dausset *et al.*, 1974); the cross with the square around it represents the value obtained with the standard stimulating cell on the two different days. The dotted line is a regression line for all values excluding the standard stimulating cell. The black dots represent the same experimental mixtures, again plotted on the two different days of the experiment, however this time expressed as a fraction of the counts per minute obtained with the standard stimulating cell. The standard stimulating cell is plotted as 1 in each of the experiments. The value of using three points is illustrated: (1) the lower MLC activation seen with some HLA haplotypes when the donors of the responding and stimulating cells, respectively, are identical for their HLA SD antigens; (2) the reproducibility of the test system; (3) a standard stimulating cell for expressing the amount of stimulation seen in any one allogeneic mixture, as discussed in the text. X, Counts per minute; ●, fraction of pool mean. (From Segall and Bach, 1976. © 1976 The Williams & Wilkins Co., Baltimore.)

on two different days. Most important is the finding that there is a highly significant correlation between the response of the individual's cells to a given allogeneic stimulating cell as compared with the response to the standard stimulating cell on one day as compared with a similar set of cultures tested on the second day.

It would thus appear that the use of standard stimulating cells provide a constant, in that the amount of stimulation found in any allogeneic mixture may be expressed as a fraction of that constant. Osoba and Falk have used a somewhat different approach to the development of a standard stimulating cell, however, with the same general rationale for its use.

D. Definition of HLA LD Determinants

Two different cellular approaches have been used to define the HLA LD determinants. First, homozygous typing cells that are either genotypically or phenotypically homozygous for the HLA-D locus have been used as stimulating cells in the MLC. The basis for using homozygous typing cells has been that responding cells of an individual carrying the HLA LD haplotype of the homozygous typing cell will not respond to that typing cell; a high degree of sharing of the HLA LD determinants between the responding cell and the homozygous typing cell will lead to markedly reduced response.

Results of experiments using the homozygous typing cells in an international workshop have suggested that six different "clusters" of LD determinants can be defined and that, on the basis of worldwide collaboration, several different homozygous cells exist to define each of these clusters. Whether the LD clusters defined are each made up of several different LD determinants is not clear, but it is suggested by the types of analysis discussed below with the PLT test. Results of one experiment using a series of homozygous typing cells defining the DW2 "cluster" are given in Table III. It is clear that some unrelated individuals respond very little to these homozygous typing cells whereas cells of others respond very strongly. The approach of using homozygous typing cells will clearly yield valuable information regarding the LD phenotype of any given individual, although it may turn out to be a relatively crude measure of that phenotype.

Second, lymphocytes primed *in vitro* to the LD determinants associated with a given HLA haplotype have been used in terms of their "secondary response," *in vitro* to define HLA LD determinants. This test has been termed the primed LD typing, or PLT, test. The basis of the PLT test is

TABLE III
PRIMARY MIXED LEUKOCYTE CULTURE (MLC) WITH
HOMOZYGOUS CELLS[a]

Responding cells	Stimulating cells	
	HB (DW2/DW2)	RR (DW2/DW2)
NK (DW2 neg.)	42,030	21,057
BB (DW2 neg.)	79,713	41,223
BKJ (DW2 hetero.)	11,185	6,202
MT (DW2 hetero.)	4,863	3,251
RR (DW2 homo.)	1,073	364
HB (DW2 homo.)	667	447

PLT–HTC CORRELATION[b]

Restimulating cells	Responding PLT
	$\left[\begin{array}{c} \text{Primary MLC A (RR)}_m \\ \text{(DW2 neg.)(DW2 homo.)}_m \end{array} \right]$
A (DW2 neg.)	588
BB (DW2 neg.)	3,097
BKJ (DW2 hetero.)	13,059
MT (DW2 hetero.)	12,997
RR (DW2 homo.)	20,778
KJ (DW2 homo.)	21,110

[a] Data obtained in collaboration with Drs. Thompson and Svegaard.
[b] PLT, primed LD typing; HTC, homozygous typing cells.

the following. Lymphocytes stimulated in MLC with allogeneic cells differing by single HLA haplotype, and left beyond their peak proliferative phase, can be restimulated 9–14 days after primary "sensitization" in MLC. In contrast to the relatively slow response seen in a primary MLC, where little significant thymidine incorporation is detected until 48 or even 72 hours after the initiation of culture, the "primed" lymphocytes will show an accelerated response to the LD antigens associated with the "priming" haplotype, a response that can be detected by studying thymidine incorporation within 24 hours or by studying the incorporation of other radioactive labels, such as uridine, within a few hours after initiation of the secondary response.

The preliminary data available with the PLT test suggest that the proliferation seen after restimulation (1) is dependent on the degree of HLA LD sharing between the initial MLC-sensitizing (stimulating) cell and the restimulating cell; (2) is a reflection of disparity at the major histocompatibility complex and does not measure factors determined by genes outside the HLA complex; and (3) can be used to define specific HLA LD determinants. A correlative study using homozygous typing cells and PLT is given in Table III.

An example of an experiment using the PLT test to look for an unrelated donor whose cells are compatible with the cells of a given patient is given in Table IV. Two different PLT cells are developed within the

TABLE IV
PRIMED LD TYPE (PLT) MATCHING[a]

	PLT cells vs. haplotypes of patient	
Haplotype recognized MLC combination	d $bc(cd)_m$	a $bc(ac)_m$
Restimulating cells		
Fx		
ab	6061	4636
father		
Mx		
cd	9185	3423
mother		
Sx		
bc	461	353
sister		
Bx		
ac	5233	3313
brother		
L	8450	3675
Y	2764	2021
Q	9715	3935
R	940	961

[a] The patient carried haplotypes a (from the father) and d (from the mother). The anti-d PLT cell was produced by sensitizing cells of a sister (carrying the b and c haplotype) to cells of the mother (carrying the c and d haplotype) as shown. The anti-a PLT is also shown. The two PLT cells were restimulated with cells of the father, mother, sister, brother, and four unrelated individuals (L, Y, Q, and R). Note that cells of L and Q appear to carry LD antigens of the d haplotype (their cells restimulate as much as those of the mother) as well as being a good match for the a haplotype. All four unrelated individuals were HLA-B identical with the patient.

family of the patient. These two cells are used to define the two HLA haplotypes of the patient. Cells of a series of unrelated individuals are used to restimulate these two PLT cells. Presumably any unrelated individual sharing the LD determinants of the patient would restimulate these two PLT cells to approximately the same degree as do the cells of the patient. In fact, individuals L and Q do restimulate to approximately the same degree as do cells of the initial sensitizing individual. Both the homozygous typing cell approach and the PLT approach are valuable in that "compatibility" as determined by these procedures is predictive of a low primary MLC—the definition of HLA LD compatibility.

In addition to these two cellular approaches, evidence has recently been obtained by van Rood and his collaborators, and subsequently several other laboratories, that genes of the HLA complex determine cell surface antigens that are detectable serologically but have a markedly different tissue distribution from the HLA SD antigens. These antigens have not been given a formal designation, but are referred to either as HLA "Ia-like" antigens or "B-cell" antigens. It may be that antisera directed at these antigens will be useful in defining the LD determinants although this has not been definitively established at the present time.

IV. Clinical Usefulness of Mixed Leukocyte Culture Testing

It has been mentioned that there is evidence from several sources that HLA LD compatibility is of prime importance in determining the success of any bone marrow transplant and appears to influence the survival of kidney grafts. In addition, as reviewed in this volume by Albert, there appears to be a stronger association between certain HLA LD determinants and given diseases (such as multiple sclerosis) than between the HLA SD antigens and that same disease. The methods of determining LD compatibility by MLC testing, or the more recent approaches to the direct definition of the HLA LD determinants, can therefore be used for these various problems.

For transplantation purposes one would ideally look for the HLA LD identical individual, i.e., no stimulation in a primary MLC test. Such an individual could be found following homozygous typing cell or PLT testing in the unrelated population. If an HLA LD identical individual is not found, then a minimum amount of HLA LD disparity is presumably most desirable. How much disparity can be allowed before unwanted clinical results evolve in a given transplant situation is not well established.

To define the specific HLA LD determinants with homozygous typing cells or PLT testing will no doubt lead to extensive testing of a number of disease states. The questions regarding both the genetic complexity (? the number of loci involved in coding for the LD determinants and the polymorphism at each of these loci) and the antigenic complexity (? the number of determinants associated with a single haplotype) has yet to be determined. Preliminary data suggest that great complexity will exist.

V. Addendum

This chapter has reviewed the MLC test as a method of determining HLA LD disparity. It has not included the other tests of cell-mediated immunity that relate to HLA antigens other than the HLA LD antigens. Primary among these tests is the cell-mediated lympholysis (CML) test, which appears to use the HLA SD antigens, or the phenotypic products of loci very closely linked to those determining the SD antigens, as the targets for cytotoxic T lymphocytes. The extent to which CML testing will be useful in clinical histocompatibility is yet to be determined.

References

Bach, F. H., Sondel, P. M., Sheehy, M. J., Wank, B. J., and Bach, M. L. (1975). In "Histocompatibility Testing 1975" (F. Kissmeyer-Nielsen, ed.), pp. 576–580. Munksgaard, Copenhagen.

Bach, F. H., and Bach, M. L. (1972). In "Clinical Immunobiology" (F. H. Bach and R. A. Good, eds.), Vol. I, pp. 157–178. Academic Press, New York.

Bach, F. H., and van Rood, J. J. (1976). N. Engl. J. Med. (in press).

Dausset, J., Hors, J., Busson, M., Festenstein, H., Oliver, R. T. D., Sach, J. A., and Paris, A. M. I. (1974). N. Engl. J. Med. 18, 979.

Eijsvoogel, V. P., du Bois, M. J. G. J., Melief, C. J. H., De Groot-Kooy, M. L., Koning, C., van Rood, J. J., van Leeuwen, A., du Toit, E. D., and Schellekens, P. T. A. (1973). In "Histocompatibility Testing 1972" (J. Dausset and J. Colombani, eds.), pp. 501–508. Munksgaard, Copenhagen.

Eijsvoogel, V. P., du Bois, M. J. G. J., Melief, C. H., and Kooy, L. (1973). Transplant. Proc. 5, 1301.

Osoba, D., and Falk, J. (1974). Cell. Immunol. 10, 117.

Segall, M., and Bach, F. H. (1976). Transplantation 22, 79.

Sheehy, M. J., Sondel, P. M., Bach, M. L., Wank, R., and Bach, F. H. (1975). Science 188, 1308–1310.

Thorsby, E., and Piazza, A. (eds.) (1976). In "Histocompatibility Testing 1975" (F. Kissmeyer-Nielsen, ed.), pp. 414–458. Munksgaard, Copenhagen.

van Rood, J. J. (1974). Semin. Hematol. 11, No. 3, 253–262.

van Rood, J. J., and Ceppellini, R. (1974). Semin. Hematol. 11, No. 3, 233–251.

The Reticuloendothelial System

W. F. CUNNINGHAM-RUNDLES

Memorial Sloan-Kettering Cancer Center, New York, New York

I. Introduction

The reticuloendothelial system (RES) is closely involved in the immune response. Macrophages, the cells of the RES, come into contact with antigens and modify it for effective presentation to lymphocytes. In response to this presentation, the lymphocytes may respond with secretion of specific antibodies or with production of lymphokines, whose effects are not antigen-specific. These lymphokines may attract other macrophages equipped to phagocytize, enzymically destroy, or merely further metabolize the original antigen. The function of the RES has classically been assessed by measuring phagocytosis of colloids; recently more specific functions of macrophages have been measured.

[1] This study was supported by Grants CA-08748-09 and CA-05826 of the National Cancer Institute.

II. Clearance Testing

The RES is composed of varieties of macrophages, which are derived from peripheral monocytes. Of the macrophages, 85% are hepatic, namely, Küpffer cells, 10% are splenic (spleen histiocytes), 2% are bone marrow macrophages, and the remainder are specific tissue phagocytes, such as the alveolar macrophages and the wandering tissue macrophages. When a colloid such as India ink (carbon) is injected intravenously in experimental animals the degree of phagocytosis by tissue macrophages depends upon (1) the degree to which each phagocyte is exposed to colloid, (2) the type and size particles of colloid, (3) the existence of specific and nonspecific opsonins for the colloid, and, (4) the number and functional state of the phagocytes. Classical experiments of Biozzi and Benacerraf indicated that at low concentrations of colloid, the variable factor in phagocytosis is the degree of perfusion of macrophage-rich beds such as the liver. At higher concentrations, uptake has been related to the number and functional state of tissue macrophages. For instance, when India ink is injected into the venous circulation of the mouse, the material disappears exponentially as judged by colorimetric measurement of the concentration of ink in the blood (Fig. 1).

If C_1 = concentration at $T = 1$ and C_2 = concentration at $T = 2$, then one can calculate a constant

$$K = (C_2 - C_1)/(T_2 - T_1)$$

And where $T_{1/2}$ is the time required for the concentration to drop by one-half,

$$K = \frac{\ln 2}{T_{1/2}}$$

since the disappearance is exponential with respect to time. At low concentrations, K is very large because the material disappears rapidly into the highly vascularized liver. At high concentrations, however, K becomes much lower, then becomes constant; this has been said to reflect the peak

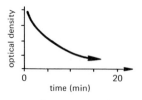
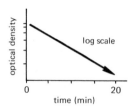

Fig. 1. Colorimetric measurement in mouse blood of the concentration of India ink injected into the venous circulation.

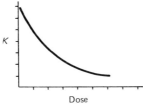

Fig. 2. Decrease of K, with increase in concentration until the value of K becomes constant, probably at the peak capacity of phagocytic function of the animal.

capacity of phagocytic function of the animal (Fig. 2), since higher doses of colloid are not absorbed. Thus, high concentrations of colloid are necessary for gauging RES phagocytosis.

In humans, the feasibility of such a test becomes dependent upon the dose of a particular colloid that can be given safely. To circumvent this potential problem, Iio and Wagner have suggested that one may extrapolate from the "K" derived from low doses of colloid to the constant that would be derived at higher, more toxic concentrations. By considering colloid–macrophage interaction in the same manner as the enzyme-substrate kinetics of Michaelis and Menten, they calculated the formula

$$\frac{1}{K} \cdot \frac{1}{D} = \frac{K_3}{K_1} \cdot \frac{1}{V_{max}} \cdot \frac{1}{D} + \frac{1}{V_{max}}$$

where K_1 = rate of phagocytosis; K_3 = rate of secretion of metabolized colloid; and D = dose of colloid. Since, as before $K = \ln 2/T_{1/2} = K_1$, one can plot $1/K_1 \cdot 1/D[f(x)]$ versus $1/D[f(y)]$, and in this graphic determination, the Y intercept is equal to $1/V_{max}$, or the reciprocal of the rate of phagocytosis at infinite dose. Despite theoretical objections to this type of analysis, the formula remains the best means of deriving meaningful data in human colloid clearance tests. A large number of materials have been used as shown in Table I. With each of the materials, the same basic technique is used. A certain dose of colloid is injected intravenously, and after 2–5 minutes of mixing time, blood concentrations of colloid are measured for 15–30 minutes. The $T_{1/2}$, K, or V_{max} derived from these tests varies with the material used.

Of the two materials used, macroaggregated albumin (MAA) and lipofundin-S, clearly the MAA is less toxic. At present, MAA is not available commercially in the United States, and lipofundin-S has just become so. A material available for liver–spleen scanning in the United States, sulfur colloid, is nontoxic, but unfortunately our own results suggest that extremely large volumes are necessary to obtain low "K" values reflecting phagocytosis (rather than liver blood flow).

TABLE I

VALUES DERIVED BY FORMULA FROM HUMAN COLLOID CLEARANCE TESTS[a]

Material	Means of measuring blood concentration	Advantage	Disadvantage	Dose (mg/kg)	Condition	$T_{1/2}$ (min)	V_{max} (mg/kg/min)	Author
Lipofundin-S (soy oil, soy phosphatide, xylite, cottonseed oil)	Serum turbidity	—	Primary hypersensitivity, especially in patients with lung pathology	150	Normal	5.0 ± 1.2	—[b]	Lemperle et al. (1900)
				150	Shock	14.2	—	
				150	Fever	9.0	—	
				150	Diabetes	7.9	—	
				150	Uremia	7.2	—	
				150	Brain injury	5.0	—	
				150	Fluothane, barbiturate	6.5	—	
				150	Post-fluothane, post-barbiturate	2.0	—	
				150	Carcinoma	2.0	—	
				150	Appendicitis	1.3	—	
Macroaggregated albumin (MAA)	Serum ^{131}I	Nonantigenic, nontoxic	No longer available in U.S.	5	Normal	6.0	—	Palmer et al. (1971)
				5	Leukemia, acute and chronic	6.2	—	
				5	Azathiaprine	7.0		
				5	Normal	4.2 ± 14.3%	1.07	Iio and Wagner (1963)
				2	Normal	5.9 ± 11.9	1.07	
				5	Pneumococcal pneumonia	4.4-4.8	1.82	

5	Day 10, experimental typhoid fever	4.3–5	1.50	
5	Day 5, experimental sand fly fever	7.5–8	—	
5	Days, tularemia	4.5–5	1.50	Berken and Sherman (1972)
2.5	Olive oil ingestion	Reduced	—	Cooksley (1973)
5	Normal	8.5 ± 0.6	—	
5	Acute infections and alcoholic hepatitis	7.4 ± 1.3	—	
5	Cirrhosis	10.2 ± 3.0	—	
5	Normal	—	—	Magarey and Baum (1900)
5	Large primary tumor	Elevated	—	
5	Distant severe metastatic disease	Elevated	—	
5	Cytoxan, 5-FU, radiotherapy	Elevated	—	
5	Small tumors, negative lymph nodes	Reduced	—	
5	Stilbestrol, estradiol	Reduced	—	
5	Chronic infection	Elevated	—	

(Continued)

TABLE I (Continued)

Material	Means of measuring blood concentration	Advantage	Disadvantage	Dose (mg/kg)	Condition	$T_{1/2}$ (min)	V_{max} (mg/ kg/min)	Author
Carbon (India ink)	Colorimeter	Volume of data in the mouse	Severe prolonged RES depression; probably carcinogenic	—	—	—	—	—
[³²p]Chromium phosphate	Blood radioactivity	—	Human pharmacology not known; remains indefinitely in macrophages	—	—	—	—	—

[a] For details of formula calculations, see text. 5-FU, 5-fluorouracil.
[b] — = Not calculated by authors.

Even more important are theoretical objections. Many investigators have felt that extrapolation from the clearance rates measured at low doses of colloid to that at higher doses may not be valid. Aside from this argument are classical problems that have recently been resolved. When large doses of colloid are given to an animal, further doses may not be absorbed at all. This had been ascribed to "saturation" or "blockade" of the cells of the RES. More recently, it has been shown that serum opsonins mediate the uptake of colloid by the RES, and that the uptake may be higher or lower depending upon the serum levels of opsonins. The opsonins have been shown to be α_2-globulins, and indeed deficiency has been described in premature infants. Thus, data derived from previous experimentation may well be descriptive only of the concentration of serum opsonins under certain circumstances, rather than of changes in the functional level of the RES per se.

III. Rebuck Skin Windows

Attempts at measurements of RES function are now being made by direct evaluation of the cellular components. A classic means is the Rebuck skin window, which is a semiquantitative test that describes the relative numbers of polymorphonuclear (PMN) leukocytes and mononuclear phagocytes in an abraded area. In this test, a small area of an individual's skin is abraded to the dermis and a cover slip is taped over the site. At intervals, the cover slip is removed, stained, and replaced with a fresh slip. The cells on the slips are identified and counted. A graph of cell types versus time may then be constructed (Fig. 3).

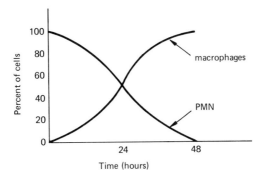

Fig. 3. Graph of cell types versus time constructed from counts of cells made by the Rebuck skin window test. PMN, polymorphonuclear leukocytes.

Characteristically PMN leukocytes and mononuclear phagocytes are the two cell types present, yet occasionally other cell types are seen. Results in a variety of clinical situations are shown in Table II. The factors underlying this series of events are under investigation.

IV. Cellular Studies

Evaluation of the cellular components of the RES has been hampered by the lack of suitable macrophage preparations. Recently, however, techniques have been devised for the isolation of certain macrophages and of macrophage precursors.

A. PULMONARY MACROPHAGES

Human alveolar macrophages have been isolated according to a technique devised by Finley *et al.* (1967). A small balloon-tipped catheter or a bronchoscope is introduced into a bronchus under local anesthesia, and the balloon is inflated. Saline, 100 ml, is injected into the catheter and subsequently removed by suction. The resulting wash contains approximately 8×10^7 pulmonary cells of which 90–95% are viable macrophages morphologically and functionally. After isolation of the macrophages, a variety of assays can be performed.

1. Phagocytosis. This is basically a variation of an assay devised for leukocytes. Macrophages are incubated at a ratio of 5 cells to 1 bacterium with a viable culture of bacteria (such as *Staphylococcus* 502A) in the presence of 15–20% serum. At the beginning and the end of incubation, aliquots of the mixture are taken and streaked on agar plates and colony counts are made.

The results are graphed (Fig. 4), and the results are expressed as

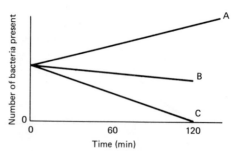

Fig. 4. Graph of results of phagocytosis assay from human alveolar macrophages. Curves: A, phagocytosis absent, bacteria grow normally; B, reduced phagocytosis; C, normal phagocytosis.

TABLE II

PRESENCE AND TIMING OF CELL TYPES IN VARIOUS CLINICAL SITUATIONS[a]

Condition	Macrophages		PMNs		Others	Comments
	Timing	Numbers	Timing	Numbers		
ALL, remission	N	N	—	—	—	—
ALL, relapse	D	↓	—	—	—	—
ALL with 6-mercaptopurine	D	↓	—	—	—	Proportional to amount of chemotherapy
All with methotrexate	D	↓	—	—	—	Reduced effect if given intermittently
Actinomycin D	D	↓↓	—	—	—	—
Cytoxan	N	N	—	—	—	—
5-FU	N	N	—	—	—	—
ACTH therapy	D	↓	N or D	—	—	—
CML, CLL untreated	D	↓ or ↑	—	—	—	—
Myeloma	N	N	D	↓	—	—
Lymphosarcoma	D	↓↓	—	—	—	—
Advanced solid tumor	D	↓	—	—	—	
Cyclic neutropemia	—	↓	—	↓	—	PMS necessary for monocyte appearance
Irradiation (distant to site)	D	↓	—	—	—	—
↓ Complement	D	↓	↓	↓	—	—
↓ γ-Globulin	D	↓	—	—	—	—
Agent of delayed hypersensitivity	D	N	—	—	—	—
Denervation of skin window	N	N	P	P	Occasional	—
Eosinophilia	N	N	N	N	—	Proportional to degree of eosinophilia
Local histamine	N	N	N	N	Eosinophilia	—
Local bradykinin	N	N	N	N	Eosinophilia	—
Local serotonin	N	N	N	N	Eosinophilia	—
Felty's syndrome	N	N	N	N	Eosinophilia	—
Newborns	N	N	N	N	Eosinophilia	—
Premature infants	D	↓↓	D	↓↓	Eosinophilia	—
Heparin	D	↓↓	D	↓	—	—
Chediak-Higasi	D	N	D	N	—	—
Ulcerative colitis	N	N	N	N	Basophilia	—

[a] N, normal; D, delayed; P, prolonged; —, not described in literature; 5-FU, 5-fluorouracil; PMNs, polymorphonuclear leukocytes; CML, chronic myelogenous leukemia; CLL, chronic lymphocytic leukemia; ALL, acute lymphocytic leukemia.

number of bacteria present. If measurement of bactericidal activity is desired, each aliquot may be lysed in water prior to streaking so that phagocytized but viable bacteria are released. Diminished phagocytosis has been demonstrated in alveolar macrophages from smokers, although the actual numbers of macrophages are higher in smokers.

2. Glucose utilization may be measured by the formation of $^{14}CO_2$ from ^{14}C-labeled glucose in the medium. Macrophages of smokers have been shown to have a higher rate of glucose utilization than those of non-smokers.

3. Mitotic activity of pulmonary macrophages may be measured by measuring the incorporation of precursors into DNA. After incubation for 1 hour with ^3H-labeled thymidine, incorporation is assayed by radio-autography. Normally thymidine is incorporated by 1% of the cells; abnormalities have not been described. Pulmonary macrophages from a small number of patients with acute leukemia were reported as normal in this respect.

4. Aryl hydrocarbon hydrolase is an inducible enzyme that acts upon the carcinogenic polycyclic hydrocarbons. The activity of the enzyme can be measured by adding a hydrocarbon such as 3,4-DP and measuring spectrophotometrically the amount of 3-hydroxybenzo [a] pyrene produced. This enzyme has been shown to be present in elevated amounts in the pulmonary macrophages of smokers.

B. KUPFFER CELLS

These hepatic macrophages have been isolated from whole rabbit livers via Pronase digestion. Contamination by polymorphonuclear cells (10–15%) and hepatocytes (5%) is eliminated on the basis of stronger adherence of the macrophages to glass or plastic in the presence of serum. Phagocytosis of latex particles by these cells has been demonstrated. This technique has not yet been applied to human liver biopsy specimens.

C. SPLENIC MACROPHAGES

These cells can be isolated directly from splenic pulp on the basis of this strong adherence to glass and plastic. However, since splenic biopsy is rarely performed, splenic macrophages are usually not available for assay here.

D. Tissue Macrophages

A variation on the Rebuck skin window can be used for the isolation of macrophages as described by Southam and Levin (1966). After abrasion of forearm skin in an area of approximately 1 cm², sterile Sykes–Moore tissue culture chambers are cupped over the site and filled with culture medium. The culture medium is removed at regular intervals and replaced with fresh medium, such that at 48 hours the cell population consists mainly of macrophages isolated on the basis of glass adherence. Subsequently, the macrophages may be resuspended (by gentle agitation with a rubber spatula in 0.15% EDTA) for counting and incubated with bacteria for measurement of phagocytosis as described above. Magliulo *et al.* (1973) have presented evidence that macrophages from convalescent tuberculous patients may phagocytize more rapidly than control macrophages; this observation should be extended and confirmed.

E. Monocytes

Substantial evidence suggests that all cellular components of the reticuloendothelial system are derived from the peripheral blood monocyte. There is evidence that alveolar macrophages may proliferate independently, but presumably this mitotic activity contributes a lesser number of cells than replenishment by circulating monocytes. *In vitro*, the monocyte can phagocytize, and in culture these cells elongate and come to resemble typical macrophages. Thus at present considerable effort is being made in investigation of the monocyte.

These cells can be separated along with lymphocytes by density gradients. Originally Cohn and Hirsch described separation of these "mononuclear" cells on the basis of density by layering of the supernatant of dextran-sedimented blood on 28% albumin. Upon centrifugation, mononuclear cells form a band separate from denser polymorphonuclear cells. The mononuclear cells are aspirated and washed; monocytes are subsequently separated by glass adherence. More recently, dextran sedimentation and albumin gradients have been superseded by Ficoll–Hypaque (or Isopaque) gradients, which may be used to separate mononuclear cells from blood in one step. Monocytes can then be studied in a variety of ways.

1. Attachment rate. This study is performed using the mononuclear cell population. The concentration of monocytes is determined morphologically with a hemacytometer. The mononuclear cells are then incu-

bated in petri dishes with serum for a specific length of time, and the nonadherent cells are vigorously washed off. A known area within the petri dish is counted for number of adherent cells (monocytes) and calculation of the number of adherent monocytes per number of monocytes incubated is made. When monocytes of tuberculous patients receiving Rifampin were compared with monocytes from normal individuals, the proportion of adherent monocytes was found to be greater by 50% in the tuberculous patients.

2. Spreading activity. In the system described above under method 1, after monocytes have attached to a surface and have been incubated for 60–90 minutes, the cells are photographed. Subsequently, the areas covered by individual cells are calculated. One study has shown that the surface area of cells from the tuberculous patients as in method 1 is greater than that of controls. On the other hand, it has been shown that surface area varies considerably from cell to cell, and thus there may be considerable error. It can also be demonstrated that in the presence of tuberculin, the number of spreading cells is markedly diminished in tuberculin-positive individuals when compared with controls.

3. Monocytes can undergo phagocytosis, apparently mediated by immunoglobulin receptors on the surface of these cells. Phagocytosis is serum dependent and nonspecific. Bacteria and latex particles are rapidly absorbed whereas erythrophagocytosis occurs only sluggishly. Uptake of bacteria is measured as previously described whereas inert particles are scored visually. It can be shown that monocytes of patients with chronic granulomatous disease have the same metabolic defect as the polymorphonuclear leukocytes of such patients: phagocytosis is normal, but killing of catalase-positive organisms is poor. In contrast, monocytes from patients with Chediak–Higashi syndrome show normal phagocytosis and reduced killing of many organisims regardless of catalase activity. A poor killing capacity seems to be particularly evident in the first 20 minutes after phagocytosis. Poor monocyte phagocytosis occurs in myelomonocytic leukemia and lymphomas. A drug administered for leprosy, clofazimine, has been shown to increase monocyte phagocytosis of yeast. Monocytes from patients with sarcoidosis were shown to phagocytize greater numbers of yeast particles than control monocytes in one study.

4. Chemotaxis. Human monocytes can be assayed for response to chemotactic factors in an assay developed by Snyderman et al. (1972) from the method of Boyden. This assay uses mononuclear cells (i.e., lymphocytes and monocytes) derived from Ficoll–Hypaque density gradients. Two chambers are separated by a Millipore or similar filter; the upper chamber is filled with a test suspension of cells, and the lower with a chemotactic agent. After a period of time, the filter is removed

and mounted on a slide and the number of cells which have migrated completely through the filter is counted. The cells have been shown to be 95% typical monocytes. Known chemotactic agents include C'5A and the supernatant of phytohemagglutinin-stimulated mononuclear cells. A syndrome has been described in which a patient with chronic mucocutaneous candidiasis was found to have monocytes that failed to respond to these agents; this defect was reversible with transfer factor. In addition, it has been reported that patients treated with bacillus calmette-Guérin have elevated chemotaxis to C'5A.

The pulmonary macrophage is also responsive to this assay. The macrophages from smokers have been shown to be more responsive to chemotactic substances than those of normals.

5. Participation in the mixed leukocyte culture (MLC) reaction. Twomey and Sharkey (1972) have shown that monocytes or macrophages are necessary for the MLC reaction: Normally, if the mononuclear cells (lymphocytes and monocytes) of two individuals are mixed, a blastogenic response occurs in each set of lymphocytes. If the cells of A are mixed with the irradiated cells of B, then only the lymphocytes of A respond. Yet if the monocytes of A and B are absorbed out with glass wool or beads, the resulting cells, which are almost exclusively lymphocytes, will not respond. This monocyte function is detected in the scheme shown in Fig. 5. As shown, monocytes may be irradiated without loss of activity provided the concentration of monocytes in the reaction is not below 1%. Clearly, this variation of the MLC can detect monocyte deficiencies and also, by including serum in the reaction, can detect circulating monocyte inhibitors. Unfortunately, enhanced monocyte function cannot be demonstrated by this method. Poor monocyte function has been described in patients with herpes zoster, and other patients are now being investigated.

6. Colony-stimulating factor (CSF). This factor has been described by a number of different authors as a protein found in serum and urine which is capable of stimulating the formation of active colonies in bone marrow culture. Evidence has accumulated that monocytes are the circulating cells that produce this factor. Clinical situations in which concentration of CSF may be abnormal are now under study.

7. Migratory inhibitory factor (MIF). This soluble factor is produced by sensitized lymphocytes in response to the relevant antigen. In the classic assay, supernatants rich in MIF prevent normal migration of guinea pig peritoneal exudate cells from capillary tubes. The concentration of MIF is calculated as the degree of migration of cells compared to migration in culture medium.

Claussen (1973) has devised a variation on this assay. Agarose plates

L, l = pure lymphocytes

L + M, l + m = lymphocytes and monocytes (from Ficoll–Hypaque or via dextran and albumin gradient)

$(L + M)_x$, $(l + m)_x$ = irradiated L + M, etc.

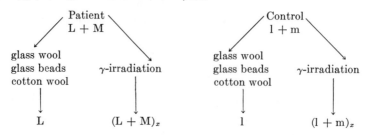

(1) L + l: No [³H]thymidine incorporation because monocytes are not present.

(2) L + $(l + m)_x$: [³H]thymidine incorporation if L, l, and m are normal.

(3) L + $(l + m)_x$: No [³H]thymidine incorporation if L cannot respond even when l and m are normal.

(4) $(L + M)_x$ + l: [³H]thymidine incorporation of M and l are normal.

(5) $(L + M)_x$ + l: No [³H]thymidine incorpration if M are deficient even when l are normal.

(6) If (2) and (5) are true and (1) is normal, then patient has normal lymphocytes and deficient monocytes.

Fig. 5. Scheme for detection of monocyte function.

supplemented with serum are allowed to harden, and subsequently 2.6-mm holes are punched in the material. Mononuclear cells, pure monocytes, or pulmonary macrophages are then suspended in MIF-rich supernatants or in solutions to be tested for MIF activity, and 7 μl of the material are placed in the cells. Over 24–48 hours the indicator cells migrate through the agarose, and by measuring with a planimeter the area of cells that have migrated, an indication of MIF activity or of indicator cell MIF responsiveness can be obtained.

This resting migratory activity of the pulmonary macrophages of smokers has been shown to be higher than that of controls, whereas the MIF response has been shown to be depressed. Monocytes of nonsmokers are the more responsive than those of smokers.

In summary, in recent years, measurement of reticuloendothelial function has progressed from assaying total body phagocytosis to evaluation of the *in vitro* functions of various distinct cell populations. Further research into macrophage function is clearly needed and will be rewarding.

References

Benacerraf, B., Biozzi, G., Halpern, B. N., Stiffel, C., and Mouton, D. (1957). *Brit. J. Exp. Pathol.* 38, 35–48.

Bennett, W. E., and Cohn, Z. A. (1966). *J. Exp. Med.* 123, 145–158.

Berken, A., and Sherman, A. A. (1972). *Proc. Soc. Exp. Biol. Med.* 141, 656–658.

Claussen, J. E. (1973). *J. Immunol.* 110, 546–551.

Cline, M. J., and Lehrer, R. J. (1968). *Blood* 32, 423–435.

Cooksley, W. G. (1973). *Brit. J. Haematol.* 25, 147–164.

Davis, W. C., Huber, H., Douglas, S. D., and Fudenberg, H. H. (1968). *J. Immunol.* 101, 1093–1095.

Dekaris, D., Silobrcic, V., Mazwian, R., and Kadrnka-Lovrencic, M. (1974). *Clin. Exp. Immunol.* 16, 311–320.

Finley, T. N., Swenson, E. W., Curran, W. S., Hubir, G. L., and Ladman, A. J. (1967). *Ann. Intern. Med.* 66, 651.

Golde, D. W., Finley, T. N., and Cline, M. J. (1974). *N. Engl. J. Med.* 290, 875–877.

Iio, M., and Wagner, H. N. (1963). *J. Clin. Invest.* 42, 417–434.

Jansa, P. (1973). *Folia Haemotol.* (*Leipzig*) 99, 121–130.

Lemperle, G., Reichelt, M., and Dink, S. (1971). *Advan. Exp. Med. Biol.* 15, 137–143.

Magarey, C. T., and Baum, M. (1970). *Brit. J. Surg.* 57, 748–752.

Magliulo, V., DeFeo, V., Stirpe, A., Riva, C., and Scevola, D. (1973). *Clin. Exp. Immunol.* 14, 371–376.

Melly, M. A., Duke, L. J., and Koenig, M. G. (1972). *J. Reticuloendothel. Soc.* 12, 1–15.

Palmer, D. L., Rifkind, D., and Brown, D. W. (1971). *J. Infec. Dis.* 123, 457–469.

Rocklin, R. E., Winston, C. T., and David, J. R. (1974). *J. Clin. Invest.* 53, 559–564.

Root, R. K., Rosenthal, A. S., and Balestra, D. J. (1972). *J. Clin. Invest.* 51, 649–665.

Saba, T. (1970). *Arch. Intern. Med.* 126, 1031.

Snyderman, R. *et al.* (1972). *J. Immunol.* 108, 857–860.

Southam, C. M., and Levin, A. G. (1966). *Blood* 27, 734.

Twomey, J. J., and Sharkey, O. (1972). *J. Immunol.* 108, 984–990.

Urbanitz, D. *et al.* (1974). *Klin. Wochenschr.* 52, 544–548.

Warr, G. A., and Martin, R. R. (1974). *Infect. Immun.* 9, 769–771.

Assessment of Allergic States: IgE Methodology and the Measurement of Allergen-Specific IgG Antibody[1,2]

N. FRANKLIN ADKINSON, JR.[3] and LAWRENCE M. LICHTENSTEIN

Division of Clinical Immunology, Department of Medicine of the Johns Hopkins University School of Medicine at The Good Samaritan Hospital, Baltimore, Maryland

I. Introduction

Clinical allergy has traditionally placed heavy emphasis on clinical history as opposed to laboratory evaluations in assessing the degree of

[1] Publication No. 173 of the O'Neill Research Laboratories, The Good Samaritan Hospital.

[2] Supported in part by Grants AI 08270 and AI 71026 from the National Institute of Allergy and Infectious Diseases, The National Institutes of Health.

[3] Recipient of an Allergic Diseases Academic Award from the National Institute of Allergy and Infectious Diseases, The National Institutes of Health.

anaphylactic sensitivity in patients with allergic diseases. Since the identification of reaginic activity with a unique class of immunoglobulins (IgE) by the Ishizakas in 1967 (Ishizaka *et al.*, 1967), the methodology for quantitative estimates of reaginic sensitivity has accelerated considerably. In this chapter we have described the most commonly employed immunological tests that may have some usefulness for research in and practice of clinical allergy. We have omitted consideration of some assays discussed elsewhere in this volume (such as lymphocyte transformation) for which clinical utility relevant to allergic diseases has not been clearly demonstrated. In addition, we have excluded from consideration other legitimate methodologies for the assessment of hypersensitivity diseases that are not principally IgE-mediated (e.g., precipitin titer determinations in hypersensitivity pneumonitis).

The chapter considers three major areas in some detail: the determination of total serum IgE levels; allergen-specific IgE determinations; and allergen-specific IgG antibody determinations. We have presented experimental procedures for methods of choice for six assays, which we consider generally most useful for the study of allergic disease.

II. Total Serum IgE

A. PRINCIPLES OF AVAILABLE METHODS

Circulating IgE is present in such low levels in normal serum that new methodology has been required for its quantification. This methodology was dependent upon the availability of IgE myeloma protein for use in producing the epsilon-chain specific antisera required by all techniques. Such antiserum is now commercially available. Methods that have proved to be satisfactory in reliably detecting less than 100 ng of IgE per milliliter can be divided into three groups: (a) gel diffusion methods; (b) solid-phase radioimmunoassays; and (c) double antibody radioimmunoassays.

The *single radial diffusion* methods as described by Mancini and by Fahey are currently in common use for the routine detection of serum immunoglobulins of the G, A, M, and D classes. The sensitivity of these methods is at best 1 μg/ml. A modification that employs in addition a ^{125}I-labeled antiserum directed against the anti-IgE molecules improves the sensitivity to about 100 ng/ml. However, this method requires contact autoradiography for development of the antigen–antibody complex bands; it may take 10 days or more to complete the test. Because of the greater sensitivity and rapidity of the radioimmunoassay methods, gel diffusion techniques are no longer in routine use.

Solid-phase radioimmunoassay methods have in common some technique of insolubilizing a highly specific anti-IgE antibody, which is then employed in a competitive binding assay using radioiodinated IgE and standards of known IgE content. Porous beads, such as cellulose particles, Sephadex, or agarose, have been used most commonly to insolubilize the IgE antibody by a variety of chemical techniques. The antibody-coated particles are then incubated with a radiolabeled IgE and unlabeled IgE preparations, either standards or unknowns. Orbital or vertical rotation of the tubes is generally employed to achieve dispersal of the immunosorbent. Incubation times of 4–24 hours are generally required. After the incubation period, the immunosorbent is washed by centrifugation, then counted by gamma scintillation (Fig. 1, A). This technique is often called the radioimmunosorbent test (RIST), and the reagents are now commercially available in kit form. As for all radioimmunoassays, the sensitivity of the RIST is dependent upon several factors, not the least of which is antibody affinity. As generally performed in major laboratories, however, a sensitivity of 5 ng/ml can be expected. The coefficient of variation is estimated to be about 18%.

A more sensitive variant of the RIST involves a direct assay sandwich technique (Fig. 1, B). As in the RIST, standard and unknown sera are first incubated with anti-IgE coated immunosorbent, but without the addition of a radiolabeled IgE. After washing, a second incubation with radiolabeled anti-IgE is employed to quantitate the degree of binding. The counts bound are directly proportional to the IgE content of the original sera. This assay is the most sensitive of all total IgE techniques; the lower limit of sensitivity is reported to be 10 pg of IgE. Such exquisite sensitivity is rarely if ever needed for clinical purposes, however, and the necessity for a second incubation doubles the time required to complete the test. The method is extensively employed for the assay of hormones and other biological substances where this degree of sensitivity is essential, but it has not been widely employed as an assay for serum IgE levels.

The anti-IgE antibody may also be adsorbed at alkaline pH to the walls of plastic tubes. The binding capacity of antisera so adsorbed is considerably less than for covalently coupled antigen-coated particles, but with a high specific activity IgE label and an avid antiserum, the technique can be used to quantitate IgE with sensitivity and precision comparable to the RIST. The advantages of the coated-tube method include a greatly facilitated washing procedure performed by repeated rinsing of the tubes in flowing tap water, and greatly reduced incubation

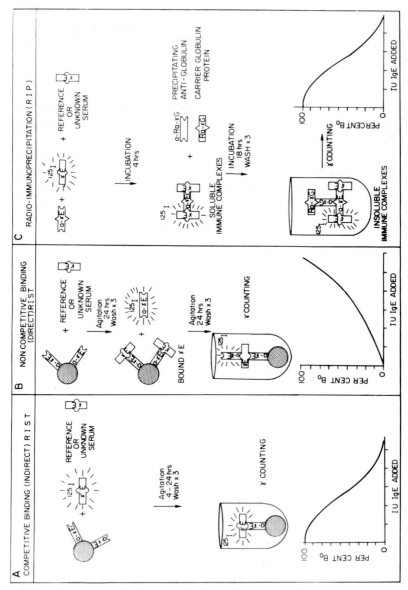

Fig. 1. Determination of total serum IgE by radioimmunoassay techniques. Schematic representation of three commonly employed methods for routine assay of total serum IgE. Technical procedures are described in the text.

time as short as 1 hour. More antibody can be adsorbed by using an indirect technique. The first step consists of adsorption of purified myeloma E protein to the polystyrene or polycarbonate tube. This is followed by washing and then incubation of the IgE-coated tubes with an antihuman IgE antiserum in great excess. The resultant insolubilized antigen–antibody complexes may then be used in a competitive binding assay as in the direct method. This indirect method is simple and precise, but its usefulness is limited by the fact that rather large quantities of purified myeloma E protein are required.

Solid-phase radioimmunoassays, particularly the RIST, have as an attractive advantage the fact that they do not require the addition of a second reagent after the completion of the competitive binding assay in order to separate bound from free antigen (i.e., IgE). In the double antibody assay described below, this second reagent is a precipitating antiserum that must be available in large quantities, often at considerable expense.[4] The double antibody radioimmunoassay, however, is unsurpassed in precision and reproducibility, and we feel it to be the current method of choice in laboratories where these features are of paramount importance.

Method of Choice: Double Antibody Radioimmunoassay for Total Serum IgE

a. Materials and Reagents. 1. Radiolabeled IgE myeloma protein or its Fc fragment if available. The chloramine T method is generally employed to radioiodinate the IgE; 25 μg of radiolabeled protein is generally sufficient for several months' work.

2. Rabbit antihuman IgE that has been rendered Fcε specific by immunizing the animals either directly with Fcε or with whole IgE myeloma followed by absorption of the antisera with Fab fragments, light chains, and other immunoglobulin classes (usually employing affinity chromatography) as needed to render the antiserum specific. Antiserum raised in sheep or goats is said to be unsatisfactory owing to heterophile antibodies in many normal human sera which cross-react with sheep and goat γ-globulin. Such antisera will give falsely elevated IgE values in these patients.

3. Goat antirabbit γ-globulin as the precipitating antibody and normal rabbit serum or rabbit γ-globulin as a carrier protein antigen. A precipitin curve or radioimmunoprecipitation technique, such as the Farr technique,

---

[4] Carson *et al.* (1975) have recently reported that use of 33% saturated ammonium sulfate to insolubilize IgG (and thus bound IgE) while leaving unbound IgE in solution. This method for separation of bound and free IgE may prove equally satisfactory to a second antibody, with the added advantages of simplicity and economy.

is employed to determine the dilution of the antiserum required for optimal precipitation of approximately 50 μg of rabbit γ-globulin.

4. A reference serum of known IgE content, preferably the WHO reference standard 68/341.

5. Plastic tubes, micropipettes, refrigerated centrifuge, and a gamma scintillation counter.

6. Buffer for washing and diluting. A widely used assay buffer is phosphate buffered saline, pH 7.5, which includes 0.5% sodium azide, 0.5% (v/v) Tween-20, and 0.2% (w/v) bovine serum albumin.

b. Procedures. 1. To a disposable plastic tube (polystyrene, 12 mm $\times$ 75 mm) the following reagents are added in sequence: 0.5 ml of standard or unknown serum diluted as desired in assay buffer, 0.1 ml of the appropriate dilution of rabbit antihuman IgE, and 0.1 ml of radiolabeled IgE myeloma (1–5 ng of [^{125}I]IgE per tube).

2. After gentle mixing, the tubes are incubated at 37°C for 3 hours.

3. The following reagents are then added to each tube in order to precipitate the bound label: 0.2 ml of diluted normal rabbit serum or rabbit γ-globulin (approximately 50 μg) and 0.2 ml of goat antirabbit γ-globulin at a dilution predetermined to produce optimal precipitation.

4. Incubation is continued at 37°C for 1 hour, after which the tubes are centrifuged at 2000 g for 30 minutes at 4°C, decanted, and washed twice with 3 ml of assay buffer. Alternatively, the second incubation may be allowed to continue overnight at 4°C and then centrifuged and washed with equivalent results.

5. The tubes are then counted in a gamma counter and the standard curve plotted with the logarithm of added IgE as a function of a percent of maximal binding (B_0). The unknown serum values are then interpolated from the standard curve, either visually or by calculation after linearization of the standard curve by suitable transformation, such as the logit (see Fig. 2).

c. Range, Accuracy, and Sensitivity. The working range of the assay will be determined by the dilution of the rabbit anti-IgE employed in the assay. For clinical purposes, a useful anti-IgE dilution is that which results in 50% inhibition of maximal binding by 50–100 ng of IgE per milliliter. The ultimate sensitivity of the assay depends primarily upon the affinity of the anti-IgE antibody. In general, one may expect to achieve a lower limit of 1–5 ng/ml with most antisera. The precision of the double antibody technique is excellent. It is generally possible to achieve a coefficient of variation of 5% or less.

d. Special Considerations. The standardization of quantitative determinations of serum IgE has been uneven at best. The use of the WHO

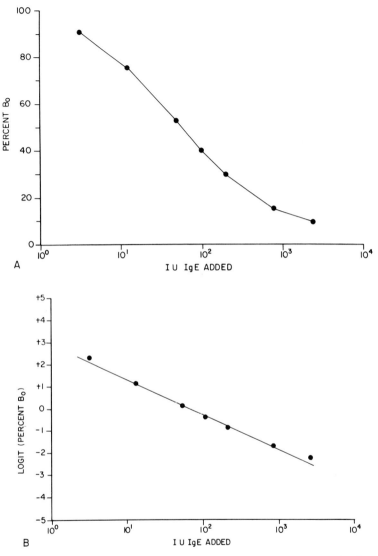

Fig. 2. Double antibody radioimmunoassay for total serum IgE. (A) The standard curve is derived from competitive inhibition of ^{125}I-labeled IgE myeloma protein binding to ra-a-IgE antisera by increasing amounts of an unlabeled IgE reference standard (see text and Fig. 1, C). B_0 represents the binding of labeled IgE when no unlabeled IgE is added. An appropriate dilution of rabbit anti-IgE is chosen to give the desired range of sensitivity. In this assay 1 ng of [^{125}I]IgE with a specific activity of 13 μCi/μg (23,500 cpm/ng) was used. (B) The dose-response curve may be linearized by logit transformation in order to allow direct calculation of IgE content: $\hat{x} = \log_{10} x = -0.627$ (logit Y) $+ 1.83$.

international reference standard for IgE (No. 68/341) as a primary standard is highly recommended. The best available data indicate that 1 IU is equivalent to approximately 2.4 ng of IgE.

In validating the assay system it is essential to establish the specificity of the antiserum for Fc$_\varepsilon$ by demonstrating that cord sera and purified human immunoglobulins at a concentration of 1 mg/ml will not significantly inhibit maximal binding. The most common cause of failure to achieve good agreement between determinations of different dilutions of a single serum is residual cross-reactivity of the antisera with human IgG.

B. Interpretation of Results

The IgE level of cord sera is quite low, probably less than 5 ng/ml. The cord sera IgE from infants of mothers with high serum IgE levels is not elevated, suggesting that IgE does not cross the placental barrier. Serum IgE undergoes a marked increase during the first year of life, after which the yearly mean increase is less impressive, adult levels being reached by about 12 years of age (see Fig. 3).

Serum IgE concentrations in nonatopic healthy adults average approximately 179 ng/ml with a range of 1 to 2700 ng/ml. After the age of 12, a serum IgE level exceeding 800 ng/ml is generally considered to be abnormally elevated. The great majority of patients with elevated serum IgE levels have atopic diseases, such as allergic rhinitis, extrinsic asthma,

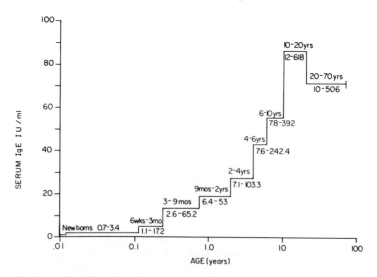

Fig. 3. Normal serum IgE values as a function of age. Horizontal plateaus represent geometric mean values; the ± SD range is shown below each plateau. (Data abstracted from Aas, 1973.)

and atopic dermatitis. One study of adults with extrinsic or allergic asthma reported a mean serum IgE value of 1589 ng/ml, with a range of 55 to 12,750 ng/ml. It should be emphasized that only about half of these patients had serum IgE levels above 800 ng/ml, the upper limit of normal for the nonatopic population. Thus, although the mean serum IgE levels for atopic and nonatopic groups differ markedly, there is considerable overlap of the two groups, up to half of allergic asthmatics having serum IgE levels that fall within the normal range. Atopic dermatitis, on the other hand, is associated with very high levels of serum IgE, and only 20% of these patients have serum IgE levels that fall within the normal range. Allergic urticaria and anaphylactic reactions, on the other hand, are not associated with elevated serum IgE concentrations.

The serum IgE level in the allergic individual may fluctuate as a function of exposure to relevant allergens. Patients with asthma and hay fever to pollen allergens may increase their basal serum IgE levels severalfold during the relevant pollen seasons. Likewise, immunotherapy with allergen extracts will stimulate IgE production during the early phase of treatment.

The basal level of serum IgE appears to be under direct genetic control, high IgE levels being inherited as a simple Mendelian recessive trait. There are in addition numerous conditions and disease states that are recognized to alter the basal level of serum IgE. Table I lists some of the clinical states in which abnormal serum IgE levels have been reported.

Pharmacological modulation of basal serum IgE levels has not been reported. Even large doses of corticosteroids over a period of many weeks do not appear to alter IgE levels.

In summary, total serum IgE can now be measured with considerable ease and accuracy. Serum IgE levels can provide a useful adjunct to other methods of assessing allergic states. The significant overlap between serum IgE levels of normal and atopic individuals precludes the use of this assay to determine the atopic status of any given individual. Of greater diagnostic significance in assessing allergic disease are determinations of the "reagin" levels, i.e., the allergen-specific IgE.

III. Allergen-Specific IgE

A. SERUM ANTIBODY

1. Passive Sensitization of Nonsensitive Skin in Vivo

The detection of serum reagins by the *passive sensitization of normal skin* has been, historically, a most useful procedure. Indeed, the first

Elevated IgE Levels
   Allergic asthma
   Allergic rhinoconjunctivitis
   Parasitic infestations: ascariasis, visceral larva migrans, roundworm infestation
     (capillariasis), schistosomiasis, echinococcosis
   Wiskott–Aldrich syndrome (in association with eczema)
   Bronchopulmonary aspergillosis
   Hyperimmunoglobulinemia E syndrome (elevated IgE, increased susceptibility to
     infection, and dermatitis)
   Hodgkin's disease (late stages)
   Drug-induced interstitial nephritis
   Pulmonary hemosiderosis[a]
   Rheumatoid arthritis[a]
   Dermatitis associated with gold therapy in rheumatoid arthritis patients[a]
Normal IgE Levels
   Drug-induced urticaria or anaphylaxis
   Recurrent urticaria
   Cancer
   Inflammatory bowel diseases
   Malaria[a]
   Hepatitis[a]
Low IgE Levels
   Hypogammaglobulinemia (congenital and some forms of acquired)
   Ataxia telangiectasia
   Multiple myeloma (with G or A paraproteins)[a]
   Chronic lymphocytic leukemia[a]

[a] Unconfirmed reports.

realization that allergy was mediated by a special class of antibody came with the report by Prausnitz and Küstner in 1921 of passive transfer of reagins in the serum of a patient sensitive to fish to the skin of a normal individual. In recognition of this achievement, the passive transfer test in man is called the Prausnitz–Küstner test or simply the P–K test. Passive sensitization is based on the well-known ability of IgE to "fix" firmly to tissue mast cells and thereby sensitize them for antigen-triggered mediator release. It has been clearly demonstrated that IgE antibodies persist in skin sites for a considerably longer period than other immunoglobulins. The inability of human IgE antibody to fix to the skin of heterologous species limits the utility of the passive transfer test, since it can be carried out only in man, or, with decreased sensitivity, in monkeys. The P–K technique is generally used when the patient, either for reasons of skin disease or young age is not suitable for direct skin tests.

The assay requires a small amount of serum, which should be handled

in a sterile fashion. Because of the possibility of transmitting serum hepatitis the patients from whom the serum is derived must not have had this
disease; in addition, serological assay for Au antigen (hepatitis B antigen) should be negative. For routine diagnostic use, a series of dilutions
of serum (e.g., 1:1, 1:10, 1:100, and 1:1000) are injected intradermally on
the recipient's back with one series of sites necessary for testing with
each antigen. It has been demonstrated that when the IgE antibody titer
is sufficiently high, challenge of the site with antigen will be positive
within a few hours of passive transfer. Usually, however, the site is
challenged at the time of maximum fixation: 24–48 hours later. Antigen
challenge is carried out with a relatively high concentration of antigen,
so that the limiting factor in determining the level of response is the
antibody concentration. The optimal antigen concentration will vary
among antigens. However, challenge preparations in the range of 1000
protein nitrogen units per milliliter (PNU/ml) are generally used. A
positive test is graded in the same fashion as the direct skin test (see
Section III,B,1). As controls, challenge of unprepared sites with antigen
is necessary. The last dilution of serum that provides a wheal and flare
reaction greater than that observed in the control is taken as the (end
point) titer. Virtually all patients with clinically significant allergy will
have a positive P–K reaction of 1:10 or greater when challenged with an
appropriate antigen. Most will have a titer of 1:100, some a titer of 1:1000,
and a very few individuals a titer of 1:10,000. As carried out in routine
diagnostic fashion, this test is imprecise; i.e., endpoint titers are reproducible only to about ±10-fold. For experimental purposes, when replicates of multiple 2- or 3-fold dilutions are placed on the back in a
variable sequence of sites, a precision of 3- to 5-fold may be achieved.

The P–K reaction can also be carried out by *passive transfer of human
serum to the skin of monkeys*. In this instance, it is similar to passive
cutaneous anaphylaxis (PCA) reactions in other species and is usually
referred to in these terms. In the monkey, the general procedure is to
plant the dilutions of serum onto the shaved abdomen of the monkey
and 24 hours later to administer the antigen intravenously together with
a dye that will bind albumin and extravasate in areas of increased capillary permeability. The sensitivity of the monkey PCA test for human
reagin is 10-fold less than that of the direct P–K reaction. However, less
experimental manipulation of the skin site is necessary, owing to the
intravenous infusion, and, for the same reason, the antigen delivered to
each site is more uniform. Therefore, this procedure has a greater degree
of precision than the P–K test.

In vivo passive sensitization tests for human IgE antibody levels are
not generally used today. They have multiple disadvantages: the possi-

bility of transmission of serum hepatitis, the lack of precision, and ethical considerations with respect to human volunteers or the expense of maintaining monkeys all preclude its general utility. More important, there are more precise, equally sensitive and less expensive tests available. So, in spite of its importance in the development of the field of allergy, the P–K test has seen its day.

2. Passive Sensitization of Human and Animal Tissues and Cells in Vitro

The basis for our ability to use *in vitro* methods to detect IgE antibody is the same principle that underlies the P–K reactions; that is, IgE antibody will bind to basophiles or mast cells from human or monkey donors and can then be detected by its ability, in the presence of appropriate antigen, to trigger the cells or tissues to respond, usually measured by the release of histamine.

There are a number of systems that can be used for assays of this type: passive sensitization of human leukocyte (basophil) preparations or of chopped skin or lung either of primate or human origin. In each instance, the cells or chopped tissue fragments are prepared, incubated with the allergic serum in appropriate dilutions for periods ranging from 30 minutes to several hours (or in the case of lung tissue, often overnight), washed free of serum, and challenged with appropriate concentrations of antigen. The fact that passive sensitization has taken place is measured indirectly; that is, by the release of one or more of the mediators of the allergic response. In practice, this is usually histamine since it can be measured most precisely. A variety of other mediators such as SRS-A or ECF-A can also be measured. These assays are less sensitive but more precise than P–K titer determination. The endpoint, or titer, is usually taken as that dilution of serum which leads to 50% of the total or maximum response at optimal antigen concentration.

Over the years, a number of claims have been made regarding the ability to diagnose human allergic conditions by using passive sensitization of mast cells or basophils from other species or of human cells of other types. Recent examples of this genre are a so-called "toxic" reaction manifested in human polymorphonuclear cells exposed to the serum of allergic individuals and the appropriate antigen, and the degranulation of or histamine release from rat mast cells passively sensitized with human serum. These techniques are at best difficult to establish and reproduce. Even if accurate, they offer no advantage over more easily reproducible tests. Human basophil degranulation tests have also been described. However, they offer no advantage since they are more laborious and less accurate than the direct assay of mediator release.

The method of choice for determining human reaginic antibody titers by passive sensitization *in vitro* employs human leukocyte preparations; basic techniques have been published by Levy and Osler (1966). An abbreviated version is presented here.

Method of Choice: Passive Sensitization of Human Leukocytes

a. Materials and Methods. The reagents required are precisely those specified for the antigen-mediated histamine release and histamine assay (see Section III,B,2 below).

b. Procedure. This procedure allows for histamine determinations in 50 tubes; depending upon experimental design, a large number of variables (i.e., sera or serum dilutions) can be studied. Using other techniques for histamine assay (see Section III,B,2,d), smaller volumes of blood (1–10 ml) are required.

1. Blood (50–100 ml) is drawn from suitable nonatopic donors (see below) as described for the direct histamine release assay. The blood is allowed to sediment in dextran for 60–90 minutes and the supernatant is centrifuged; the platelet-rich plasma is discarded, and the sedimented cells are washed once in cold Tris-A buffer.

2. Sensitizing mixtures with dilutions of test sera in Tris-A buffer with EDTA (4×10^{-3} M) and heparin (10 $\mu g/ml$) are added to tubes containing about 10^7 leukocytes.

3. The sensitizing mixtures are incubated for 120 minutes at 37°C with gentle agitation every 15 minutes. At the end of this period, the cells are pelletted (8 minutes at 365 g). The supernatant may be discarded or saved for re-use if desired, since only a small preparation of the IgE has fixed to the cells. The cell button is washed twice with cold Tris-A buffer.

4. The sensitized cells are suspended in Tris-ACM buffer, an appropriate antigen dilution is added, and the cells are incubated an additional 30–60 minutes at 37°C, during which histamine release occurs. The histamine released is assayed fluorometrically as described below (Section III,B,2).

5. Estimation of the reaginic potency of a serum usually requires a minimum of two experiments (Fig. 4). In the first experiment, four or five antigen concentrations are evaluated after passive sensitization with undiluted serum in order to choose the optimal antigen concentration giving maximum histamine release. In a subsequent experiment, the percentage of histamine release is assessed for multiple dilutions of the reaginic serum employing the optimal antigen concentration as deter-

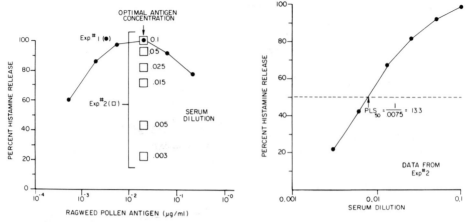

Fig. 4. Determination of PLS$_{50}$. In experiment 1 (left), the test serum is used to passively sensitize leukocytes; these cells are subsequently challenged with antigen over a broad range of concentration in order to determine the optimal antigen concentration for maximum histamine release. In a subsequent experiment (No. 2), aliquots of leukocytes are passively sensitized with increasing dilutions of the unknown serum and then challenged with antigen at the previously determined optimum concentration. The percentage of histamine release is plotted as a function of serum dilution (right), and the dilution required for 50% histamine release is interpolated. The reciprocal of this dilution is the index of the reaginic potency, PLS$_{50}$.

mined previously. That serum concentration required to sensitize normal human leukocytes for 50% histamine release with optimal antigen levels has been designated the PLS$_{50}$. The reciprocal of that dilution is taken as the titer of reaginic antibody.

c. *Precision, Accuracy, and Sensitivity.* The PLS$_{50}$ correlates highly with P–K titers in ragweed reaginic sera (Fig. 5). Although the passive leukocyte sensitization assay is about 5-fold less sensitive than the P–K test, the sensitivity can be increased markedly by carrying out the histamine release in 50% deuterium oxide (D$_2$O). On the other hand, the precision and reproducibility of the *in vitro* assay far exceed those of the P–K test.

d. *Special Considerations.* This assay, although useful for certain studies, has a number of drawbacks. First, it is too laborious for routine diagnostic purposes and large quantities of normal human cells are required in order to obtain the PLS$_{50}$ value for any one serum. Second, the method requires the availability of a group of donors who have been demonstrated to be "good recipients" since only about one in five normal individuals can be adequately passively sensitized. The reasons for this are unknown. Finally, since each passive recipient is somewhat different

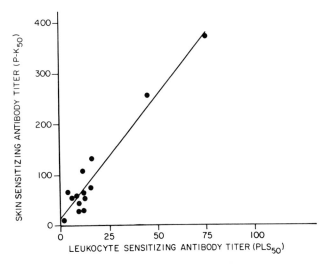

Fig. 5. Correlation of PLS₅₀ and PK₅₀ titers. PK₅₀ titer is the reciprocal of the serum dilution required to induce a reaction that is half of the maximum response observed. PLS₅₀ titer was determined as shown in Fig. 4. $r = +0.92$; $p < 0.001$; slope = .47. (Data from Levy and Osler, 1967.)

in his responsiveness, the same donor must be accessible for repeated experiments, or a reference serum must be employed for standardization—a requirement that further complicates the assay.

For some special research purposes, however, this assay has distinct advantages. It must be remembered that the serological methods discussed below assess only the affinity of IgE antibody for antigen. They provide no information about the interaction between cell surface IgE receptors and the Fc portions of the IgE molecule. At the moment, this distinction is of little clinical importance, but as knowledge about allergic disease processes improves, the differentiation between serological determinations and biological determinations may prove to be of some value.

3. In Vitro Methods: Serological Assays

The traditional serological techniques of immunology that have been used to characterize specific antibody of the immunoglobulin classes that exist in much higher serum concentrations cannot be successfully applied to the *in vitro* study of reagins. This is due to the fact that circulating IgE antibody specific for a given allergen is present in nanograms, or even picograms, per milliliter quantities. These levels are of the order of a thousandfold less than is found in the major immunoglobulin class, IgG. Thus development of serological assays for allergen-specific IgE was hampered for technical reasons.

The first method capable of demonstrating in a semiquantitative manner the union of IgE antibody with a known allergen *in vitro* was the radioimmunodiffusion method. It is essentially a technique for visualizing minute amounts of antigen–antibody complexes in agar gels. In the first step, the IgE-containing serum under evaluation is allowed to diffuse toward nearby wells that contain anti-IgE. This results in the formation of IgE–anti-IgE complexes that concentrate in a line between the two wells although there is no visible precipitation. The gel is then thoroughly washed to remove antibody of other classes capable of combining with the allergen. The former anti-IgE is then filled with radiolabeled allergen, which is allowed to diffuse toward and combine with the precipitated IgE band. The gel is again washed, and autoradiography is applied to visualize the allergen-specific IgE antibody. This technique is cumbersome and at best semiquantitative. Its most serious drawback is that it requires about 3 weeks for completion of one set of assays. The sensitivity of the assay has not been rigorously defined, but it is probably less sensitive than the Prausnitz–Küstner reaction. Because of these difficulties and the development of a much more satisfactory serological assay for specific IgE antibody, this radioimmunodiffusion method is no longer in common use.

The radioallergosorbent test (RAST) was first introduced in 1968 and is now widely employed as the method of choice for serological determination of specific IgE antibody. The assay is basically a solid-phase radioimmunoassay, a variant of the RIST in which allergen rather than antibody is coupled to an insoluble matrix. These allergen-coated polymers are incubated with agitation in the serum under study, during which time antibodies of *all classes* with suitable affinity for the allergens are bound. The particles are then washed and undergo a second incubation with the radiolabeled, highly specific anti-Fc$_\varepsilon$ antibody. The bound radioactivity is measured and is directly related to the specific IgE antibody content of the serum. The insolubilized allergen, as well as the radiolabeled anti-IgE antibody, must be present in moderate excess, although their precise concentrations are not critical. Results are generally available within 24–48 hours. Since this method is highly sensitive and displays a satisfactory correlation with biological tests for specific IgE, it has been widely used in research and more recently in clinical laboratories as the reagents are now commercially available. It will be described in some detail below.

Method of Choice: Radioallergosorbent Test (RAST)

a. Materials and Reagents. 1. Materials required for the preparation of solid-phase allergens: Sephadex G-25 superfine particles, microcrystalline cellulose particles, or Sepharose 4B particles; cyanogen bromide; ethanolamine, high and low pH buffers.

2. Rabbit antisera specific for the Fc fragment of IgE (Fcε), preferably purified by affinity chromatography.

3. Radioiodinated rabbit anti-Fcε usually performed by the chloramine-T method; however, other methods are satisfactory. The radioiodinated antibody should have a specific activity in the range of 50–100 μCi/mmole.

4. Plastic tubes (12 × 75 mm), a slowly rotating orbital rotator for the tubes, micropipettes, centrifuge, aspiration bottles, a gamma scintillation counter, and assay buffer—usually phosphate-buffered physiological saline at pH 7.4 containing 0.2% sodium azide, 0.5 % (v/v) Tween-20, and 0.2% (w/v) bovine serum albumin.

b. Procedures. 1. Preparation of allergen-coated particles is usually carried out by the cyanogen bromide activation method now widely in use (see Cuatrecasas and Anfinsen, 1971).

2. Preparation of rabbit anti-IgE myeloma protein. The antiserum is usually rendered specific for the Fc fragment by absorption with the Fab fragments of IgE myeloma and with normal human serum. These absorptions are best accomplished by solid-phase immunoabsorption although they may also be undertaken in fluid phase. After absorption, the specific antibody is purified by affinity chromatography using Sepharose-coupled IgE myeloma.

3. Assay procedure (see Fig. 6). Using a serum known to have reaginic activity against the allergen under study as a standard, preliminary experiments are run to determine the appropriate dilutions of the allergen-coupled particles and the radioiodinated anti-Fcε. Both of these reagents must be demonstrated to be in ample excess in order that the radioactivity bound be proportional to the specific IgE antibody of the sera. A 0.5-ml sample of appropriately diluted allergen-coated particles (usually 0.5–3.0% v/v) and 0.1 ml of the serum under test are incubated in 12 × 75 mm disposable plastic tubes, which are capped and subjected to orbital rotation at room temperature for 4–18 hours. Particles are then washed four times with the assay buffer using brief centrifugation to sediment the particles and a collared aspirator tube to remove the supernate. After three washes, 0.5 ml of the ^{125}I-labeled anti-IgE is added to each tube, and incubation with orbital agitation is continued for 18–24 hours at room temperature. Particles are again washed three times, and bound radioactivity is counted to statistical precision. Nonallergic sera and buffer controls should be less than 0.5% of the maximum counts bound.

The potent serum to be used as a standard is assayed in duplicate in

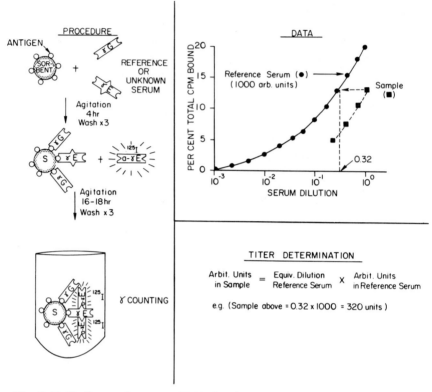

Fig. 6. Radioallergosorbent test (RAST). The procedure is schematically represented (left) and described in the text. Data from the binding of multiple dilutions of a reference serum, as well as a sample of unknown potency, is illustrated (upper right). Note that serum dilution curves of the reference and sample sera are approximately parallel. Assuming 1000 arbitrary units in the reference serum, the calculation of relative sample potency can be performed at any sample dilution in the parallel portion of the curve (lower right).

serial 2-fold dilutions from neat through a dilution whose binding is equivalent to the reagent blank. Unknown sera are assayed with reference to the dilution curve provided by the reference serum. Potency can be expressed as the reciprocal of the dilution of the standard serum that gives equivalent results to the serum under evaluation (see Fig. 6).

c. Interpretation of Results. The RAST is at best a semiquantitative assay. Antibody assays utilizing a reference serum always depend for their quantitation upon parallelism between the dilution curves of the reference serum and the sera under study. The slopes of the dilution curves are a function of the average antibody affinity. Insofar as the average antibody affinity of a test serum differs from that of the reference sera, the slopes of the two lines will not be parallel and the titer derived will be dependent upon the dilution of the test serum taken for assay. In practice, most sera from allergic patients who have not undergone immunotherapy display roughly equivalent dilution curve slopes. Active immunization may be expected to alter average antibody affinity, potentially making less quantitatively reliable the distinctions which can be drawn between sera from immunized and nonimmunized individuals, or among sera from an immunized individual at various points during his course of immunotherapy. Clinically, this problem may have little significance. The good correlation between the RAST and other tests of reaginic activity (see below) suggests that this may be true.

Recently it has become possible to quantitate on a weight basis the specific IgE content of reference sera in order to provide a quantitative estimate of the absolute IgE antibody content of test sera (Schellenburg and Adkinson, 1975). However, it must be remembered that each assay is tied to its own reference standard whose reaginic antibody titers vary considerably. Thus, in terms of absolute antibody content, a high titer of antibody against one antigen may be equivalent to a relatively low titer against an independent antigen. Thus for clinical use, each laboratory must provide from its own evaluation the data necessary to give a clinical interpretation to the outcome of the tests. This is obviously unsatisfactory. To date no international reference sera for interlaboratory standardization of the RAST tests have come into use although the matter is currently under active consideration.

d. Precision, Accuracy, and Sensitivity. The RAST is a highly sensitive test, said to be capable of measuring picogram quantities of IgE antibodies. It approximates the sensitivity of the Prausnitz–Küstner reaction, which is about 10-fold less sensitive than direct skin tests. The coefficient of variation for replicates when all reagents remain constant is 10–15%.

B. Tissue-Fixed Antibody

1. In Vivo Methods: Direct Challenge of Sensitized Tissue

By far the most common, and still the most useful, diagnostic test in human allergic disorders is direct skin testing. The procedure is based upon the fact that the skin contains mast cells sensitized with IgE antibody. When the appropriate antigen is injected into the skin, the mast cells release histamine and other mediators, causing a wheal and flare reaction. A variety of techniques for administering the antigen intradermally have been devised but do not alter the basic mechanism. On the other hand, it is often claimed that for nasal, conjunctival, or bronchial symptomatology taking the antigen directly to these tissues yields a higher incidence of appropriately positive reactions. Thus, antigen solutions have been dropped into the conjunctival sac, applied to the nose, or blown into the lungs. Recent work has shown, however, that when appropriately and quantitatively done, these tests all indicate similar levels of sensitivity. For example, the correlation coefficient between the quantity of ragweed antigen required for a 2+ skin test and that required to increase airway resistance by a specific amount is approximately 0.6 ($p < 0.001$) (Fig. 7). Patients with ragweed hay fever alone and those with ragweed hayfever and asthma demonstrate the same correlation between bronchoprovocation and skin testing. Therefore, for most clinical needs, we need not consider the methodology of bronchial, nasal, or conjunctival challenges. Instead, we shall concentrate on direct skin testing, which offers a simple, straightforward, and relatively safe method for *in vivo* assessment of reaginic sensitivity.

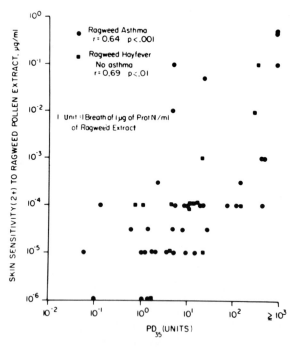

Fig. 7. Correlation of bronchial and skin reactivity to pollen extract. Provocation dose (PD_{35}) of ragweed extract causing 35% decrease in airway conductance (abscissa) vs antigen concentration required for 2+ skin test response to ragweed pollen extract (ordinate) in ragweed asthmatic patients (●) and ragweed hay fever patients without asthma (■).

Method of Choice: Direct Intradermal Skin Testing

a. Materials and Methods. Freshly prepared serial 10-fold dilutions of aqueous extracts of allergenic materials; tuberculin-type 1-ml syringes with 25- or 26-gauge needles; a mild antiseptic solution for skin cleansing; a millimeter rule.

b. Procedures. Beginning with the most dilute solution (usually 1 PNU/ml, 1:10,000 (w/v) or 10^{-5} to 10^{-6} μg of a purified allergen per milliliter), 0.02–0.05 ml is injected *intradermally* so as to raise a 2–5-mm wheal. At 15–20 minutes the skin response is measured in terms of wheal and erythema, and the skin test response is judged as shown in the tabulation.

Grade	Erythema (mm diameter)	Wheal (mm diameter)
Negative	<5	<5
1+	5–10	5–10
2+	10–20	5–10
3+	20–30	5–10
4+	30–40	10–15 with or without
	>40	pseudopodia
		>15 with pseudopodia

If there is no noticeable skin response in 10–15 minutes, a 10-fold higher dilution may then be injected. Serially increasing dilutions are employed until a $\geq 2+$ skin reaction is obtained. This midpoint titer is taken as an index of reaginic sensitivity.

c. Precision, Accuracy, and Sensitivity. By the use of precise volume injections and directly measured skin test responses, skin testing endpoints or midpoints can be determined to a precision of ± 3-fold. The good correlation between serological estimates of serum reagins and the results of direct skin tests suggests that this assay accurately reflects the quantity of allergen-specific IgE antibody being produced by the organism. The sensitivity of direct skin testing for tissue-fixed allergen-specific IgE is unexcelled. The minimal amount of cell-fixed IgE required for a positive test is not known.

d. Special Considerations. In addition to intradermal skin testing, skin testing by other means, including the prick test and the scratch test, has advocates. In the prick test, a small drop of concentrated antigen solution is placed upon the skin, and a needle is advanced through the drop into the dermis. This reproducibly deposits about 3 nl intradermally. After 15–20 minutes the skin response is graded as for the intradermal test. The scratch test is a cruder technique, in which a superficial scratch into the dermis is made and a drop of antigen solution is placed on the scratch. Whealing and erythema around the scratch after 15–20 minutes is judged positive if greater than for the saline control. In our hands, the intradermal test is more precise and reproducible and is, thus, the method of choice for routine clinical procedures. In a pediatric age group, the somewhat less traumatic and more easily performed prick or scratch test can be appropriately used. When carefully done, it can be shown that the results of each of these tests correlate with one another in a reasonable fashion.

The major difficulty with the interpretation of skin test results is that the allergen preparations that are commercially available are completely nonstandardized. We have, for example, assayed different preparations of ragweed antigen and found them to vary in skin test potency or activity in the leukocyte histamine release assay in excess of 100-fold. This has been the experience in a number of other laboratories. Pollens and other allergenic solutions are provided in terms of weight per volume or in protein nitrogen units (PNU). Even the claimed PNU, which bear no relationship to allergenicity, are often not accurately determined. This is an unfortunate situation, since for several of the major allergen extracts the dominant protein antigen is known, and it is possible to assay the materials for potency by simple immunodiffusion techniques. With the exception of antigen E determinations for ragweed extracts, this is not done for commercial preparations. The clinician who wishes to purchase standardized skin testing materials cannot do so. One possible hedge against this unhappy situation is the purchase of lyophilized materials in rather large batches. Appropriate dilutions of these materials can then be made and evaluated on patients of known stable sensitivity prior to their introduction to the diagnostic testing laboratory.

It is also important to remember that in very dilute concentrations, such as those required for skin testing, many proteins tend to adhere to glass or to become denatured. It has been demonstrated, for example, that ragweed antigen E in dilute solution loses 99% of its potency during 24 hours at room temperature. This problem can be solved by making dilutions of allergens in a protein-containing buffer. We routinely use 0.3% human serum albumin. Even so, for maximum reproducibility, a fresh series of dilutions should ideally be prepared once weekly.

Because of these difficulties with allergen standardization, appropriate clinical interpretations of skin test results is difficult. In terms of the protein concentration of purified allergens, however, examples may be provided. Highly clinically allergic individuals often have a 2+ response to 10^{-5} or 10^{-6} μg of purified allergen per milliliter. The average allergic individual responds to a solution containing 10^{-4} to 10^{-3} μg/ml. If a 0.01 μg/ml or higher concentration of antigen is needed to elicit a significant positive response, the likelihood of a clinically important sensitivity is markedly reduced.

If sufficient attention is paid to avoid contamination by irritating materials, false positives or negatives are rare. With high concentrations of allergens, it is possible to obtain positive reactions that do not correlate with clinical disease upon exposure to the allergens. This fact is often overlooked, and skin test results are questioned. The skin tests remain accurate in the sense that they are detecting small amounts of allergen-specific IgE antibody, but in these cases the results are clinically irrelevant. On the other hand, certain extracts, for example, house dust, contain large amounts of extraneous materials that are irritating. In high concentrations, such extracts will cause positive reactions in virtually everyone tested. These reactions may reflect nonspecific irritation rather than low levels of irrelevant IgE antibody.

2. In Vitro Methods: Direct Challenge of Sensitized Tissue or Cells

Although skin testing remains the standard diagnostic procedure in allergy, there is an increasing tendency to develop *in vitro* methods that do not involve as much patient and physician time and can be standardized. As noted above the RAST technique can be used for diagnostic purposes. It is also possible to use direct *in vitro* histamine release from sensitized cells and tissues of allergic donors for the same purpose.

The basophilic leukocytes of allergic individuals, when challenged with appropriate antigen, release histamine in a dose-dependent fashion. Similar techniques have been developed to measure histamine release from other actively sensitized tissues, such as lung, skin, and nasal polyp tissue. However, leukocyte histamine release is the only feasible technique for general diagnostic purposes.

Method of Choice: Histamine Release from Human Leukocytes

a. Methods and Materials. 1. Anticoagulant solution: 12.5 ml of 6% clinical dextran plus 5.0 ml of 0.1 M EDTA plus 375 mg of dextrose in a polycarbonate tube or siliconized glass tube for each 50 ml of blood drawn; 10$\times$ Tris buffer: 140.3 gm of NaCl, 7.45 gm of KCl, 74.5 gm of

Trizma (Tris preset pH 7.6 at 25°C from Sigma Chemical Company, St. Louis, Missouri) dissolved in 2000 ml of distilled water in a volumetric flask. Human serum albumin is used at 30 mg/ml in distilled water. Stock calcium and magnesium solutions ($0.075\ M$ and $0.5\ M$, respectively) are prepared with calcium chloride and magnesium chloride salts. Tris-A buffer is prepared by diluting 10 ml of $10\times$ Tris and 1.0 ml of 3% HSA to 100 ml with distilled water. Tris-ACM buffer contains 10 ml of $10\times$ Tris, 1 ml of 3% HSA, 0.8 ml of $0.075\ M$ calcium chloride, and 0.2 ml of $0.5\ M$ magnesium chloride, diluted to 100 ml with distilled water.

2. Reagent grade materials and solutions as follows: $3\ N$ and $1\ N$ NaOH, o-phthalaldehyde (recrystallized), $2\ M$ phosphoric acid, $0.12\ N$ HCl, $0.1\ M$ EDTA, 8% perchloric acid ($HClO_4$), N-butanol, histamine dihydrochloride, sodium chloride, N-heptane.

3. Equipment: plastic syringes or blood donor sets, polycarbonate or siliconized glass reaction tubes, refrigerated centrifuge, serological centrifuge, syringe microburettes, 15-ml glass culture tubes for extraction, glass cuvettes, fluorometer, pipettes, routine laboratory glassware.

b. Procedures. 1. Venipuncture of an allergic individual is performed by drawing blood into a mixture of dextran, glucose, and EDTA (see materials above). The cells are allowed to sediment 60–90 minutes, and the supernatant containing plasma, platelets, and leukocytes is aspirated and spun for 8 minutes at 110 g at 4°C. The cell button is washed twice in Tris-A buffer.

2. After washing, the cell pellet is resuspended at a concentration of approximately 10^7 cells/ml in Tris-ACM buffer; 1 ml of cells is added to each reaction tube.

3. Appropriate antigens, 0.2 ml at multiple dilutions, is added to a series of reaction tubes in duplicate. Some reaction tubes are challenged only with Tris-A buffer and serve as blanks, whereas other tubes are lysed with 8% perchloric acid to provide a "complete" or total amount of histamine in the cell preparation.

4. The reaction tubes are incubated at 37°C and swirled several times during the 45–60-minute incubation, during which histamine is released.

5. When the reaction is complete, the tubes are centrifuged in a desktop serological centrifuge for 5 minutes. The supernatant is decanted into 15-ml glass tubes containing 300 mg of sodium chloride and 1.25 ml of N-butanol. The butanol–water mixture is alkalinized by adding 100 μl of $3\ N$ NaOH and vortexing vigorously. Centrifugation at 1500 g for 5 minutes at 4°C is performed, after which 1 ml of the top (butanol) layer is removed and added to another 15-ml glass culture tube containing

0.6 ml of 0.12 N HCl and 1.9 ml of N-heptane. The tubes are capped and shaken vigorously. After the development of the interface, an 0.5-ml aliquot from the bottom (acid) layer is removed and placed into a cuvette suitable for the fluorometer to be used.

6. Cuvettes are placed in a 4°C water bath. To each cuvette, 100 μl of 1 N NaOH is added with a syringe microburette, after which the preparation is vortexed and 25 μl of 0.2% o-phthalaldehyde solution (OPT) is rapidly added and mixed, and the condensation reaction between OPT and histamine is allowed to proceed for 40 minutes at 4°C. The reaction is stopped by the addition of 50 μl of 2 M phosphoric acid. The tubes are then warmed to room temperature and read in a fluorometer with 350 nm activation and 450 nm emission.

7. Histamine standards are carried through the entire procedure, and "external standards" (i.e., not extracted) are also run. Results are usually presented in terms of the percentage of total histamine released by any given antigen concentration, although results can as well be represented in terms of nanograms of histamine released per tube. Dose-response curves are constructed for each antigen. A patient's *cell sensitivity* to a particular antigen is defined as the interpolated value that produces 50% histamine release (Fig. 8).

c. Precision, Accuracy, and Sensitivity. In the hands of an experienced technician, the coefficient of variation for within-assay duplicates is generally less than 10%. In addition, between-assay reproducibility of a given result is usually ±3% histamine release. Estimates of sensitivity are difficult to achieve, since the number of cell-bound IgE molecules necessary to elicit 50% histamine release is not known. However, when the assay is compared with direct skin testing using purified allergens, the sensitivity of direct histamine release from human leukocytes is approximately equivalent to skin testing. In those patients who require high concentrations of antigen to induce a positive skin test, (i.e., >0.1 μg/ml), histamine release often occurs to a limited extent (i.e., 30–50% total) or not at all. Many of these individuals do not display clinical symptoms correlating with environmental exposure to these antigens. On the other hand, histamine release can be obtained with dilute concentrations of appropriate antigen in the vast majority of clinically sensitive individuals.

d. Special Considerations. Histamine release from human leukocytes is a precise, reproducible laboratory evaluation that correlates well with the state of clinical allergy (see Section III,C and Fig. 12 below). As described above, it remains largely a research tool, since it is too laborious

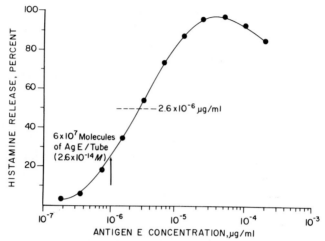

Fig. 8. Histamine release dose-response curve. The peripheral leukocytes of a ragweed-sensitive individual were challenged *in vitro* with antigen E, the purified principal allergen of ragweed pollen. The dose of antigen required for 50% histamine release (in this case 2.6×10^{-6} µg/ml, ---) is taken as an index of cell sensitivity to the antigen. This dose-response curve is typical for a sensitive individual and illustrates two consistent observations: inhibition of maximum histamine release in antigen excess, and the exquisite sensitivity of the *in vitro* assay.

for routine clinical work. Of importance in this regard is the recent publication by Siraganian (1974) describing an automated histamine release apparatus that processes 40 reaction tubes per hour. This automated technique can be performed using whole blood as well as isolated cells. Sensitivity of the histamine assay involved is about 10-fold greater than the manual extraction procedure with a coefficient of variation of about 1%. Automated technology may open up the histamine release technique to more widespread clinical and research use.

C. CORRELATION AND COMPARISON OF ALLERGEN-SPECIFIC IgE METHODS

The conventional test for the presence of reaginic antibodies in a putatively allergic individual has been the direct skin test, either intradermal or prick. Its correlation with clinical symptomatology is well established, and its sensitivity is unexcelled. When properly performed, however, it is laborious, semiquantitative and observer-dependent, and is not entirely without morbidity. Practical considerations, especially in research protocols, often necessitate its limited use. Provocative tests, such as bronchial challenge with allergen, generally correlate well qualitatively with direct skin tests, but are more cumbersome and entail greater risk than skin testing. Bronchial challenge remains a valuable research tool in the investigation of asthmatic states, but its clinical usefulness as an indicator of reaginic hypersensitivity remains controversial. A third assay for tissue-fixed IgE antibody, which can be readily performed on most patients, is *in vitro* histamine release from allergen-challenged peripheral leukocyte preparations. This method has a satisfactory correlation with both direct skin testing and bronchial challenge techniques (see Figs. 9 and 10). It is less sensitive than direct skin testing and requires rather large specimens of freshly drawn blood together with specialized equipment. It remains a valuable research tool for the investigation of mechanisms of allergy, but without automated methodology it has less utility as a potential screening procedure for reaginic hypersensitivity to a large number of allergens.

The clinical significance of circulating IgE antibodies as opposed to the tissue-fixed reagins measured by the assays mentioned above has recently been given careful study. The standard method for the quantita-

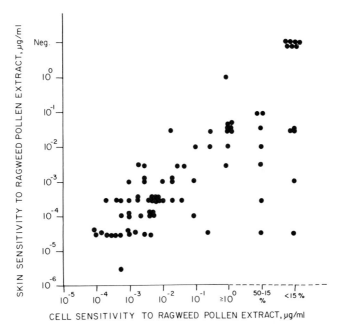

Fig. 9. Correlation of cell sensitivity and skin test reactivity to whole ragweed pollen extract in 87 unselected patients with both fall and spring hay fever symptoms. Twelve patients with varying degrees of skin reactivity had less than 50% histamine release with *in vitro* challenge of their leukocytes. Seven of these patients were subsequently shown to have poor correlation between ragweed pollen count and daily symptom scores during the ragweed season.

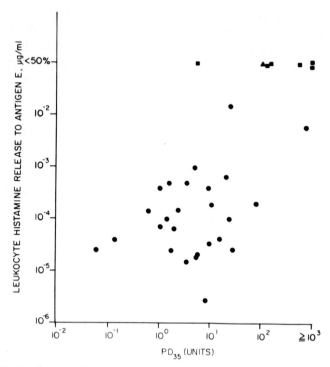

Fig. 10. Correlation of bronchial and leukocyte reactivity to antigen. Provocation dose of crude ragweed extract causing 35% decrease in airway conductance (abscissa) vs. leukocyte histamine release to antigen E (ordinate) in 33 patients with history of asthma during the ragweed season. PD = provocation dose; 1 unit = 1 breath of 1μg of protein N per milliliter of ragweed extract. $r = 0.69$, $p < 0.001$. ▲, 50% histamine release to crude ragweed, but not to antigen E; ■, patients releasing less than 50% histamine; ●, 50% histamine release to antigen E.

tion of circulating IgE antibodies has been the Prausnitz–Küstner reaction. The P–K technique correlates very well with the results of direct skin tests, although it is about 10-fold less sensitive than the latter. Because of the risk of serum hepatitis and the need for human volunteers, current use of the P–K test is restricted to special circumstances. The demonstrated correlation between the P–K titer and the skin sensitivity to direct allergen challenge gave rise to the hope that other assays of circulating reagin might provide the same useful information without the necessity of passive sensitization of tissues either *in vivo* or *in vitro*. With the development of the radioallergosorbent test (RAST), extensive studies of allergic populations have been undertaken in an attempt to establish the correlation of RAST titers and assays of tissue-fixed reagins. In general, 75–95% agreement between the results of RAST determinations and direct skin tests and/or provocative tests has been reported. The agreement approaches 100% in profound hypersensitivity states. The most common discrepancy reported is that of a negative provocative test or skin test and a positive RAST assay (see Fig. 11). Because of its simplicity, ease of performance, semiquantitative nature, and good correlation with additional assays of tissue-fixed IgE antibodies known to reflect clinical hypersensitivity states, the RAST assay has promise of becoming a standard allergy evaluation technique.

D. Clinical Relevance of Specific IgE Determinations

Using an allergic rhinitis model, it has been possible to demonstrate good agreement between symptom index scores and a variety of assays for specific IgE in untreated allergic individuals. In multiple patient groups, such a clinical correlation holds up well for direct skin testing

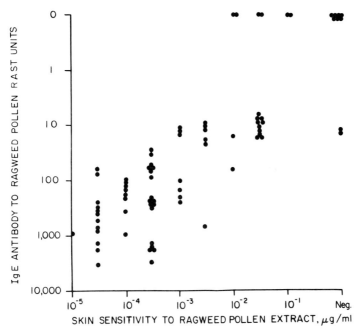

Fig. 11. Correlation between skin testing and RAST assay. Skin sensitivity to crude ragweed pollen extract is expressed in terms of the concentration required for a 2+ midpoint skin response. Circulating IgE antiragweed antibodies were determined in a radioallergosorbent test employing a purified ragweed antigen preparation coupled to cellulose particles; a reference serum designated to have 4000 arbitrary units was used for standardization.

and for direct histamine release from human leukocytes (see Fig. 12). These correlations can also be demonstrated in populations of allergic asthmatic individuals. The results of bronchial challenge also correlate well with skin testing, not only for patients with allergic asthma, but for patients with allergic rhinitis alone. This finding suggests that bronchial provocation is simply an indication of the presence of IgE antibody on sensitized mast cell and does not as such relate to the clinical state of asthma. In a recently completed study of ragweed allergic patients with a clinical history of ragweed asthma, we were not able to demonstrate a correlation between symptom severity on a day-to-day basis and the ragweed pollen count. It may be that symptom quantitation in asthma is in such a state that disease severity–diagnostic procedure correlations cannot yet be made. In all these assays (histamine release, bronchial challenge, direct skin tests, RAST), there is a small but significant number of false-positive tests while very few false negatives. That is, individuals who are entirely asymptomatic clinically may sometimes have positive skin tests, weakly positive RAST titers, or low-level histamine release at high allergen concentrations.

Increases in the concentration of reaginic antibody, as well as total serum IgE, have been found to occur during the appropriate season in seasonally allergic patients. One group of grass allergic children demonstrated greater than a 4-fold increase in IgE antigrass antibodies during the grass pollen season. During the same interval the mean total serum IgE increased 75%.

Specific immunotherapy with allergen extracts also increases the serum levels of specific IgE antibody during the early weeks of treatment. In several series of patients studied, there was a 2- to 8-fold increase in specific IgE antibody during the first month of immunotherapy as compared to pretreatment base lines. Over subsequent months, if treatment is continued, the specific IgE level gradually falls. It now appears that after two years of treatment more than 90% of patients show a modest decline of allergen-specific serum IgE. Whatever symptomatic benefit can be attributed to specific immunotherapy cannot be correlated with the effect of therapy on specific reagin levels. In a minority of patients more dramatic changes are sometimes observed in which the peripheral leukocytes of treated patients become completely unreactive to antigen. This appears to be the result of a biochemical alteration (?desensitization) which is currently not explained. It occurs in the absence of similar changes in the serum IgE antibody level or in skin-test sensitivity. When this decrease in cell sensitivity occurs, it is highly correlated with the disappearance of severe clinical symptoms. Unfortunately, this occurs in very few patients. Other reported fluctuations of specific IgE antibodies

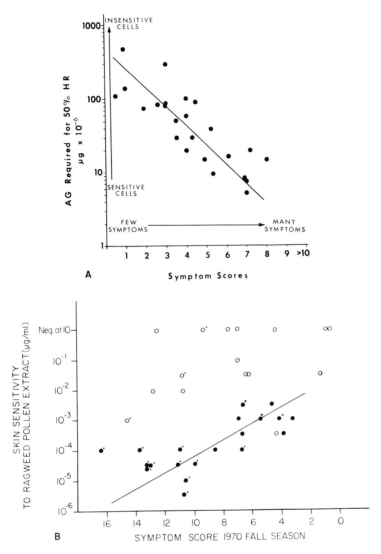

Fig. 12. Correlation of leukocyte cell sensitivity and skin-test reactivity with symptom scores in ragweed hay fever patients. (A) Symptom scores drawn from daily diaries maintained by patients during the ragweed pollen season vs antigen concentration (AG) required for 50% histamine release (HR) in 25 untreated highly sensitive ragweed hay fever patients. Rank correlation coefficient = 0.75; $p < 0.01$. (B) The skin test response to ragweed pollen extract and average daily symptom scores in untreated ragweed hay fever patients. ●, Group highly sensitive by histamine release and skin test; ○, patients of low sensitivity by histamine release and skin test; asterisks indicate patients with significant correlation between daily pollen counts and daily symptom scores.

in serum include a decrease in both total serum IgE and parasite-specific IgE antibody in patients successfully treated for a variety of parasitic infestations.

Finally, at least for the special case of urticarial and anaphylactic reactions to penicillin, the presence of specific IgE antibodies as demonstrated by direct skin tests with penicillin antigens has been shown to be superior to clinical history of prior reactivity in identifying currently hypersensitive patients. Whether this predictive value for penicillin skin tests will also apply to serological assays of specific IgE, such as the RAST test, is currently under study. Similar studies are underway in Hymenoptera-hypersensitive patients, where there is a similar need to identify those currently at risk for serious allergic reactions.

IV. Allergen-Specific IgG Antibodies

A. IgG REAGINS

Accumulating experimental evidence, recently from animal studies of rat and mouse mast cell systems, in addition to the well-studied guinea pig γ_1 antibody model, suggests that a certain subset of IgG antibodies will fix to tissue mast cells and may function as a reagin. In contrast to IgE reagin, the binding of IgG reagin to its Fc receptor on target cells is apparently labile and of low affinity. In man, these IgG reagins have been demonstrated by reverse anaphylaxis experiments utilizing a highly specific anti-IgG antisera to initiate histamine release from peripheral leukocytes, and by passive sensitization of monkey skin by purified human IgG preparations. The functional role played by IgG reaginic antibody in the pathogenesis of allergic disease is at present obscure but appears minimal. The clinical significance of IgG reagin in man is totally unevaluated.

B. IgG "BLOCKING" ANTIBODIES

That there are at least two types of allergen-specific serum antibody has been appreciated since the classic work of Cooke and associates. They defined a heat-stable antibody, which does not fix to skin but when mixed with allergen decreases the skin test endpoint. It was widely supposed that this so-called "blocking" antibody was involved in the mechanism of protection provided by immunotherapy, and therefore many studies of the changes in this antibody with immunotherapy have been carried out. Most early studies employed the ability of this antibody to block skin test, but since this technique is highly variable and laborious, and since like the P–K test it carries the risk of serum hepatitis, it has not been used for many years. Unfortunately, the first alternative technique chosen was hemagglutination, which measures IgM antibodies preferentially. With hemagglutination assays no relationship could be found between an increase in blocking antibodies and clinical protection following immunotherapy.

About 10 years ago the histamine-release technique was employed to study blocking antibody levels *in vitro*. The principle is that IgG antibodies do not fix to the cells but can bind allergen in the fluid phase and thereby impair its interaction with cell-bound IgE. The result is the inhibition of release of histamine.

With the histamine-release technique, blocking antibody was measured in two ways. First, dose-response curves were carried out in normal serum and in the patient's serum before and after immunotherapy. It was found that all allergic individuals have some naturally occurring blocking antibody (sufficient to shift the dose-response curve to antigen about 3-fold, on the average). This antibody level is increased many thousand-fold by immunotherapy. This "blocking antibody" is predominantly if not exclusively of the IgG class. The quantity of blocking antibody can be assessed by the increase in the concentration of antigen required to release 50% of the histamine in allergic as opposed to normal serum. Alternatively, the blocking antibody assay can be run with a constant amount of antigen but increasing dilutions of the allergic serum. Percentage inhibition of histamine release versus serum dilution is plotted, and that serum concentration which inhibits 50% is taken as the antibody titer.

More recently, we have used a modified radioimmunoprecipitation technique for the measurement of IgG "blocking" antibodies. Because of its relative simplicity and its excellent correlation with the inhibition of histamine-release technique (see Fig. 14 below), we now consider it to be the method of choice.

Method of Choice: Modified Radioimmunoprecipitation Test for IgG "Blocking" Antibody

This modified radioimmunoprecipitation assay is a further modification of the standard allergen binding-capacity technique in immunology in which class-specific antisera are used to precipitate antigen–antibody complexes, the antigen of which has been radiolabeled. The adaptation described here involves a nonsaturation technique whereby antibody estimates are made relative to a reference serum rather than determined in absolute amounts. In doing so, the assay time can be greatly shortened and relatively small amounts of radiolabeled allergen are required.

a. Materials and Reagents. 1. Radiolabeled allergens of interest. Radio-iodination with ^{125}I by the chloramine-T method is generally employed, although other coupling methods are satisfactory, 100 μg of radiolabeled allergen is sufficient for a large volume of work over several months time.

2. Rabbit or goat antihuman IgG which has been rendered Fcγ specific by Fab adsorption or by immunization with purified Fcγ. Depending upon the potency of the crude antisera, 0.05–0.3 ml *per assay tube* may be required for maximum precipitation of the IgG content of the diluted human serum together with the carrier IgG protein. For most investigations this requires large volumes of goat antisera, which can be pro-hibitively expensive if purchased commercially. If the sera under study are known or can be shown to possess insignificant quantities of antibodies of the IgA and IgM class (as is shown to be the case for ragweed-sensitive patients on immunotherapy), then absorption of the crude antisera to render it gamma-chain specific may not significantly alter the results and thus may be unnecessary.

3. Carrier IgG protein. For most purposes, serum from a nonallergic individual known not to contain antibody against the allergen under study can be utilized as a source for the IgG protein used in the diluent to boost the IgG content of dilute serum specimens to a common level.

4. Plastic tubes, micropipettes, refrigerated centrifuge, gamma scintil-lation counter, and borate-buffered saline (BBS), pH 8.0, as a diluent.

b. Procedures. 1. A suitable reference serum must be chosen. Ideally, this should be the most potent human serum available, usually chosen from among allergic individuals undergoing immunotherapy with the allergen of interest. To prepare the standard curve the reference serum is first diluted 1:30 in BBS, pH 8.0. Subsequent 2-fold dilutions are made in BBS containing 300 μg of human IgG per milliliter of buffer (about a 1:30 dilution of a nonallergic serum or sera pool). An appropriate dilu-tion of the radiolabeled allergen is chosen such that maximum plateau binding using the reference serum continues through a dilution of about 1:100 (see Fig. 13). The amount of labeled allergen required will be small (usually nanograms per tube) but will vary depending on potency of the standard sera, immunoreactivity of the radioiodinated allergens, and the exact conditions employed in the assay. Twofold dilutions of the reference serum are continued until the counts bound approach the serum blank count (nonallergic serum pool). The standard set of dilutions

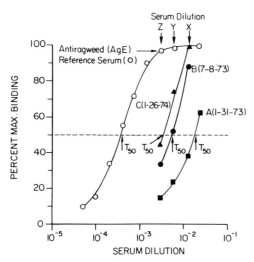

Fig. 13. Radioimmunoprecipitation assay for allergen-specific IgG antibody. See text for technical procedure. Open circles (○) illustrate reference serum dilution. Filled symbols (■, ●, ▲) illustrate dilution curves for the same patient undergoing progressive injection therapy with ragweed extract. (A, initial bleed; B, 6 months later; C, 6 months following.) Two methods for calculation of relative IgG antiragweed antibody potency are illustrated. Using arbitrary serum dilutions (indicated X, Y, and Z), the relative potency of the three sera to each other and the reference serum (A:B:C:R), is 1:5.2:40:50) for dilution X; (1:2.5:5.3:40) for dilution Y; and (1:2:3:30) for dilution Z. Thus relative potencies vary considerably when a single arbitrary dilution is evaluated. Alternatively, sera may be compared at that dilution which produces 50% reduction of maximum binding (T_{50}); the relative potencies by this method are (1:3.4:5.0:54).

of the reference serum provide the standard curve and are included in each assay.

2. In 12×75 mm plastic or glass tubes, the following reagents are added: 0.1 ml of serum dilution of reference serum or unknown serum, diluted as for the reference serum; and 0.1 ml of radioiodinated allergen at the appropriate dilution. The serum and antigen are mixed gently by shaking the test tube rack, which is then incubated for 4 hours at room temperature.

3. Of the goat antihuman Fcγ (at the dilution required for maximum precipitation of about 30 μg of human IgG), 0.1 ml is added to the serum–allergen mixture. Tubes are again mixed by gently shaking test tube racks and incubated at 4°C for about 16 hours (overnight). Alternatively, the tubes may be incubated for 1 hour at 37°C and then processed without significant alteration of precipitated readioactivity.

4. Assay tubes are centrifuged at 3000 *g* for 30 minutes at 0°C, and

supernatants are decanted. The precipitates are then washed three times with 3-ml volumes of cold BBS. Radioactive counts in the precipitates are then determined with a gamma counter.

5. Results may be expressed in one of two ways (Fig. 13). Unknown sera may be evaluated at a single arbitrary dilution and potency expressed as a dilution titer relative to the reference serum dilution curve. This method makes assumptions about the homogeneity of average antibody affinity in the reference and unknown sera that may not be justified. Alternatively, the effects of differing average antibody affinities may be minimized by comparing the dilutions required for 50% inhibition of maximum binding of the unknown serum and the reference serum, much as is done for the assay of blocking antibodies by inhibition of histamine release. The second method of reference is always preferable, but it involves evaluating each unknown serum in three or more dilutions.

c. *Precision, Accuracy, and Sensitivity.* The method is quite precise, with coefficients of variation in the range of 2–5% usually achievable. For this reason duplicate determinations are generally adequate. The accuracy of this method has never been determined by direct comparison with quantitative estimates of specific antibody. The estimates of antibody potency obtained with this method will be influenced more or less by the variance of the average antibody affinity among the sera studied. This is not an important variable in the antigen binding-capacity assays where the available antibody is saturated by excess allergen. However, these methods require large amounts of allergen (micrograms per tube) and as long as 5–6 days to approach equilibrium in dilute solutions. The sensitivity of the method is unknown, but it equals or exceeds that of the inhibition of histamine release assay.

d. *Special Considerations.* This assay for allergen-specific IgG is precise, rapid, and technically easy to perform, and it requires relatively small amounts of purified allergens. The results obtained are relative unless the amount of antibody in the reference serum is known, but they are adequate for most clinical study purposes. In principle as well as in fact, the assay results are parallel to those obtained by the inhibition of histamine release assay, which is much more cumbersome to perform. The estimates of IgG "blocking" antiragweed antibody obtained by the two methods are highly correlated (Fig. 14).

C. Clinical Relevance of "Blocking" Antibodies

It is now well established that immunotherapy with the appropriate antigen can lead to the clinical amelioration of hay fever. It also results in

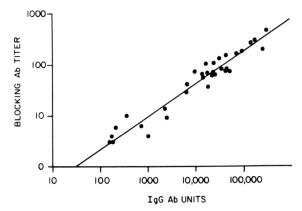

Fig. 14. Correlation of two methods for determining blocking antibody. IgG anti-ragweed antibody as determined by the radioimmunoprecipitation assay and employing the T_{50} method of titration (see Fig. 13) vs blocking antibody titer stated as the reciprocal of the serum dilution required for 50% inhibition of histamine release *in vitro* in 32 sera from ragweed-sensitive patients with a wide range of antibody titers. $r_s = 0.96$; $p < 0.001$.

an increase in allergen-specific antibody in essentially all immunoglobulin classes. Of these, only the so-called "blocking" antibody of the IgG class and the IgE antibody have been studied in detail. With either radio-immunoassays or the inhibition of histamine release, blocking (IgG) antibody can be detected in all allergic individuals, even those who have not been treated. With intensive preseasonal or perennial therapy, blocking antibody levels may rise about 30- to 3000-fold, depending upon the immunotherapy regimen and the individual treated. Although there have been some reports showing a close correlation between the rise in blocking antibody and the degree of clinical relief, we have not observed this in our clinical studies. Certainly, there is no direct quantitative relationship between improvement in clinical symptoms and the increment in blocking antibody following immunotherapy. However, if immunotherapy patients are roughly divided into two groups along clinical improvement lines and again by IgG blocking-antibody response, there is an association of clinical improvement with blocking antibody production. This relationship is statistically significant but occurs in only two-thirds of patients (Fig. 15).

Blocking antibodies have been postulated to be of some importance in providing protection against penicillin anaphylaxis although, obviously, this has not been subjected to controlled clinical investigations. Recent studies of immunotherapy in patients with sensitivity to Hymenoptera suggests a clear relationship between blocking antibody level and

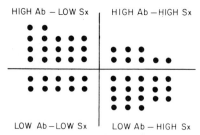

Fig. 15. Correlation between blocking antibody levels (Ab) and symptom (Sx) scores. Fifty-three patients who underwent immunotherapy for ragweed hay fever were divided into two groups by two different criteria: high and low blocking antibody and high and low symptoms after therapy. If high antibody is related to low symtom scores and vice versa, all individuals should fall in the appropriate quadrants. About two-thirds do so, which is a significant correlation but not one that suggests causality. Question: Is Ab level related to Sx? Data: 35 yes/18 no; $p < 0.02$.

clinical risk of anaphylaxis. This result might have been expected, since in this instance the allergen (bee venom antigens) must pass through the blood stream before reaching the target organs to produce the anaphylactic symptomatology. This is quite different from the introduction of airborne allergens into the nasal mucosa, where they can reach tissue mast cells without exposure to serum immunoglobulins. While only a small number of individuals have been studied, immunization with Hymenoptera venoms leads to a several thousandfold rise in blocking antibody which is associated with complete clinical protection against in-hospital stings; previous stings in the same patients had caused severe reactions.

Inasmuch as the correlation between serum-blocking antibodies and clinical relief in hay fever patients is weak, a number of investigators have studied blocking antibodies in nasal secretions. The secretory antibodies, theoretically at least, stand immediately between the target cells and the inciting allergen. Allergen-binding antibodies of the IgA and IgG class can be found in nasal washings of all patients with ragweed hay fever, but not in normal controls. (Secretory antibodies can be measured by a radioimmunoprecipitation assay similar to that described in Section IV,B for serum IgG antibodies.) Most of this naturally occurring secretory antibody is of the IgG class, but almost all individuals have, as well, antibody of the IgA class, which is the locally produced 11 S IgA dimer containing secretory piece. No definite rise and fall in the level of secretory antibody can be demonstrated during seasonal exposure to ragweed pollen. Immunotherapy, however, causes a severalfold rise in both the IgA and IgG allergen-binding capacity of nasal secretion. There is no quantitative relationship between the rise in serum IgG antibody and that in nasal secretions. Insofar as we have been able to ascertain, no blocking activity is found in serum IgA. After immunotherapy the serum IgG antibody may rise on the average over 100-fold, whereas the rise in nasal IgG antibody is less than 10-fold. Moreover in individual cases, there is no correlation between the magnitude of IgG antibody rise in nasal secretions and that in the serum. It therefore seems likely that the IgG noted in nasal secretions is produced locally rather than representing a "spillover" from serum. It can be concluded, therefore, that immunotherapy for allergic disorders will lead to a modest increase in specific secretory antibody of both the IgA and IgG classes. However, such studies have failed to demonstrate a relationship between clinical improvement and the level of either secretory IgA or IgG antibody.

V. Conclusions

As a result of the advancing methodology of the last decade, allergen-specific human IgE can now be measured in picogram quantities in serum, in exocrine secretions, and on cells in a variety of organs. As outlined in this chapter, numerous methods of sufficient sensitivity are available for the measurement of clinically relevant amounts of IgE antibody. Choice of appropriate methods for clinical diagnosis or research in allergic mechanisms depends largely on considerations other than sensitivity. On the other hand, there is considerable room for advancement in the precise quantitation of absolute amounts of specific IgE antibody. The role of the level of "irrelevant" IgE antibody in serum and on mast cells and basophils has not been explored, principally because of our ignorance of the precise ratio of irrelevant to allergen-specific IgE in the preparations under study.

By and large, the correlations of cell-fixed reagins and circulating reagins are quite good and indeed much better than might have been anticipated. This finding, coupled with rapidly advancing solid-phase radioimmunoassay technology, has allowed for the ascendancy of serological techniques for the determination of reaginic sensitivity. Such techniques as the RAST, if problems of standardization can be solved, may in the future provide quantitative, clinically useful, and easily obtainable information about the allergic status of patients with hypersensitivity diseases.

Future research on allergy must also give due consideration to possible biological importance of IgG reagins, serum-blocking IgG antibodies, and the allergen-specific IgG and IgA antibodies in the exocrine secretions. And, too, the biological role of IgE antibody in general is still an unsolved problem. One can hope that IgE methodology has now advanced to the point where it is sufficient to the task required of it.

Selected References

Aas, K. (1973). *Farmakoteropie* **4**, 85.

Augustin, R. (1973). The techniques for the study and assay of reagins in allergic subjects. *In* "Handbook of Experimental Immunology" (D. M. Weir, ed.). p. 42 ISR. *Blackwell, Oxford.*

Carson, D., Metzger, H., and Bazin, H. (1975). Simple radio-immunoassay for the measurement of human and rat IgE levels by ammonium sulfate precipitation. *J. Immunol.* **115**, 561.

Cooke, R. A., Barnard, J. H., Hebald, S., and Stull, A. (1935). Serological evidence of immunity with co-existing sensitization in a type of human allergy (hay fever). *J. Exp. Med.* **62**, 733.

Cuatrecasas, P., and Anfinsen, C. B. (1971). Affinity chromatography. *Methods Enzymol.* **22**, 345 (see p. 352).

Gleich, G. J., Averbeck, A. K., and Svedlund, H. A. (1971). Measurement of IgE in normal and allergic serum by radioimmunoassay. *J. Lab. Clin. Med.* **77**, 690.

Ishizaka, K., Ishizaka, T., and Hornbrook, M. M. (1967). The identification of γE-antibodies as a carrier of reaginic activity. *J. Immunol* **99**, 1187.

Johansson, S. G. O., Bennich, H. H., and Berg, T. (1972). The clinical significance of IgE. *In* "Progress in Clinical Immunology" R. S. Schwartz, ed.), Vol. I, p. 157. Grune & Stratton, New York.

Levy, D. A., and Osler, A. (1966). Studies on the mechanism of hypersensitivity phenomena. XIV. Passive sensitization *in vitro* of human leukocytes to ragweed pollen antigen. *J. Immunol.* **97**, 203.

Levy, D. A., and Osler, A. G. (1967). *J. Immunol.* **99**, 1074.

Lichtenstein, L. M., Ishizaka, K., Norman, P. S., Sobotka, A., and Hill, B. M. (1973). IgE antibody measurement in ragweed hay fever: Relationship to clinical severity and the results of immunotherapy. *J. Clin. Invest.* **52**, 472.

May, C. D., Lyman, M., Alberto, R., and Cheng, J. (1970). Procedures for immunochemical study of histamine release from leukocytes with small volumes of blood. *J. Allergy* **46**, 12.

Osler, A. G., Lichtenstein, L. M., and Levy, D. A. (1968). *In vitro* studies of human reaginic allergy. *Adv. Immunol.* **8**, 183.

Rowe, D. S., Grab, B., and Anderson, S. G. (1973). An international reference preparation for human serum immunoglobulin E. *Bull. W. H. O.,* **49**, 320.

Schellenberg, R. R., and Adkinson, N. F. (1975). Measurement of absolute amounts of antigen-specific human IgE by a radioallergosorbent test (RAST) elution technique. *J. Immunol.* **115**, 1577.

Siraganian, R. P. (1974). An automated continuous flow system for the extraction and fluorometric analysis of histamine. *Anal. Biochem.* **57**, 383.

Autoantibodies in Hematological Disorders

C. P. ENGELFRIET

Central Laboratory of the Netherlands Red Cross Blood Transfusion Service, Amsterdam, The Netherlands

I. Introduction

In some important hematological disorders, autoantibodies may be formed against elements other than those of the blood, such as autoantibodies against nuclear antigens and autoantibodies against tissues. However, the techniques for the detection of these antibodies are treated elsewhere in this volume; in this chapter, I shall deal only with autoantibodies against blood cells and their significance for shortening the lifespan of these cells. It will be seen that the techniques designed for the detection of these autoantibodies are directly related to their serological and immunochemical characteristics.

Autoantibodies against red cells were the first autoantibodies to be discovered, by Donath and Landsteiner in 1904, in a patient with paroxysmal cold hemoglobinuria. For that reason, and because our knowledge

345

of red cell autoantibodies is most advanced, I shall first discuss the detection of red cell autoantibodies, then that of platelet autoantibodies, and finally the problems of leukocyte-autoantibody detection.

It must be realized that the essential characteristic of autoantibodies is their autoreactivity. Most of the techniques used for their detection serve equally well to detect isoantibodies against blood cells.

II. Autoimmune Hemolytic Anemia

In the demonstration of red cell autoantibodies we are dealing with four kinds of autoantibodies, each with a different serological behavior. In order to detect these various antibodies, we must therefore adapt our techniques. These antibodies, in accord with their serological behavior, are grouped as follows:

1. Incomplete warm autoantibodies: antibodies not capable of agglutinating red cells suspended in saline; optimal activity at about 37°C.

2. Warm hemolysins: antibodies capable of hemolyzing red cells *in vitro* by activation of complement; optimal activity at about 37°C.

3. Cold agglutinins/hemolysins: antibodies capable of agglutinating red cells in saline and of hemolyzing these cells *in vitro;* optimal activity at temperatures below 37°C.

4. Biphasic hemolysins: cold hemolysins with optimal *in vitro* activity at 0°C. As activation of complement is incomplete at that temperature, a second-phase incubation at 37°C is necessary to obtain hemolysis.

Although several techniques are essential for the detection of these various kinds of antibodies, one test, the direct antiglobulin test is of key importance. Not only is it the only technique by which incomplete warm autoantibodies can be detected on patients' red cells, but also it reveals the presence on the red cells of complement factors, and such factors are present on the red cells of all patients with hemolysins. Our investigation of the blood of a patient suspected of having autoimmune hemolytic anemia thus begins with the direct antiglobulin test on the red cells. If the result is negative, there are no autoantibodies detectable in the patients' blood; if it is positive, then a full serological examination must follow.

A. Testing for Autoimmune Hemolytic Anemia

1. Direct Antiglobulin Test (DAGT) on Red Cells

This test is based on a principle described by Moreschi in 1904 and rediscovered and introduced into clinical medicine by Coombs, Mourant, and Race in 1945. The principle is that red cells coated with incomplete antibody will be agglutinated by an animal serum containing hetero-antibodies against human immunoglobulins. Coombs *et al.* first applied this principal for the detection of incomplete isoantibodies in serum (indirect antiglobulin test), but Boorman *et al.* and Loutit and Mollison discovered in 1946 that the red cells of some patients with hemolytic anemia are agglutinated directly by antiglobulin serum, thus demon-strating *in vivo* sensitization. Further investigations by Dacie (1967) showed that the agglutination of a patient's red cells by antiglobulin serum may be due to the presence on the red cells of immunoglobulin G (IgG) and/or non-IgG; Harboe and Müller-Eberhard showed that the presence of complement factors on the red cells is responsible for the non-IgG reactions. However, the rapidly increasing knowledge of the im-munoglobulins necessitated a more sophisticated evaluation of the posi-tive DAGT. The application of antisera specific for the various classes of immunoglobulins revealed (Engelfriet *et al.*, 1975) that, apart from IgG, incomplete autoantibodies present on a patient's red cells may also be IgA or IgM, and the use of antisera specific for the subclasses of IgG showed that there is a wide variation in IgG incomplete warm anti-bodies as far as subclasses are concerned. As we shall see the Ig class and IgG subclass of incomplete warm antibodies are of great significance because of their biological behavior.

In the DAGT the red cells of the patient are first submitted to a multi-specific antiglobulin serum, which recognizes antibodies of all classes and also has anticomplement activity. In case of a positive result the cells must be tested with class-specific, and if possible IgG subclass-specific, reagents as well as with anticomplement serum. If incomplete warm autoantibodies are detected, an eluate from the patient's red cells is prepared by any of the methods currently in use. The eluate is ex-amined in the indirect antiglobulin test to establish the possible blood-group specificity of the autoantibodies, using a suitable cell panel. As most of the incomplete warm autoantibodies show a higher activity with enzyme-treated cells, the eluate is also examined in an enzyme technique for the same purpose.

a. Test Procedures. i. DAGT. Red cells are recovered from the clot, washed three times in large volumes of saline to remove aspecifically adherent plasmaproteins, and made up to a 5% suspension in saline. In agglutination tubes (7 × 45 mm) 1 drop of the antiglobulin reagent (whatever its specificity) or a two fold dilution thereof is mixed thor-oughly with 1 drop of the red cell suspension. Incubation is for 1 hour at 37°C; the results are read microscopically.

ii. Indirect Antiglobulin Test. One drop of the eluate and 1:2 and 1:4 dilutions thereof are incubated with 1 drop of a 5% suspension of "panel" red cells for 1 hour at 37°C. The cells are then washed thrice and incubated with 1 drop of a proper dilution of the antiglobulin reagent (anti-IgG when the direct AGT is positive with anti-IgG, etc.). The dilution must be chosen to avoid possible prozone effects. Results are read microscopically after incubation at 37°C for 0.5 hour.

iii. Enzyme Technique. One drop of the eluate and 1:2 and 1:4 dilutions thereof are incubated with 1 drop of a 5% suspension of enzyme-treated "panel" red cells and incubated for 1 hour at 37°C. Results are then read microscopically.

b. Results of DAGT and Their Implication. In evaluating the results of the DAGT, we can assume that red cells not sensitized by antibody and not coated by complement factors are not agglutinated by antiglobulin serum if the latter is made properly free of heteroagglutinins by absorption. Therefore any agglutination seen in this test must be regarded as a positive result, which must then be further evaluated by testing with class-specific antiglobulin reagents and specific anticomplement serum. I shall now discuss the patterns that may be found and the investigations that these imply. It must be realized that the value of all results entirely depends on the quality, particularly the specificity, of the antiglobulin reagents and that it is difficult to prepare class-specific reagents and very difficult indeed to prepare IgG subclass-specific reagents. The specificity control of the antiglobulin reagents used is therefore most essential.

Reaction Patterns. Pattern 1: A positive result is found only with anti-IgG and/or anti-IgA serum. This indicates that only noncomplement-binding IgG and/or IgA incomplete warm autoantibodies are present. An eluate is examined in the indirect AGT using anti-IgG and/or anti-IgA, and in an enzyme technique to establish blood-group specificity of the antibodies (see below). If IgG antibodies are present, the DAGT is, if possible, done with subclass-specific antisera.

Pattern 2: A positive result is obtained with anti-IgG and/or anti-IgA and anticomplement serum. Although *in vitro* complement activation by IgG incomplete warm autoantibodies has been reported in the literature, these antibodies, like IgA incomplete warm autoantibodies, are in our hands noncomplement binding. In some of the patients, the presence of complement on the red cells can be explained by the presence of warm hemolysins in the patient's blood, which frequently occur together with incomplete warm autoantibodies. In these cases, the patient's serum must be examined for the presence of such hemolysins by the appropriate technique (see below). Why complement is detectable on the red cells of patients without hemolysins is not clear, as it is unlikely that complement can be activated via the alternative pathway by antibody that has reacted with antigen on cell membranes. A possibility, suggested by van Loghem, is that in these cases a virus is bound to the cell membrane, which reacts there with an antivirus antibody and which then activates complement. This leads to the fixation of activated complement on the cell membrane.

Pattern 3: The DAGT is positive with anti-IgM and anticomplement. Incomplete IgM warm antibodies are complement-binding, and complement is always found on the cells of these patients. In our experience, for unknown reasons, incomplete IgM antibodies cannot be eluted from the red cells. Instead of an eluate, the patient's serum must be examined in the indirect AGT with anti-IgM and anticomplement serum, but the antibodies are present in the serum of only some of the patients. The serum must also be examined for warm hemolysins.

Pattern 4: The DAGT is positive with anticomplement serum only. This may mean that the patient's blood contains warm hemolysins, cold autoagglutinins/hemolysins, or biphasic hemolysins; the serum of these patients must be tested by the appropriate techniques (see below). However, in some cases no autoantibodies can be detected in the blood of these patients. Although the red cell survival is then nearly always normal, the finding is without clinical significance as it may indicate *in vivo* activation of complement. Activated complement factors may be bound to the red cell membrane also when the complement is not activated by the action of red cell antibodies.

If IgG incomplete warm autoantibodies are detectable on the patient's red cells, the cells must if possible be tested with subclass-specific antisera. Any of the patterns in Table I may be found. The significance of these findings will be discussed later.

2. Tests for Detection of Autoantibodies in the Patient's Serum

a. Procedure for the Detection of Autoagglutinins. One drop of the patient's serum is incubated with 1 drop of a 5% suspension of the patient's red cells for 1 hour at 16°C; the result is read microscopically. If the result is positive, the titer and possible specificity of the antibodies must be determined using a suitable cell panel.

b. Procedures for the Detection of Warm and of Cold Hemolysins. Five drops of a mixture of equal parts of the patient's serum and fresh AB serum, brought to pH 6.5, are mixed with 1 drop of a 20% suspension of normal and of bromelinized cells and incubated for 1.5 hours, each

TABLE I

PATTERNS DETECTED WITH SUBCLASS-SPECIFIC ANTISERA

Anti-IgG	Anti-IgG₁	Anti-IgG₂	Anti-IgG₃	Anti-IgG₄
+	+	−	−	−
+	+	+	−	−
+	+	+	+	−
+	+	+	+	+
+	−	+	−	−
+	−	+	+	−
+	−	+	+	+
+	−	−	+	−
+	−	−	+	+
+	−	−	−	+

combination separately, at 16°C and 37°C. The tubes are then centrifuged, and the presence of hemoglobin in the supernatant is determined
either with the naked eye or, more accurately, by a photospectrometric
method. The sera are brought to pH 6.5 by mixing 13 volumes of serum
with 1 volume of a 0.25 N solution of HCl. As some warm hemolysins
have the specificity anti-i, it is advisable to use both I-positive cells and
ii-cells if the presence of warm hemolysins is suspected. As a control,
each combination is also tested with normal serum instead of the patient's
serum. If a positive reaction is obtained, the test must first be repeated
in the same combination, but without complement, to demonstrate that
the hemolysis is complement dependent. The titer and possible specificity
of each hemolysin is determined using a suitable cell panel.

c. *Procedure for the Detection of Biphasic Hemolysins.* Five drops of a
mixture of equal parts of the patient's serum and fresh AB serum are
incubated for 1.5 hours in melting ice. After careful centrifugation for
1 minute at 1000 rpm, the supernatant is removed and replaced by
guinea pig complement. After mixing, the tubes are incubated at 37°C
for 20 minutes, centrifuged, and the presence of hemoglobin in the
supernatant is determined. Controls are as for warm and cold hemolysins.
The titer and possible blood-group specificity of biphasic hemolysins
are determined using a suitable cell panel.

B. CLINICAL SIGNIFICANCE OF RED CELL AUTOANTIBODIES

It is impossible to treat this subject extensively. Only a short survey
of the diseases in which red cell autoantibodies occur can be given. The

main emphasis will be given to the significance of the various autoantibodies for red cell survival.

1. Occurrence of the Various Red Cell Autoantibodies

Groups 1 and 2. Incomplete warm antibodies and/or warm hemolysins: (a) solitary; (b) secondary to idiopathic autoimmune disease (mainly systemic lupus erythematosus and pernicious anemia), malignant disease of the lymphoid system, and miscellaneous disorders

Group 3. Cold agglutinins (hemolysins): (a) chronic → monoclonal rarely biclonal paraproteinemia; (b) transient → infectious disease (*Mycoplasma pneumoniae*, listeriosis, viral)

Group 4. Biphasic hemolysins: (a) chronic → monoclonal paraproteinemia, syphilis; (b) transient → viral infection

2. Significance of the Red Cell Autoantibodies for Red Cell Survival

There is no doubt that red cell antibodies capable of hemolyzing red cells *in vitro* by activation of the complement system also do so *in vivo*, thus causing intravascular hemolysis. In fact, complement lysis is the most effective method of red cell destruction. Thus, when hemolysins are most active at body temperature and capable of reacting with cells that are not enzyme-treated, as is very rarely the case with warm hemolysins, then *in vivo* hemolysis is very severe indeed, and, in all cases studied by us, leads to the patient's death in a few days. Most warm hemolysins react only with enzyme-treated cells, but in spite of this fact, they shorten red cell survival *in vivo*, be it only moderately. How these antibodies react with red cells *in vivo* is not known.

Luckily for many patients, most of the hemolysins reactive with cells that are not enzyme-treated are cold antibodies with no, or only slight, activity at body temperature, i.e., cold autoagglutinins/hemolysins and biphasic hemolysins. These antibodies can react only with red cells in the small vessels of the exposed skin, particularly in the cold, in which the temperature of the blood may drop considerably below 37°C. Therefore hemolysis will increase considerably when the temperature of the surroundings drops, hence the symptom of paroxysmal cold hemoglobinuria. In many patients there is a constant, be it slightly, increased hemolysis. In chronic cold agglutinin disease, nature has provided a natural defense mechanism: for unknown reasons, the antibody–red cell–complement interaction does not always lead to hemolysis, both *in vitro* and *in vivo*, presumably because the activation of complement is not completed. However, as a C_3 antigenic determinant is detectable on the red cells of all patients with complement-binding autoantibodies, the activation must have progressed as far as C_3. The C_3 inactivators present in the plasma very soon split the activated C_3 present on these cells that thus escape immediate complement hemolysis, leaving an inactive part of C_3 on the cell membrane. As no new activated C_3 molecules can be bound to the membrane sites occupied by the inactive part of C_3, the cell becomes resistant against complement hemolysis. The dual cell population formed in these patients is reflected in the biphasic survival curve obtained when measuring the ^{51}Cr survival time of the red cells of these patients. Red cells, escaped from direct complement hemolysis, but coated with activated C_3 will adhere to the C_3 receptor on monocytes-macrophages, which even *in vitro* leads to cell destruction. It has been shown that such cells are destroyed *in vivo* by this process, at least until the activated C_3 molecule is split by C_3 inactivators, and this process therefore is another mechanism of cell destruction by the activity of complement-binding antibodies. Part of the lymphocyte population also carry a C_3 receptor. Whether attachment to this receptor also leads to red cell destruction has not yet been convincingly shown.

Whereas little doubt is felt about the harmful effect on the red cell life-span of hemolysins, there is much less certainty about the red cell-destroying power of incomplete warm autoantibodies. In the first place these antibodies themselves do not hasten red cell death *in vitro* and, second, there are patients with such antibodies in abundance without hemolytic anemia and in whom the ^{51}Cr survival time of the red cells is actually normal. This has lead to much doubt about the nocive effect of these autoantibodies. The last word about this subject has not yet been said, but there is hope for a full understanding of the role of these antibodies.

Briefly the situation is as follows: IgM incomplete warm autoantibodies, though not *in vitro* hemolysins, activate complement, also *in vitro*, at least as far as C_3, and it seems certain that these antibodies cause destruction of red cells by means of adherence to the C_3 receptor on monocytes-macrophages, mainly in the liver, as there are many such cells present in this organ and the blood flow is extensive. IgG antibody-coated red cells adhere to the Fc receptor present on the monocyte-macrophage membrane, and this attachment also leads to red cell destruction *in vitro* by phagocytosis or extracellular destruction. This seems an attractive mechanism for red cell destruction by IgG incomplete warm autoantibodies *in vivo*, but there are some snags. In the first place adherence of red cells coated with IgG incomplete antibodies to monocytes-macrophages is readily inhibited *in vitro* by the addition of IgG, for example in plasma, and plasma is present wherever red cells come in contact with monocytes-macrophages *in vivo*. Also IgA incomplete warm antibodies seem to destroy red cells *in vivo* by the same mechanisms as IgG antibodies (circumstantial evidence), and it has been shown that IgA antibodies do not adhere to the Fc receptor.

However, there also are a number of arguments for the assumption that adherence to the Fc receptor on monocytes-macrophages is responsible, and these are as follows: it was shown by LoBuglio that if *in vitro* IgG-coated red cells are incubated with monocytes and plasma, no adherence takes place unless the hematocrit of the mixture is over 85%, and this was confirmed by us. Now *in vivo* such hemoconcentration takes place in the spleen, the hematocrit does reach values of over 85%, and in most patients with IgG incomplete warm autoantibodies red cell destruction is confirmed to this organ. Furthermore LoBuglio showed that red cells attached to the Fc receptor on monocytes *in vitro* become spherocytic, and spherocytosis is a typical symptom of patients with this kind of autoantibodies.

Finally only IgG_1 and IgG_3 were found to be able to adhere to the monocyte-macrophage Fc receptor, but not IgG_2 and IgG_4, and it was therefore interesting to determine the subclass specificity of IgG incomplete warm autoantibodies. We did indeed find that in patients with only IgG_2 or IgG_4 autoantibodies there are no signs of hemolysis, while patients with IgG_3 autoantibodies always have overt hemolytic anemia. The only discrepant finding was that among patients with only IgG_1-incomplete warm autoantibodies there are some in whom severe hemolytic anemia is present, but others in whom no signs of increased red cell destruction are found and in whom the ^{51}Cr red cell survival is in fact normal. This may mean that IgG_1 may or may not be capable of adherence to the Fc receptor. We have in fact been able to show that the red cells of those patients with only IgG_1 antibodies who have hemolytic anemia adhere to monocytes *in vitro*, while the red cells of patients with only IgG_1 antibodies without signs of increased hemolysis do not adhere to monocytes (Meulen *et al.*, in preparation). A part of the lymphocyte population also carry an Fc receptor, but whether attachment to this leads to cytotoxicity *in vitro* has not been shown satisfactorily.

If it could be demonstrated that adherence to the Fc receptor is indeed the essential mechanism, then the explanation for the fact that IgG incomplete warm autoantibodies may have such very different effects in different patients lies in the different efficacy of the subclasses of IgG in this mechanism. It is clear that establishing the subclass specificity of IgG incomplete warm autoantibodies is relevant. As IgM incomplete warm antibodies cause red cell destruction mainly in the liver, and IgG and IgA antibodies nearly always only in the spleen, the determination of class specificity also is important.

A last word about the significance of the determination of possible blood group specificity of red cell autoantibodies is appropriate. It has been clearly shown that in patients with specific autoantibodies compatible donor red cells survive normally and, should transfusion be necessary, compatible blood must be given, even in patients with mixtures of specific and "aspecific" antibodies when donors compatible for the specific antibodies must be chosen. Unfortunately the specificity of autoantibodies is often such that compatible donors are extremely difficult to find (e.g., anti-P, anti-I), but the foundation of national and international banks of frozen blood make compatible transfusions increasingly possible, even in such cases.

3. Additional Remarks

1. Our knowledge of the serological and immunochemical characteristics of red cell antibodies is such that when the results of all our techniques are negative, we may be pretty sure that no red cell autoantibodies are present in the patient. However, this does not definitely exclude the possibility of autoimmune hemolytic anemia. Theoretically, it must be considered possible that in some patients autoimmunity against red cells is wholly of the cellular type. No reliable techniques are available to demonstrate the presence or the absence of cellular immunity against red cells and, although in some patients there is circumstantial evidence that this form of autoimmunity is implicated, we have no way of confirming this at present.

2. Some evidence has appeared that in pure red cell anemia the dysfunction of the bone marrow may be due to the presence of autoantibodies against proerythroblasts. However, as this problem is still in the experimental stage, I have not included this subject in this section.

3. No mention has so far been made of red cell autoantibodies formed under the influence of treatment with a drug. Either of the following mechanisms may be encountered. (a) Red cell autoantibodies are formed during treatment with certain drugs, but the antigen against which the autoantibodies are directed has nothing to do with the drug, which was responsible for the autoantibody formation. Example: α-methyldopa. A high percentage of patients on this drug form IgG incomplete warm autoantibodies against red cells, which are indistinguishable from other IgG incomplete warm autoantibodies except that frequently they do not seem to increase hemolysis. No satisfactory explanation has as yet been found for this, but the detection of the autoantibodies is as aforemen-

tioned. (b) IgG or IgA incomplete antibodies against penicillin may be responsible for hemolytic anemia. In this case the antigen against which the antibodies are directed has nothing to do with the red cell. They are purely antipenicillin; penicillin is fixed on the red cell membrane, the red cell being destroyed secondarily to the penicillin–Antipenicillin reaction on its surface. These antibodies are easily detected in the indirect antiglobulin test using penicillin-treated red cells. (c) The antibodies are formed against a combination of the drug and a red cell antigen, both the drug and the red cells being necessary for the detection of the antibodies. To detect these antibodies, the usual techniques for red cell autoantibody detection must be performed after addition of an isotonic solution of the drug.

III. Autoantibodies against Thrombocytes

Our knowledge about platelet autoantibodies is much less advanced than that about red cell autoantibodies. This is partly due to the fact that serologically speaking platelets are much more difficult cells, as they tend to adhere to each other and aspecifically bind immunoglobulin to a much greater extent than do red cells. This, however, cannot be the only explanation because platelet isoantibodies can be detected by several techniques, including the platelet agglutination test, the complement-binding technique, and the antiglobulin consumption and mixed antiglobulin tests, the use of which to detect autoantibodies has not been productive. A more elusive character of the platelet autoantibodies must be another important factor. Owing to strong circumstantial evidence, most immunohematologists have, however, kept their faith in the existence of platelet autoantibodies and their importance in idiopathic thrombocytopenia. The most important arguments for their existence are that the plasma of patients with idiopathic thrombocytopenia (ITP) induces thrombocytopenia in normal "volunteers," that the IgG fraction of such plasma is equally effective, and that only specific absorption with platelets removes this thrombocytopenia-inducing capacity. This tenacious faith in the reality of platelet autoantibodies has induced serologists to try any new technique that came on the market for the detection of these elusive antibodies. That the disappointments were many is reflected in the length of the list of techniques, and a full review of this matter is not possible in this section.

The most important new techniques applied in recent years are, in my opinion, cell electrophoresis, platelet-factor 3 release, ^{14}C-labeled serotonin release, and immunofluorescence techniques. Cell electrophoresis is based on a reduction in the mobility in an electric field of antibody-coated platelets as compared to normal ones. With this technique we have not been able to detect autoantibodies in the serum of patients with ITP, nor could we demonstrate that platelets of such patients moved more slowly than normal platelets. The techniques based on the release of platelet-factor 3 and ^{14}C-labeled serotonin measure a secondary effect of the platelet-antibody interaction. However, these factors may also be released from platelets by nonimmunological causes; the techniques therefore are not as specific for antibody activity as one would wish. Good results with these techniques have been described, but in our hands the ^{14}C-labeled serotonin release technique gave most erratic results with the most reliable HLA antisera from our panel. The best possibilities seem to be offered by the different varieties of the immunofluorescence technique, although the aspecific fluorescence of normal platelets, incubated with normal serum, is a drawback. Therefore, in our opinion (van Boxtel, 1973a,b, 1975), the most promising technique was fluorescence microphotometry as first applied to platelet serology by Denk et al., it allows for the objective measuring of quantitative differences between specific and aspecific fluorescence, for the measuring of the fluorescence of single cells, and for the application of statistical methods to calculate which values may be considered to represent a positive result. Finally, few platelets are necessary for the technique; this makes possible the actual demonstration of the autoreactivity of detected antibodies. In our hands, this technique was the first to allow us the demonstration of platelet autoantibodies in some patients with idiopathic thrombocytopenia, and I shall restrict myself in this section to a description of this technique and an evaluation of the results obtained with it, fully aware of the fact that this is a most subjective choice.

A. TESTING FOR AUTOANTIBODIES AGAINST THROMBOCYTES

1. Procedure

The detailed description of the test is given in the Appendix. The principle of the technique is as follows: a drop of a thrice-washed platelet suspension, prepared from EDTA blood, is dried on a slide and fixed with acetone, unless otherwise stated. The platelets are incubated with 3 drops of the patient's serum in a plexiglass moist chamber for 30 minutes at 37°C and subsequently washed for 15 minutes in phosphate-buffered saline (PBS) at room temperature and then dried. Three drops of a conjugated antiglobulin reagent is then added or, when a double sandwich technique is done, 3 drops of an unconjugated antiglobulin reagent. Incubation is again done for 30 minutes, but at room temperature followed by a 5-minute wash in PBS. In the case of a double sandwich method, this is followed by a similar incubation with 3 drops of conjugated antiglobulin serum directed against the immunoglobulins of the unconjugated reagent first used, followed by a final 5-minute wash. The fluorescence is then measured of 20 platelets in the middle of the preparation, which is indicated by drawing a 1.5 mm line with a glass pencil and choosing 10 cells at each side of this mark. The mean of the fluorescence value of 20 platelets is calculated and compared with the mean fluorescence value obtained with 10 different normal sera tested on the platelets prepared on the same day. When the patient's platelets are examined, the mean fluorescence value of 20 platelets of the patient is compared with that of 20 platelets of a normal control.

2. Methods for Evaluation of the Results

In evaluating the results of immunofluorescence microphotometry (IFMP), we are less fortunate than in evaluating results obtained by the various techniques for the detection of red cell autoantibodies. In these techniques the control values are 0, but in the IFMP with platelets the mere measuring of fluorescence does not necessarily indicate a positive result. In other words, because aspecifically adhered plasma proteins cannot sufficiently be removed from the platelet surface by washing, we must work against background values.

Statistical calculations are necessary to decide which values may be safely considered to represent a positive result. When testing patient's serum, the values obtained are compared with the mean value obtained with 10 normal sera. The variability obtained with 10 normal sera was calculated to be 13%. The mean fluorescence of normal sera is taken as the 100% value and fluorescence values more than twice the variation coefficient above the mean normal value of the day is called positive, i.e., values of over +126%. It can be calculated that the probability of rejection for values over +126% is $p \leq 0.055$. The level of the mean fluorescence values obtained with normal sera appear sometimes to differ on different days, even when platelets from the same donor are used. This is probably caused by small variations in the technical procedures, but the results with patient's serum must therefore always be compared with the mean value of 10 normal sera, measured on the same day. It could further be calculated statistically that, presuming 100% to be the fluorescence value of a normal platelet preparation, the values with other platelets must be between the limits —31% and +45% to be called normal with 95% probability. These values become —40% and +60% for a 99% confidence interval.

Another difficulty in evaluating the results obtained with the IFMP is that so many patients with ITP have been isoimmunized by pregnancy and/or transfusions. Unless the possibility of isoimmunization can be excluded with certainty (and this is often very difficult or impossible), an examination of the patient's serum alone does not allow the conclusion that autoantibodies against platelets are present, only the actual demonstration of the autoreactivity of the antibodies offering a conclusion.

B. RESULTS AND SIGNIFICANCE OF TESTS

So far, after a great number of preliminary experiments to evaluate the usefulness and practicability of this technique, a full investigation—including the patient's own platelets—has been done in 24 patients with ITP. In 14 of these patients clear evidence of *in vivo* sensitization of the platelets was obtained (i.e., in 56%). In the serum of 10 of these patients autoantibodies against platelets were also detectable in the patient's serum. The serum of 3 patients, whose platelets did not give positive results, did produce a positive reaction not only with donor platelets, but also after incubation with the patient's own platelets. These results show that examination of the patient's platelets is essential for a proper diagnosis. The explanation for the results in the last 3 patients may be either that we are dealing with antibodies with low avidity which insufficiently sensitize the platelets *in vivo* or that, on the contrary, the antibodies are so effective *in vivo* that sufficiently sensitized platelets are immediately removed from the circulation. In view of the thrombocytopenia in these patients, the latter seems the more logical explanation.

The question now arises what is the significance of these findings. We are confident that with this technique in about 60% of these patients the presence of autoantibodies against platelets has been detected. Does this mean that the other 40% of the patients do not suffer from immune thrombocytopenia? This question we can not answer at present. The detection of platelet autoantibodies has been so difficult that it is likely that, although the IFMP allowed us to detect autoantibodies for the first time, it is unlikely that all autoantibodies are picked up by it. Second, it is possible that in some patients the effect of the autoantibodies is such that most of the sensitized cells are immediately removed from the circulation and, as in some cases all autoantibodies present in the blood seem to be absorbed on the platelets, it could be that the combination of these two circumstances makes the demonstration of the autoantibodies impossible. Finally, it is very well possible that in an important percentage of the patients only cellular immunity is responsible for the thrombocytopenia, but as there are no reliable methods yet available to demonstrate either the presence or the absence of cellular immunity against platelets, we cannot test this possibility. It is also possible that a number of these patients suffered from nonimmune thrombocytopenia.

As already mentioned in the Introduction, our knowledge of platelet autoantibodies lags far behind that of red cell autoantibodies. However, the IFMP will allow us to study the immunochemical characteristics of the platelet autoantibodies in a fairly easy manner, provided we have at our disposal class- and subclass antiglobulin and anticomplement antisera that are specific in the IFMP. Preliminary results show that these autoantibodies, like incomplete warm autoantibodies against red cells, are nearly always IgG, but that IgA and IgM antibodies may also be found, although much less frequently. Particularly the complement-activating characteristics of these antibodies will have to be studied. The results of these studies together with those of *in vitro* adherence experiments to monocytes-macrophages and lymphocytes and *in vitro* cytotoxicity studies may teach us something about the mechanisms by which platelet autoantibodies destroy their target cells *in vivo*, and this may have consequences for a more differential treatment of patients with autoimmune thrombocytopenia.

IV. Autoantibodies against Leukocytes

Whether autoimmunity against leukocytes can be the cause of a shortage of these cells in the peripheral blood is still a subject of much doubt. The history of autoimmune leukopenia began most hopefully in the early years of leukocyte serology, but problems of interpretation soon arose. This subject has been extensively reviewed by Walford in 1960, and only some main points will be mentioned here.

In the first place it was found that most of the leukoagglutinins suspected of being autoantibodies and inductive of leukopenia were in fact isoagglutinins due to multiple transfusions and/or pregnancies. However, in some selected cases the autoreactivity of these agglutinins was demonstrated, but it must be borne in mind that the leukoagglutination technique, even today, is not a reliable method.

Between 1954 and 1961, several investigators (Miescher, Dausset and Brécy, van Loghem *et al.*, Tullis, Engelfriet and van Loghem) reported the binding of γ-globulin to leukocytes, demonstrated by means of the antiglobulin consumption test. The autoreactivity of many sera giving a positive reaction in this technique was established, and in some cases evidence of spontaneous sensitization of the patient's leukocytes was given. A very strong correlation was found between a positive LE-cell test and a positive antiglobulin consumption test, and in fact it was shown that the LE-cell factor behaved as an autoantibody against leukocytes *in vitro*. Spontaneous sensitization of the leukocytes in patients with systemic lupus erythematosus (SLE) could only rarely be detected, indicating that the LE factor does not sensitize leukocytes *in vivo*. A positive antiglobulin consumption test was also found in cases in which the LE cell test was negative, but at that time it was not realized that there are antinuclear factors of several specificities that *do not* produce LE cells. It is quite well possible, but not definitely established, that in the LE-cell test negative cases, antinuclear antibodies were still the cause of the positive antiglobulin consumption test.

Interest in autoantibodies against leukocytes has been reawakened by the finding of Mittal *et al.* of cold autolymphocytotoxins in the serum of patients with SLE. These autocytotoxins were reactive optimally in the cold, and most sera were unreactive at temperatures above 22°C. The activity was in the IgM fraction of the sera. Since then such cold autocytotoxins have been found in many diseases, such as viral disease (infectious mononucleosis, measles, rubella), autoimmune disease (SLE, rheumatoid arthritis, myasthenia gravis, etc.), Hodgkin's disease, and even after vaccination and in pregnancy. The real clinical significance of the antibodies must still be determined. Terasaki *et al.* have suggested that these antibodies are a nonspecific by-product of an immune response and may in some way act to hinder lymphoid cells from further production of an immune response.

Whether these antibodies shorten the survival of white cells *in vivo* remains to be seen. Mostly they were found to be active *in vitro* only below 22°C, and the *in vivo* activity of these antibodies must be considered doubtful. Moreover, the antibodies were only found to be cytotoxic in the presence of rabbit complement, and their *in vitro* cytotoxicity may be an artifact. However, it is not impossible that in some cases in which the antibodies are active at higher temperatures, such as is also the case with cold hemolysins, they may in fact cause the *in vivo* lysis of target cells.

This is all that can be said at present about leukocyte autoimmunity. Future investigations will undoubtedly further clarify the situation. The technique for the detection of autolymphocytotoxins is given in the Appendix.

Appendix

IMMUNOFLUORESCENCE MICROPHOTOMETRY ON PLATELETS

Equipment

A Leitz Orthoplan microscope may be used, and for measurements a phase contrast oil immersion objective (110 ×, NPL/L1.30) in combination with a Periplan GF × 10 measuring ocular in the phototube and a Zernike phase contrast condenser. The oculars in the binocular head were also Periplan GF × 10. The microscope is provided with a vertical fluorescence illuminator for incident excitation light. Excitation light for measurements is provided by a stabilized direct current Xenonarc lamp (Osram XBO 75W). In the light path of this lamp, a standard-ring field diaphragm is placed so that a field with a diameter of approximately 10 μm only is excited.

Substage illumination for phase contrast observation is obtained by means of an Osram 12V, 100W Quartz iodine lamp. The filter changers of the lamp housing are not used; instead, a revolver with four different filters or filter combinations was constructed behind the mirror used to effect the change from the light of one lamp to that of the other. Thus, there are always identical filters for both lamps; this system also prevents overheating of the filters. For narrow-band excitation for fluorescein isothiocyanate (FITC) a dichroic mirror is employed with a λH of 495nm and a double-band interference filter TAL 483. A barrier filter K515 and a substage barrier filter K530 are used, respectively, to improve contrast (with a factor 3.5) and to avoid excitation during focusing (the filters were supplied by Schott and Gen., Mainz, Germany).

A Leitz photometer attachment MPV with a Knott light-measuring device of the type MFLK, BN5001T is used (Knott Elektronik, Munich, Germany). The MPV photometer viewing telescope has an eyepiece (GF × 12) with a graticule for centering the measuring diaphragm and reading its aperture. This standard ring measuring diaphragm has a diameter of 0.8 mm. Thus a field with a diameter of only about 4 μm is measured for the magnification used. The photomultiplier is connected to an amperometer (Kipp A 13) with five ranges of sensitivity.

Antigen

Venous group O blood, 8 ml, is collected in nonsiliconized round-bottom glass test tubes containing 1 ml of a 5% solution of disodium-

EDTA. Platelet-rich plasma is obtained by centrifugation for 5 minutes at 800 g. The platelet-rich plasma is transferred to a second tube and by centrifugation in a thermostatically controlled Christ Universal/III KS centrifuge for 20 minutes at 2800 g (3500 rpm) platelet buttons are obtained. After isolation, the platelets are washed thrice in an EDTA buffer pH 6.8–7.0 (a 0.009 M solution of disodium EDTA in saline buffered with 0.0264 M $Na_2HPO_4 \cdot 2H_2O$). In order to prevent the formation of cryoprofibrin strict measures must be taken to carry out isolation and washing at room temperature.

The fluid above the last pellet is removed as completely as possible, then platelets are resuspended in phosphate-buffered saline (PBS). The final density of the routine suspension is to be $\pm 0.03 \times 10^9$ platelets per milliliter. One drop of the final suspension is dried on a slide with a fan at room temperature and, except for use with the anticomplement conjugate, when unfixed preparations must be used, it is fixed with acetone for 10 minutes at room temperature.

Procedure

The middle of the area of fixed platelets is marked by drawing a 1.5 mm line with a glass pencil. The platelets are incubated for 30 minutes at 37°C with 3 drops of serum, first brought to room temperature, in a plexiglass moist chamber. After incubation the preparations are washed for 15 minutes in PBS at room temperature. After drying of the preparations, the platelets are incubated with 3 drops of conjugated antiimmuno-globulin serum for 30 minutes at room temperature and washed again three times for 5 minutes in PBS at room temperature. It is important to note that the conjugate must be applied when the wash buffer on the fixed platelets has just evaporated.

If a double sandwich is applied, the preparations, after incubation with the patient's serum, are first incubated with a nonconjugated anti-immuno-globulin reagent, washed, and subsequently incubated with a conjugated antiserum against the immunoglobulins of the nonconjugated antiglobulin reagent. The preparations are finally mounted in glycerol, covered with a cover glass, fixed with paraffin wax, and stored at −20°C until measured.

Measuring Procedure

The equipment is standardized with a uranyl glass (Schott GG 17) as described by Ploem. The standard value of the uranyl glass is chosen in such a way that the mean fluorescence of platelets incubated with undiluted normal serum and anti-Ig conjugate gives on the graduated scale of the amperometer a deflection of about 25 scale units, or 75 scale units when a higher sensitivity of the amperometer is employed. However, this does not mean that the same average fluorescence values are obtained for standard preparations, because of minor unnoticed variations in the isolation of platelets and the fluorescence procedure. For this reason only preparations made on the same day are compared with each other. Before measurement a preparation is inspected with phase contrast illumination, and the glass pencil mark is brought into the field of inspection. The emission of 10 platelets with a normal diameter and at the same distance from each other is measured. The mean fluorescence of 20 cells is calculated.

TECHNIQUE FOR THE DETECTION OF AUTOLYMPHOCYTOTOXINS

Isolation of Lymphocytes

Heparinized blood, 10 ml, is mixed in an Erlenmeyer flask with a small quantity of iron powder (carboxyl iron powder, code 1-1-63763, General Aniline and Film Corp, Dyestuff and Chemical Division, Linden, New Jersey). The flask is shaken for 10 minutes in a water bath at 37°C. The contents are then put in a glass tube and mixed with 2.5 ml of a 5% Dextran solution in saline (MW 200,000). After sedimentation at 37°C, the supernatant is removed and carefully placed on top of 2.5 ml of Ficoll–Isopaque 75% in two tubes.

Centrifugation is carried out for 15 minutes at 2000 rpm. The lymphocytes are then removed from the interphase (i.e., from on top of the Ficoll–Isopaque solution) and mixed with heparin/saline in a centrifuge tube; the suspension is then centrifuged for 5 minutes at 1500 rpm. The cells are washed once more in heparin/saline and finally resuspended in fresh AB serum (1000 cells/ml).

Technique

In a well of a Falcon microculture plate 0.001 ml of patient's serum is mixed under oil with 0.001 ml of cell suspension for 3 hours at 15°C. Rabbit complement, 0.005 ml, is then added; a further incubation of 1 hour at 15°C is carried out, and 0.003 ml of a 5% solution of Eosine-yellow in distilled water is added. After incubation for 3 minutes at room temperature, 0.008 ml of a 1% solution of acid-free paraformaldehyde (pH 7.2) is added, and the percentage of killed cells is determined under a phase-contrast inverted microscope. As a control the test is also done with normal AB serum instead of patient's serum.

References

Dacie, J. V. (1967). The haemolytic anaemias. II. "The Auto-immune Haemolytic Anaemias." Churchill, London.

Engelfriet, C. P., von dem Borne, A. E. G. K., Beckers, D., and van Loghem, J. J. (1974). Autoimmune haemolytic anaemia: Serological and immunochemical characteristics of the antibodies; mechanism of cell destruction *Ser. Haematol.* **7**, 328.

Mollison, P. L. (1972). "Blood Transfusion in Clinical Medicine," 5th ed. Blackwell, Oxford.

van Boxtel, C. J. (1973a). Immunofluorescence microphotometry for the detection of platelet antibodies. I. Standardization of the method. *Scand. J. Immunol.* **2**, 217.

van Boxtel, C. J. (1973b). II. The sensitivity of the method, compared to that of conventional serological methods. *Scand. J. Immunol.* **2**, 531.

van Boxtel, C. J. (1975). Demonstration of autoantibodies against platelets. *Scand. J. Immunol.* **4**, 657.

Walford, R. L. (1960). "Leukocyte Antigens and Antibodies." Grune & Stratton, New York.

Rheumatoid Factors in Human Disease

HUGO E. JASIN and J. DONALD SMILEY

Department of Internal Medicine, The University of Texas,
Southwestern Medical School, Dallas, Texas

I. Introduction

Rheumatoid factors (RF) are antibodies to IgG, the major immuno-globulin class in human serum. They are not limited, as their name would seem to imply, to rheumatoid arthritis (RA), but are also found infrequently in the serum of some normal persons, and more often in the serum of patients with connective tissue diseases or infections, such as chronic hepatitis, tuberculosis, and subacute bacterial endocarditis.

Their clinical importance rests upon their measurement as a laboratory aid for the differential diagnosis of several rheumatic diseases with confusingly similar features, and in their probable role in the formation of immune complexes that may increase joint inflammation or produce vasculitis.

The very property that led to the discovery of RF by Cecil and his co-workers (1931), their ability to enhance aggregation of antigen–antibody (IgG) complexes, was used by later investigators to develop sensitive assays for their quantitation. Waaler (1940) and later Rose and his co-workers (1948), developed an antibody-sensitized sheep red cell

365

agglutination (SSCA) method, which with modifications has gained wide-spread clinical use.

The RF that are measured clinically are usually in the IgM class, but IgG and IgA antibodies directed against IgG have also been found, as will be discussed below.

II. General Test Procedures

The commonly used tests for RF may be divided into two types: the aggregation of particles coated with human IgG and the aggregation of particles coated with rabbit IgG (Table I). The heavy-chain portion of both human and rabbit IgG share several common or cross-reactive antigenic regions that react with human RF. As will be discussed, however, some of the antibodies that react with human IgG do not react with rabbit IgG, leading to qualitative and quantitative differences between the two types of RF tests depending upon the disease of the serum donor which is being tested. Each type of test has special advantages and disadvantages. For example, a disadvantage of the type using rabbit IgG as the target antigen (coated on sheep erythrocytes) is the necessity of repeated absorption of the test sera to remove heterophile (antisheep) antibodies, which many human sera contain and which obscure the correct titration of hemagglutination related to RF.

Among the tests using latex particles coated with human IgG (RA-Latex), the slide latex fixation test is a roughly quantitative screening procedure which mixes one drop of a 1:20 dilution of the decomplemented human test serum on a glass slide with an equal volume of a commercial preparation of latex particles coated with a pool of heat-

TABLE I
COMPARISON OF COMMONLY USED TESTS FOR
RHEUMATOID FACTORS

Test[a]	Coating	Titer considered positive (serum dilution)
RA-slide latex fixation	Human IgG	1 to 2+ at 1:20
RA-tube latex fixation	Human IgG	>1:160
D cell	Human IgG	>1:16
Sensitized sheep cell agglutination	Rabbit IgG	>1:16

[a] RA = rheumatoid arthritis; D cell = Rh(D)-positive human red blood cell.

aggregated human IgG. When the mixture is tilted back and forth, visible particle flocculation is produced by RF in the test serum. The rate and degree of flocculation can be graded from 1+ to 4+. The test is easily performed in a few minutes. The same human IgG-coated latex particles may be used for more accurate titration of RF by testing serial dilutions of the test serum. Alternatively, human red blood cells which are Rh (D)-positive (D cells) may be sensitized with small amounts of isologous human anti-D antiserum produced in an Rh (D)-negative person. This antibody is one of the IgG class, and when applied in subagglutinating amounts to the D cells and tested in the absence of complement, a sensitive hemagglutination assay is obtained. This latter test (D-cell test) is limited in its universal applicability by genetic variations in the allotype antigens on the IgG coat. Only certain IgG anti-D antisera provide the necessary target antigens for most RF. One such antiserum (from a patient named Ripley) has been widely used as a standard coating for the D-cell test for RF.

One of the most widely used quantitative RF tests utilizes rabbit IgG-antisheep erythrocyte antibody to lightly sensitize sheep red blood cells for agglutination (SSCA) by RF. This test has now been modified for use in microtiter plates so that as little as 0.025 ml of serum is needed for each complete titration. Details of procedure for the two commonly employed tests for RF are provided in the Appendix.

Finally, aggregated preparations of human IgG which form insoluble immunoabsorbents have been used to remove from the serum anti-IgG of all immunoglobulin classes. This latter method has been successfully applied to serum fractions to estimate IgG-RF and IgA-RF (Torrigiani et al., 1970). This latter test is not widely used because of the variation in nonspecific protein absorption obtained from one laboratory to another.

III. Clinical Significance

Serological tests, such as the SSCA, which detect antibodies to rabbit IgG are more specific for rheumatoid arthritis (RA) than tests such as the RA-Latex which detect antibodies to human IgG. On the other hand, the less specific RA-Latex is simpler to perform so that it is widely used as a preliminary screening test. Table II shows the range of frequency of positive tests in adult and juvenile RA compiled from a number of independent reports (see Vaughan, 1972). In juvenile RA, the reported incidence of positive RF tests varies widely, positive tests and the average RF titers being much lower in younger children than in adults.

TABLE II
INCIDENCE OF POSITIVE TESTS FOR
RHEUMATOID FACTOR IN ADULT AND
JUVENILE RHEUMATOID ARTHRITIS (RA)

Disease	Percent positive	
	RA-Latex	SSCA[a]
Adult RA	70–85	60–70
Juvenile RA	10–20	6–25

[a] Sensitized sheep red cell agglutination.

Positive tests approach the adult disease incidence in older children, whose clinical pattern resembles RA of adult onset. The probability of a positive test or a high titer of RF in adult RA increases with the severity of the disease, the presence of widespread erosive lesions of articular bony surfaces, a more unremitting course, and the coexistence of rheumatoid nodules or vasculitis. These points are summarized in Table III.

Although the presence of positive tests for RF are more likely to be present in patients with more severe RA, there is often a poor correlation between the level of such positive titers and observed clinical activity. Positive tests are obtained in RA patients very early in the course of the disease, and it is likely that RF is usually present before the clinical appearance of overt arthritis in the majority of patients. By the same token, negative tests obtained in patients with early RA usually remain negative throughout the course of their disease. These initial serological findings, therefore, can be used to predict the prognosis of a given patient, since seronegative RA is usually a much less severe disease. However, a small number of RF-negative patients develop severe RA when their arthritis activity continues without remission for over three years.

TABLE III
CLINICAL FEATURES
ASSOCIATED WITH HIGH TITERS
OF RHEUMATOID FACTORS IN
ADULT RHEUMATOID ARTHRITIS

Generalized, severe polyarthritis
Widespread bony erosions
Unremitting course
Rheumatoid nodules
Rheumatoid vasculitis

Although high titers of RF are often associated with severe RA, the RF titer in any given patient usually does not change with disease activity. Only a few patients initially having positive RF tests become seronegative following a remission of their arthritis, most patients whose disease becomes inactive continue to be seropositive for many years. Significant decreases in RF titer may follow treatment with gold, penicillamine, or immunosuppressive agents. In patients with Sjögren's syndrome, reversion of RF tests to negative is usually associated with the appearance of malignant lymphoma. Occasionally, patients with very high titers of RF develop a plasma hyperviscosity syndrome similar to that seen in patients with Waldenström's macroglobulinemia.

Rheumatoid factors are found in 1–4% of the general population, using the RA-Latex test; and in about 1%, using the SSCA test, with the highest incidence in sera from elderly persons over 75 years old. The distribution of positive RF in healthy individuals is equal in men and women. In most of these otherwise normal individuals whose sera are positive for RF by the RA-Latex test, the SSCA is negative. Follow-up studies of healthy individuals with positive RF tests over a 9-year period have shown that these persons are ten times more likely to develop clinically evident RA than seronegative controls in the general population.

Because IgM antibody is a more efficient agglutinator of particles coated with antigen than IgG or IgA antibodies, the RA-Latex and SSCA tests detect IgM RF preferentially. Using methods of immunoabsorption of RF on insolubilized IgG, available principally in research laboratories, IgG- and IgA-RF have been detected in the serum of otherwise seronegative RA patients, in sera from patients with juvenile RA and from a group of patients with adult RA complicated by vasculitis. The relative importance of the different immunoglobulin classes of RF in the pathogenesis of the chronic inflammatory process is unknown.

Table IV shows the incidence of positive RF tests in several other connective tissue diseases. Between 20% and 50% of the patients with systemic lupus erythematosus (SLE) have positive RF tests, although larger series have shown that the percent positive was closer to the 20% value. Unlike RA, in which high RF titers are frequently obtained, in SLE the titers are usually low and in many cases positive reactions are transient. Since some patients with SLE show prominent arthritis indistinguishable from RA, quantitation of RF level is important. As in SLE, a significant number of patients with scleroderma and dermatomyositis have positive RF tests in low titer. The clinical significance of these findings is unknown, but some of the patients with each of these three disorders also have Sjögren's syndrome. In Sjögren's syndrome, with or without associated RA, positive tests are found in the sera of most pa-

TABLE IV
RHEUMATOID FACTOR TESTS IN THE CONNECTIVE
TISSUE DISEASES[a]

	Percent positive	
Disease	RA-Latex	SSCA
Systemic lupus erythematosus	20–50	20–50
Scleroderma	15–35	15–35
Dermatomyositis	15–35	15–35
Sjögren's syndrome	96	74
Mixed cryoglobulinemia	90–100	30

[a] RA, rheumatoid arthritis; SSCA, sensitized sheep red cell agglutination.

tients. Positive RF in serum from patients with polyarteritis nodosa is no more frequent than would be found in the normal population. Because patients with essential mixed cryoglobulinemia share many of the features of SLE and RA, it is listed in Table IV with the connective tissue diseases. Mixed cryoglobulinemia is more frequent in adult females, who develop nonthrombocytopenic purpura localized to the legs, arthralgias, hepatosplenomegaly, and, in over half of the patients, rapidly progressive glomerulonephritis. Their serum contains low to moderate amounts of cryoglobulins and depleted complement levels. These cryoglobulins behave as true immune complexes and contain IgM rheumatoid factor which has reacted with IgG. Positive RA-Latex tests are found in the serum of almost every patient.

RF which react with IgG are present in many patients with chronic inflammatory processes or in diseases in which there is a sustained antigenic stimulus. For example, astute clinicians have observed that the RA-Latex is a better diagnostic test for hepatitis that for RA, and it may be also used as a diagnostic aid in the detection of subacute bacterial endocarditis, where 48% of patients have a positive test (Table V).

Table V also lists in different categories a number of other nonrheumatic diseases in which RF is frequently positive. In general, the RF titers are lower than those encountered in the sera of patients with RA and remain positive only during the active phase of the disease. It is also apparent that in most of these nonrheumatic diseases, the RA-Latex is much more often positive than the SSCA. Among the infectious diseases with high frequency of positive RF, many tropical diseases such as kala azar, leishmaniasis, and trypanosomiasis have been omitted because they are so rarely seen by medical practitioners in the United States. In the group of patients with chronic interstitial fibrosis of the lung, the highest

TABLE V

INCIDENCE OF POSITIVE RHEUMATOID FACTOR TESTS IN
OTHER DISEASES[a]

| | Percent positive | |
Disease	RA-Latex	SSCA
Infectious diseases		
Bacterial diseases	20	11
Subacute bacterial endocarditis	48	22
Viral diseases	17	14
Syphilis	13	5
Leprosy	24	15
Liver diseases		
Viral hepatitis	30–40	21
Chronic liver disease	30–80	15–25
Pulmonary diseases		
Pulmonary tuberculosis	11	6
Chronic interstitial fibrosis	20–50	5–45
Sarcoidosis	17	5
Miscellaneous		
Purpura hyperglobulinemia	100	62
Waldenström's macroglobulinemia	30	22
Renal homograft	74	8
Myocardial infarction	12	20

[a] RA-Latex, rheumatoid arthritis-latex test; SSCA, sensitized
sheep red cell agglutination test.

incidence of positive tests has been reported in serum from patients with
idiopathic pulmonary fibrosis or silicosis with massive fibrosis.

Appendix: Commonly Used Rheumatoid Factor Tests

RA-LATEX FIXATION

Reagents

Polystyrene latex particles (0.5–1% v/v) in 0.1 M glycine buffer, pH
8.2, are coated with 0.5% human IgG in the same buffer using 5 volumes
of IgG solution for each 1 volume of a latex particle suspension which
gives a light transmission of 7% at 650 nm.

Procedure

1. All sera are decomplemented for 20 minutes at 56°C, then spun.
2. Ten twofold serial dilutions of the test serum and of known posi-

tive and known negative sera are prepared in the glycine buffer beginning with a 1:20 dilution. This is achieved by starting with 1.9 ml of buffer, to which 0.1 ml of serum is added. Each subsequent tube receives 1.0 ml of buffer. After the first tube has been mixed, 1.0 ml is transferred to the second and mixed; again 1.0 ml is transferred, etc., until the tenth tube, from which 1.0 ml is discarded.

3. The coated latex reagent, 1.0 ml is added, then the tubes are shaken and placed at 56°C for 2 hours.

4. The tubes are cooled for 5 minutes at room temperature, then spun at 900 g for 2.75 minutes.

5. The procedure may be modified to a microliter plate method by reducing the above volumes. Commercially prepared latex particles coated with IgG are available and are stable for several months when refrigerated.

6. A positive result is represented by particle flocculation with serum dilutions of 1:160 or higher accompanied by confirmatory positive and negative results in the known positive and known serum controls.

Sensitized Sheep Cell Agglutination (SSCA) Test

Reagents and Materials

1. Sheep erythrocytes (SRBC) 1–3 weeks of age, which are commercially available as a suspension in citrate buffer, are washed three times in 0.9% NaCl, then resuspended to a concentration of 2% (v/v).

2. Microdiluters (0.025 ml), blotters, dropper pipettes, and microtiter U-plates (Scientific Products, McGaw Park, Illinois). The U-plates contain 8 rows of 12 wells, each with a working capacity of 0.125 ml.

3. Rabbit anti-SRBC antibody (amboceptor), 1:100 dilution in 0.2% phenol in 0.9% NaCl.

4. Positive and negative control sera.

Procedure

1. Serum absorption: To remove human anti-SRBC antibodies, adsorb the control and test sera with an equal volume of washed packed SRBC, which are suspended in the sera by gentle mixing and incubated for 60 minutes at 37°C. After spinning at 900 g for 5 minutes, the adsorbed serum is removed into a separate tube for use below.

2. Rabbit anti-SRBC titration: The amboceptor is diluted to 1:100, 1:200, 1:300 . . . 1:800 to obtain the greatest dilution that will just agglutinate a 0.5% (v/v) suspension of SRBC. Intermediate dilutions should be made to establish the base agglutination titer (BAT) between

the above dilutions. The SRBC and the amboceptor dilutions in a final volume of 1 ml would be incubated overnight at 4°C before reading the agglutination titer. Once established, the BAT is then further diluted fourfold (1:4 BAT), and this concentration is used to sensitize the SRBC to be agglutinated by RF.

3. Sensitization of SRBC: Using 1.25 ml of 1:4 BAT (diluted rabbit anti-SRBC) per microtiter plate, add an equal volume of a 2% (v/v) suspension of SRBC with continual swirling. Then incubate for 30 minutes at 37°C. Use within 30 minutes.

4. Actual test: Allowing 12 wells per specimen, place 0.025 ml of 0.9% NaCl in each well with a dropper pipette which delivers this amount per drop. Place a 0.025-ml microdiluter in each serum and transfer to well No. 1. After mixing, serially transfer to successive wells through well 9, mixing each time. Transfer 0.025 ml of the same serum to well 10 using a microdiluter and serially dilute as above through well 12. Add 0.025 ml of a 2% suspension of sensitized SRBC to wells 1–9. Add 0.025 ml of a 0.5% suspension of *unsensitized* SRBC to wells 10–12 as agglutination controls. Mix by gentle shaking, incubate overnight at 4°C, and read with a magnifying viewer lamp through the bottom of the plate.

References

Bartfeld, H., and Epstein, W. V. (1969). *Ann. N.Y. Acad. Sci.* **168**, 1–51.
Cecil, R. L., Nichols, E. E., and Stainsby, W. J. (1931). *Amer. J. Med. Sci.* **181**, 12–25.
Christian, C. L. (1967). *In* "Laboratory Diagnostic Procedures in the Rheumatic Diseases" (A. S. Cohen, ed.), pp. 96–113. Little, Brown, Boston, Massachusetts.
Rose, H. W., Ragan, C., Pearce, E., and Lipman, M. O. (1948). *Proc. Soc. Exp. Biol. Med.* **68**, 1–6.
Singer, J. M. (1961). *Amer. J. Med.* **31**, 766–779.
Torrigiani, G., Roitt, I. M., Lloyd, K. N., and Corbett, M. (1970). *Lancet* **1**, 14–16.
Vaughan, J. H. (1972). *In* "Arthritis and Allied Conditions" (J. L. Hollander and D. J. McCarty, Jr., eds.), pp. 153–171. Lea & Febiger, Philadelphia, Pennsylvania.
Waaler, E. (1940). *Acta Pathol. Microbiol. Scand.* **17**, 172–188.

Antibodies to Nucleic Acids

NORMAN TALAL

Department of Medicine, University of California, San Francisco, California

I. Introduction

Systemic lupus erythematosus (SLE) is an acute and chronic inflammatory disease in which circulating immune complexes deposit in the fine capillaries of the kidney, choroid plexus, and other tissue sites. The disease generally occurs in females of child-bearing age. An immune-complex glomerulonephritis is the most serious complication. The discovery by Hargraves in 1948 of the lupus erythematosus cell (LE cell) phenomenon was a major contribution both to the diagnosis of the disease and to its pathogenesis.

The LE cell is a polymorphonuclear leukocyte that contains a homogeneous cytoplasmic inclusion of nuclear debris. It is usually present in the peripheral blood of patients with SLE, but is not necessarily diagnostic of SLE. The formation of the LE cell depends upon the presence of antinuclear factor in the serum of lupus patients. Antinuclear factor is actually a heterogeneous group of antinuclear antibodies with varying specificity for DNA, nucleoprotein, histones, and other nuclear contents. Only the antinucleoprotein antibody is capable of inducing the LE cell phenomenon. The addition of serum containing antinuclear factor to normal peripheral blood leukocytes will result in the formation of the LE cell. Complement is fixed in this reaction. Antinuclear factor can be absorbed from serum with isolated cell nuclei, but not with intact cells.

The mechanism of LE cell formation depends upon the interaction of the antinuclear factor with the nuclear contents of degenerating leukocytes. Increasing the fragility of the leukocytes favors this interaction since it is believed that normal intact leukocytes do not engage in this reaction. After such interaction, the nuclear material separates from the cytoplasm and appears as a free "LE body." It is ingested by a phagocytic polymorphonuclear leukocyte, which then becomes recognizable as the LE cell.

Antinuclear factors themselves can be assayed directly by the method of immunofluorescence microscopy. This test is performed by using a tissue such as mouse liver as a nuclear substrate for the detection of antinuclear antibodies. The test serum is overlayered on the tissue, which is fixed to a glass microscope slide. A fluorescent antiserum to human immunoglobulins is added next, and the entire preparation is exposed to a fluorescent light source. If antibodies to nuclear constituents are present, the nucleus will appear brilliantly fluorescent. A number of different patterns of nuclear fluorescence can be detected by this method, particularly when sera are studied at various dilutions. The different patterns bear a general relationship to the chemical nature of the nuclear antigens.

One of the most important nuclear antigens is DNA itself, which under normal circumstances is a very poor immunogen. Indeed, normal animals have a remarkable tolerance to DNA and are capable of making antibodies to single-stranded DNA only when the latter is complexed to methylated albumin and presented in Freund's adjuvant. Double-stranded DNA does not produce antibodies in experimental animals under any circumstances. The greater immunogenicity of single-stranded compared to double-stranded DNA is true clinically as well. A number of disease states are associated with the formation of antibodies to single-stranded DNA. The formation of antibodies to double-stranded DNA, however, is generally confined to SLE alone. The only other situation in which antibodies to double-stranded DNA appear with any frequency is in the disease of hybrid New Zealand Black mice (NZB/NZW F_1).

The latter are an inbred strain of mice genetically predisposed to develop LE cells, antinuclear factor, and immune-complex glomerulonephritis. They are considered a laboratory model for human SLE. Immunological and virological factors, as well as genetic influences, are involved in their disease. The homozygous New Zealand Black (NZB) mouse has a Coombs' positive autoimmune hemolytic anemia as the predominant clinical manifestation. In the hybrid NZB/NZW F_1 mouse, a spontaneous immune complex glomerulonephritis with LE cell formation is the major clinical picture. As in human SLE, this disease is worse in female NZB/NZW F_1 mice who develop severe disease earlier in life compared to males.

The kidneys of patients dying from SLE and of NZB/NZW F_1 mice have been studied by immunofluorescence and by elution methods to determine the antibody nature of the immunoglobulins present in the glomerular deposits. Both in the human and mouse disease, a large percentage of these deposits are made up of antibodies to nuclear material, especially to DNA. Thus, the significance of antibodies to double-stranded DNA is 2-fold: (1) such antibodies are frequently associated with SLE and are therefore useful diagnostically, and (2) their presence is also associated with severe active lupus and the presence of immune-complex glomerulonephritis. Therefore, the development of tests to specifically identify antibodies to DNA was a major step forward in the field of antinuclear antibodies.

A wide variety of techniques are available to measure the presence and concentration of antibodies to DNA. These techniques include hemagglutination, immunoprecipitation in agar, complement fixation, counterimmunoelectrophoresis, bentonite flocculation, and radioimmunoassay. The latter is preferred because it measures the direct interaction of DNA with antibody, is extremely sensitive and reliable, yet is relatively easy to perform.

The next significant advance in this field was the discovery that patients with SLE made antibodies to RNA as well as antibodies to DNA. Despite the structural similarities between DNA and RNA, these nucleic acids are quite different immunologically, and antibodies to one tend to cross-react very little with the other. RNA is more immunogenic than DNA and can produce antibodies in the absence of carrier molecules or Freund's adjuvant. This is particularly true of double-stranded RNAs such as polyinosinic acid·polycytidylic acid [poly(I)·poly(C)] and polyadenylic acid·polyuridylic acid [poly(A)·poly(U)]. These synthetic polyribonucleotides have diverse biological effects including the ability to induce interferon and to behave as immunological adjuvants.

The spontaneous appearance of antibodies to double-stranded RNA in the sera of lupus patients raises interesting questions about the nature of the immunogenic RNA. Double-stranded RNA is most often associated with viral replication and is actually found inside the virions of some viruses, such as reovirus. The antibodies to RNA in SLE have greatest specificity for viral RNA and less specificity for mammalian RNA or for synthetic polyribonucleotides. The suggestion has been made, therefore, that viral double-stranded RNA may be the naturally occurring immunogen that provokes the formation of antibodies to RNA in SLE. If this were true, a similar mechanism of immunization to viral nucleic acids could also explain the formation of antibodies to double-stranded DNA.

The same techniques that are used to detect antibodies to DNA are also employed to measure antibodies to RNA. Here again, the radioimmunoassay method has several advantages over the other procedures.

II. Performance of the Tests

A. LUPUS ERYTHEMATOSUS (LE) CELL TEST

Venous blood is drawn into heparinized tubes containing small glass beads. The tubes are incubated and shaken in a rotator for 20 minutes. After centrifugation, the buffy coat is removed by pipette, smeared on glass slides, and stained with Wright's stain. The slides are scanned for at least 3 minutes. A true LE cell contains a homogeneous inclusion body whereas a heterogeneous inclusion is seen inside a "tart cell" or "pseudo LE cell." Neither the latter nor free extracellular material are to be considered diagnostic.

B. ANTINUCLEAR ANTIBODIES BY INDIRECT IMMUNOFLUORESCENCE

A rat liver is quick-frozen, sectioned by cryostat, and mounted on glass microscope slides. Sera to be tested are diluted 1:10 and placed over the tissue sections. Positive and negative controls are included. After washing, fluorescein-labeled antihuman γ-globulin is added. After the excess is washed off, the slides are examined under the fluorescence microscope. Positive sera should be studied at serial dilutions to determine the titer.

C. ANTIBODIES TO DNA

Antibodies to DNA can be detected by all the standard immunogenic techniques that measure an antigen–antibody interaction. Methods employing immunoprecipitation, complement fixation, hemagglutination, bentonite flocculation, and counter immunoelectrophoresis are all in use.

The ideal test should be sensitive, specific, reproducible, and quantitative. The precipitin test is generally performed as an Ouchterlony double-diffusion assay in dilute agarose gel. It is relatively insensitive and only detects antibodies to DNA in a limited number of lupus patients. The complement-fixation test is more sensitive and detects between 50 and 75% of lupus patients as positive. However, it is somewhat difficult to perform as a routine assay procedure and cannot be used with anti-complementary sera. Since many lupus sera are anticomplementary, this is a serious limitation. The passive hemagglutination test, in which DNA is adsorbed onto the surface of tanned formalinized erythrocytes, is a useful and sensitive assay procedure employed in many research laboratories. However, we favor the radioimmunoassay method because it detects the primary interaction between radioactive DNA and antibody rather than depending on a secondary phenomenon, such as hemagglutination.

The DNA can be made radioactive in one of two ways. It can be complexed with radioactive actinomycin, which binds strongly to DNA, or it can be internally labeled by growing tissue culture cells or bacteria in the presence of radioactive thymidine (labeled either with ^{14}C or ^{3}H) which gets incorporated into DNA. The cells or bacteria are then lysed, and the radioactively labeled DNA is chemically purified and isolated. A human tumor cell line called KB is frequently used for this purpose. Radioactive DNA can now also be purchased from several commercial sources.

The serum to be studied for antibodies is heated to 56°C for 30 minutes to destroy complement components, which can bind some nucleic acids nonspecifically. The serum is then incubated with the radioactive DNA at 37°C for 30 minutes and then at 4°C for at least 60 minutes. Essentially all the antigen binding and formation of radioactive immune complexes takes place during this time period, but longer incubations in the cold may be used if one wishes. An overnight incubation at this point is sometimes convenient.

The radioactive immune complex can be detected in several ways. In a Farr-type assay, the complex is precipitated by 50% saturated ammonium sulfate, which brings down the γ-globulin. Any radioactive DNA bound to γ-globulin is precipitated whereas free unbound DNA is soluble in the ammonium sulfate. The separation of precipitate and supernatant is accomplished by centrifugation. Since the volumes are generally small and the precipitate is easily disturbed, great care must be exercised in removing an aliquot of supernatant for determination of radioactivity. The amount of radioactive antigen bound can be calculated from this determination.

The Farr assay is time-consuming and cannot be used with some radioactive nucleic acids. For these reasons, it has been replaced in our laboratory by the cellulose ester filter method for detecting radioactive immune complexes. In this assay procedure, the antigen–antibody immune complexes are collected on cellulose ester (Millipore) filters whereas free DNA passes through the filter. The filters are then processed for determination of radioactivity by scintillation counting. The amount of radioactivity retained on the filter is a direct measure of serum antibody concentration. Results are generally expressed as counts per minute rather than percentage of antigen bound. The mean and two standard deviations for a panel of normal sera are determined for each new preparation of radioactive DNA. High binding is found with most lupus sera.

Antibodies to RNA or to DNA:RNA hybrid nucleic acids can be determined in much the same way using the filter radioimmunoassay method. Radioactive antigens currently used in our laboratory include ^{3}H-labeled reovirus RNA, ^{14}C-labeled poly(I)·poly(C), ^{3}H-labeled poly(A)·poly(U), ^{3}H-labeled poly(A), and ^{14}C-labeled polydeoxythymidylic·polyriboadenylic acid (dT·rA). Many of these are commercially available, and it is hoped that more will become available as these assays become more routine.

An additional advantage of the radioimmunoassay method is the ability to study the specificity of the antinucleic acid antibody by inhibition of binding using nonradioactive antigens in a competitive manner. The relative specificity of anti-RNA antibodies for viral RNA was established in part by such a procedure.

III. Results and Interpretation

A positive LE-cell test is always an abnormal finding and suggests the presence of serum antinuclear factor. It is in no way indicative of a phagocytic or other cellular abnormality, but rather is a natural consequence of serum antibodies reactive with nuclear antigens. Indeed, leukocytes from several animal species can substitute for human peripheral blood leukocytes in the assay system. The LE cell should not be confused with "tart cells" or pseudo LE cells that may appear in serum, particularly in patients with hypersensitivity reactions.

Antinuclear factor may be present in the absence of a positive LE-cell test, although most often the two are present together. Each individual laboratory should standardize its test for antinuclear factor and define the serum dilution that is to be considered positive. The interpretation of the test depends upon setting the sensitivity so as to exclude positive results with normal sera. In most laboratories, a serum dilution of 1:16 or 1:32 that still gives positive nuclear fluorescence is considered abnormal. Higher titers are generally seen in patients with severe active lupus; lower titers are associated with clinical improvement and remission.

The significance of titers lower than 1:16 or 1:32 in otherwise healthy individuals is uncertain. It clearly does not indicate the presence of lupus, but raises the interesting possibility that small amounts of antinuclear antibodies may be present in normal individuals. Whether they play some physiological role in the normal catabolism of nucleic acids and nucleoproteins is not known.

Even the presence of antinuclear factor in significant titers does not necessarily indicate the presence of disease. Antinuclear factor and rheumatoid factor may develop in 25–40% of elderly individuals (over the age of 80 years) without any signs of lupus, rheumatoid arthritis, or any other illness. Furthermore, an ever expanding number and variety of drugs can elicit the formation of antinuclear factor and LE cells without necessarily resulting in symptoms of disease. Continued administration of these drugs may result in symptoms of lupus and is therefore not advisable, particularly since discontinuation of the drugs is generally followed by disappearance of serologic abnormalities.

Several research laboratories have called attention to the pattern of nuclear fluorescence, distinguishing four main types: (1) homogeneous or diffuse, in which there is uniform staining of the entire nucleus; (2) peripheral or membranous, in which only the rim closest to the nuclear membrane is stained; (3) speckled, in which there is staining of clumps scattered throughout the nucleus; and (4) nucleolar, where only the nucleolus is stained. The peripheral or membranous pattern correlates with the presence of antibodies to DNA, particularly double-stranded DNA, and is therefore associated with active lupus nephritis. The other patterns are of limited significance.

Since there are immunologically specific tests for antibodies to DNA, it is unnecessary to depend on an immunofluorescent pattern to make this determination. Moreover, patterns can be misread easily by relatively inexperienced individuals who are not regularly performing these studies in large numbers on a daily basis. Furthermore, more than one pattern may be seen with a single serum, the picture changing with different serum dilutions. In some sera, the diffuse nuclear pattern will disappear with higher serum dilutions, and the speckled or nucleolar pattern will then be visible. This is quite understandable, since several antibodies of differing specificity are generally present simultaneously. The analysis and reporting of immunofluorescent patterns should remain a matter for the research laboratory specializing in this technique. Routine service laboratories should confine themselves to reporting positivity or negativity, and titer if antinuclear antibodies are present.

Antinuclear factor represents a heterogeneous group of antibodies reactive with various nuclear antigens. Included in this group are antibodies specific for single- or double-stranded DNA, for various nucleoproteins (in which the antigenic determinants require the presence of both nucleic acid and protein), and for various proteins found within the nucleus. A better understanding of the significance of these antibodies will come from an immunochemical approach in which antigens of defined specificity are used in the assay. An example of this approach is the determination of antibodies to DNA.

Anti-DNA antibodies are likewise heterogeneous and can show preferential specificity for single-stranded DNA or double-stranded DNA, or be equally reactive with both. Antibodies to single-stranded DNA may be inhibited by purine or pyrimidine bases, whereas antibodies to double-stranded DNA probably require a rigid double-helical structure for reactivity.

We employ a radioimmunoassay to measure the direct binding of radioactive DNA to antibody. The radioactive antigen–antibody immune complexes are collected on cellulose ester filters. The amount of radioactivity retained on the filter is a direct measure of serum antibody concentration.

One of the problems with this assay method is the source, strandedness, and specificity of the radioactive DNA. Since from an immunochemical standpoint all DNA is structurally similar, the source of the DNA should not be of great consequence. In fact, antibodies from SLE are equally reactive with DNA from human normal or leukemic leukocytes, salmon sperm, calf thymus and pneumococcus. More important, however, is the degree to which the DNA is truly double- or single-stranded. Single-stranded DNA is highly negatively charged and can bind nonspecifically to basic groups on serum proteins. Such binding, even if it occurs to γ-globulins, would not be immunologically specific (i.e., through specific antigen-binding sites on the Fab fragment of the immunoglobulin). The filter cannot distinguish specific from nonspecific binding, and so there is always some retention of radioactivity even with normal serum. This problem is minimized by working at a pH of 8.0. This "background" radioactivity can be quite high with some preparations of DNA, possibly because a large amount of single-stranded material is present.

Never the less, after determination of DNA binding by serum from a panel of normal sera, an arbitrary upper limit of normal can be established (generally two stranded deviations above the mean for the normal group). Sera from patients with SLE and from NZB/NZW F_1 mice frequently bind more DNA than this, indicative of anti-DNA antibodies. In the mice, the concentration of such antibody increases progressively with age. In patients, high binding correlates with low serum complement, active disease, and a markedly abnormal urinary sediment. These are signs of active lupus with nephritis. Low binding is associated with normal serum complement, clinical remission, improved urinary sediment, and improved renal function.

Antibodies to RNA can also be detected by the filter radioimmunoassay method using either radioactive viral or synthetic RNAs. The former is preferred but is not yet commercially available. The two most studied synthetic polyribonucleotides are poly(I)·poly(C) and poly(A)·poly(U), both of which are available commercially. We have recently studied the binding of ^{14}C-labeled poly(I)·poly(C) and ^{3}H-labeled poly(A)·poly(U) by lupus sera, which were first fractionated by sucrose density gradient ultracentrifugation. We found that poly(A)·poly(U) was always bound in the regions of the gradient corresponding to the distribution of immunoglobulins (either 7 S, 19 S, or both). However, poly(I)·poly(C) was sometimes bound to very light fractions smaller than 7 S, and presumably not immunoglobulin. For this reason, we believe that nonspecific binding may occur more readily with poly(I)·poly(C). We prefer poly(A)·poly(U) to detect anti-RNA antibodies when viral RNA is not available.

IV. Differential Diagnosis

The most important fact to remember about a positive LE cell test or assay for antinuclear factor is that these findings are not diagnostic of SLE. Although a positive LE cell test is considered one of the fourteen major diagnostic features of SLE (four of these features are required for a definite diagnosis), LE cells and antinuclear factor are also found in a number of other diseases, including rheumatoid arthritis, discoid lupus erythematosus, scleroderma, dermatomyositis, Sjögren's syndrome, and drug-induced lupus. They are occasionally seen in chronic or lupoid hepatitis.

LE cells and antinuclear factor occur in about 25% of patients with rheumatoid arthritis, particularly those with the most severe disease. LE cells and antinuclear factor are often associated with complications of rheumatoid arthritis, such as vasculitis, peripheral neuropathy, leukopenia, and splenomegaly (Felty's syndrome), and the sicca complex

(Sjögren's syndrome). The appearance of LE cells or antinuclear factor in a patient who otherwise has rheumatoid arthritis should not alter the diagnosis. Glomerulonephritis is not seen in such patients.

Discoid lupus erythematosus is part of the general spectrum of lupus in which skin manifestations predominate. About 35% of patients with the discoid variety have antinuclear factor, and about 8% have LE cells.

Drugs that are frequently associated with LE cells, antinuclear factor, and a lupuslike syndrome include procainamide, hydralazine, isoniazid, various anticonvulsants, phenothiazines, and oral contraceptives. The serological abnormalities and symptoms are generally dose and time related and reversible in days to weeks after discontinuation of the drug. Antibodies to double-stranded DNA and immune complex nephritis are generally not seen in drug-induced lupus. The mechanism of this phenomenon is not understood.

Antibodies to single-stranded DNA are only slightly more specific for SLE than is antinuclear factor. They are seen in a wide variety of related rheumatic diseases including Sjögren's syndrome and rheumatoid arthritis. By contrast, antibodies to double-stranded DNA are highly correlated with SLE. As shown in Table I, even when anti-double-stranded DNA occurs in other conditions, it is present in extremely low concentrations. A rising titer of antibodies to DNA, particularly when associated with a fall in serum complement, may be a sign of an incipient lupus crisis or episode of glomerulonephritis.

The specificity for SLE of antibodies to double-stranded RNA is intermediate between antibodies to single-stranded DNA. As shown in Table II, antibodies to reovirus RNA were most commonly seen in SLE and NZB/NZW F_1 mice. However, their frequency in rheumatoid arthritis and

TABLE I

ANTIBODIES TO ^{3}H-LABELED REOVIRUS RNA DETECTED BY THE CELLULOSE ESTER FILTER RADIOIMMUNOASSAY[a]

Sera tested	Number tested	Number positive	Percent positive	Mean (cpm)	Range (cpm)
Systemic lupus erythematosus	50	35	70	315	0–898
NZB/NZW F_1 mice	29	22	76	270	44–759
Sjögren's syndrome	46	9	19	63	0–411
Rheumatoid arthritis and Sjögren's syndrome	23	4	17	78	0–738
Rheumatoid arthritis	21	3	14	51	0–371
Normal	88	4	4	17	0–263

[a] Radioactivity added = 900 cpm (positive >100 cpm).

TABLE II
ANTIBODIES TO ^{14}C-LABELED KB DNA DETECTED BY THE CELLULOSE ESTER
FILTER RADIOIMMUNOASSAY[a]

Sera tested	Number tested	Number positive	Percent positive	Mean (cpm)	Range (cpm)
Systemic lupus erythematosus	50	38	76	119	7–269
NZB/NZW F$_1$ mice	29	15	52	64	10–143
Sjögren's syndrome	45	0	0	18	7–35
Rheumatoid arthritis and Sjögren's syndrome	24	2	8	23	10–65
Rheumatoid arthritis	21	1	5	20	8–56
Normal	44	1	2	29	16–83

[a] Radioactivity added = 280 cpm (positive >55 cpm).

Sjögren's syndrome is higher than that of anti-double-stranded DNA. This is even more striking in discoid lupus erythematosus, where the frequency of antireovirus RNA is 42% compared to 14% for anti-DNA.

Antibodies to RNA are not necessarily associated with renal disease (and are not known to be part of the immune complex deposition that occurs in SLE). They may be seen in patients with relatively mild SLE and even in asymptomatic relatives of lupus patients. They usually do not occur in drug-induced lupus.

References

Attias, M. R., Sylvester, R. A., and Talal, N. (1973). Filter radioimmunoassay for antibodies to reovirus RNA in systemic lupus erythematosus. *Arthritis Rheum.* **16**, 719–725.

Dubois, E. L., ed. (1974). *"Lupus Erythematosus:* A Review of the Current Status of Discoid and Systemic Lupus Erythematosus and Their Variants," 2nd ed. Univ. of Southern California Press, Los Angeles.

Talal, N., Steinberg, A. D., and Daley, G. (1971). Inhibition of antibodies binding polyinosinic·polycytidylic acid in human and mouse lupus sera by viral and synthetic ribonucleic acids. *J. Clin. Invest.* **50**, 1248–1252.

Complement

HARVEY R. COLTEN[1] *and CHESTER A. ALPER*

Allergy Division, Department of Medicine, Children's Hospital Medical Center, The Center for Blood Research, and the Department of Pediatrics, Harvard Medical School, Boston, Massachusetts

I. Introduction

Complement was discovered in the late nineteenth century when it was recognized that the bactericidal activity of fresh serum required the participation of at least two factors: a heat-stable factor, specific for the particular organism (antibody); and a second, nonspecific, heat-labile factor designated complement. During the two decades following its discovery, it became apparent that complement consists of several components that act in a definite sequence to effect bacteriolysis. The com-

[1] Dr. Colten is recipient of Research Career Development Award #5-KO4-HD70558.

plexity of the complement system has become apparent only in the past two decades. Nevertheless, recent advances in protein chemistry and the development of suitable functional assays for individual complement components have clarified the chemical, physical, and functional properties of the complement system. This has, in turn, led to a better understanding of the role of complement in human diseases.

II. Complement Components and Activation Sequence

The classical complement system consists of nine components designated C1, C4, C2, C3, C5, C6, C7, C8, and C9 in order of their sequential interaction. Under physiological conditions, the first component, C1, is a macromolecular complex of at least three, and possibly four, distinct proteins named C1q, C1r, C1s, and C1t. Three or four additional components comprise the alternative (properdin) pathway of complement activation. Altogether then, including the three natural inhibitors of complement, some nineteen distinct plasma proteins are considered part of the complement system. In normal serum, the concentration of these proteins is about 300 mg/100 ml, or approximately 4–5% of the total serum protein. As can be seen in Table I (pp. 388–389), several of the

Property	C1q	C1r	C1s	C1t	C2	C3	C4	C5	C6
Approximate mean normal serum concentration (mg/100 ml)	18	10	3	—	1	150	40	7	6
Relative electrophoretic mobility	γ_2	β	α_2	—	β_1	β_1–β_2[a]	β_1	β_1	β_2
Approximate molecular weight	400,000	170,000	110,000	—	117,000	185,000	240,000	200,000	95,000
Sedimentation coefficient, $s_{20,w}$(S)	11	7	4	—	6	9.5	10	9	6
Carbohydrate (%)	15	—	—	—	—	2.7	14	19	—

[a] Dependent on divalent cation concentration. [b] Cobra venom binding protein.

proteins (C3, C4, C1q, C1 inhibitor, properdin factor B) are present in rather high concentrations. C3, in fact, is visible on ordinary zone electrophoresis of fresh serum, particularly if $Ca^{2+} + Mg^{2+}$ is added to the electrophoresis buffer to slow its electrophoretic mobility in relation to transferrin and β-lipoprotein.

All the complement components studied thus far are glycoproteins, containing between 3 and 43% carbohydrate. The carbohydrate portion of these molecules may be critical for function, as has been shown for C9 and the C3 inactivator. The amino acid composition of most of the complement proteins is unremarkable except for C1q and factor B, which are unusual for their high glycine content. C1q also contains a high proportion of hydroxylysine and hydroxypropoline residues, and in this respect resembles collagen. Some of the physicochemical characteristics of the complement proteins are summarized in Table I; these have been discussed in detail elsewhere (see Müller-Eberhard, 1975).

Activation of complement via the classical pathway is initiated by binding of C1q to an antibody–antigen complex. Immunoglobulins of the IgM and IgG (subclasses $IgG_{1,2,3}$) class, but not IgE, IgA, or IgG_4, bind C1q, which then undergoes a conformational change leading to activation of the C1r enzyme. Activated C1r then cleaves C1s, revealing its enzymic sites that are capable of cleaving C4 and C2. Cleavage products of C4

TABLE I

PHYSICOCHEMICAL PROPERTIES OF HUMAN COMPLEMENT AND PROPERDIN PROTEINS

C7	C8	C9	C1 inhibitor	C3 inactivator	C6 inactivator	Properdin	Factor B	Factor D	CoF binding protein[b]
6.5	5	0.2	18	1	—	2.5	35	—	<2
β_2	β_1	α_2	α_2	β	β	γ_1	β_2	α_2	β_2
120,000	150,000	79,000	90,000	100,000	—	185,000[c]	100,000	—	—
5	8	4.5	4	5	6	5[c]	6	3	5
—	—	—	42	—	—	9.8[c]	10.6	—	—

[c] These values are for properdin isolated in activated form. Native properdin is a β-globulin.

and C2 then associate to form an unstable enzyme $\overline{C42}$, which facilitates the enzymic cleavage of C3 into C3a, a relatively small fragment with anaphylatoxic and chemotactic activity, and a large fragment, C3b, which in addition to other activities participates in further complement activation. C3b is degraded to C3c and C3d in whole serum, largely as a result of the action of the C3b inactivator. The fifth component, C5, is cleaved by the action of $\overline{C423}$ into C5a and C5b fragments, which have functions similar to the corresponding fragments of C3. Subsequent sequential activation of C6 and C7 allows the formation of a stable trimolecular complex, C567 in the fluid phase and presumably on cell surfaces as well. The addition of C8 to red cells sensitized by antibody and the first seven complement components may result in slow lysis of such cells. More rapid lysis accompanies the addition of C9 to EAC1–8.

Conceptually, this reaction sequence has been divided into two distinct phases; an activation phase consisting of the interaction of the first four components and an attack phase involving the sequential activation of C5–9. It appears that specific limited proteolysis occurs only in the activation steps and in the action of $\overline{C423}$ on native C5. A stable fluid phase complex of C56789 can be generated, and a similar complex forms on cell surfaces as well. The mechanism by which the fully activated complement system produces membrane damage and cell lysis is not yet understood.

The properdin proteins have been intensively restudied in the past few years. As originally defined, the properdin system consisted of properdin itself and two other proteins, designated factors A and B. It is now clear that factor A is C3 and that *activated* factor A is probably the major cleavage fragment of C3 (C3b). Factor B has also been isolated and characterized. Another protein, designated factor D, which has the capacity to cleave factor B, has recently been found to be part of the system. One of the fragments of factor B has the ability, probably through its action on an unidentified intermediary protein(s) to cleave C3 into C3a and C3b. Remarkably, C3b is necessary for the activation of factor D. Thus, a positive feedback loop is formed by which generation of a product (C3b) activates a system capable of producing further cleavage of C3 and generation of more C3b. The C3 inactivator acts as a brake on this process by cleaving C3b in such a fashion that it is no longer able to activate factor D. The presence of a positive feedback loop in the form of the alternative pathway has many important implications for our understanding of the function of complement in the amplification of immune reactions.

A theoretical framework for the mechanism of complement action has been developed in studies of complement-mediated cytolysis. These concepts have allowed the design of tests for the functional measurement of both antibodies and individual complement components on a molecular basis. Of fundamental importance in this regard is the "one-hit" theory of immune hemolysis, which states that a single effective site resulting from the sequential action of antibody and complement is a necessary and sufficient condition for lysis of the erythrocyte. This theory now has considerable experimental support. Simply put, the degree of hemolysis (as a decimal fraction) of a suspension of erythrocyte indicator cells increases asymptotically as a function of the average number of effective sites per cell. This relationship, known as the Poisson distribution, makes it possible to calculate the number of effective molecules of a complement component from the proportion of cells lysed in a standard hemolytic assay, as will be described below.

III. Biological Activities of Complement

Complement contributes to the inflammatory response and to host defense against invasion by pathogenic organisms. In certain pathologic states, complement appears to play a role in mediating tissue injury. Although earlier studies of complement emphasized immune cell lysis with its requirements for all components, it is now established that many of the important biological activities of the complement system become manifest early in the activation sequence. These functions are mediated for the most part by cleavage fragments of complement proteins.

Neutralization of certain viruses may be accomplished by the properdin pathway or by IgM antibody with C1 and C4 or by IgM antibody, C1, C4, C2, and C3. The properdin pathway, the classical pathway, and all the proteins of the common pathway are probably required for the bactericidal properties of serum for smooth gram-negative bacteria.

Both C3a and C5a are anaphylatoxins; that is to say, they both cause contraction of smooth muscle and an increase in vascular permeability. They both cause degranulation of mast cells with attendant histamine release. It appears likely that it is the released histamine which mediates the smooth muscle contraction and vascular permeability change. Both C3a and C5a are also chemotactic for leukocytes. The anaphylatoxin properties of these fragments are rapidly destroyed in whole serum by the action of an enzyme called anaphylatoxin inactivator, probably identical with carboxypeptidase B. There is evidence that another enzyme, chemotactic factor inactivator, destroys the chemotactic activity of C3a and C5a. C3a and C5a may be generated by noncomplement proteolytic enzymes, such as plasmin, trypsin, and tissue and bacterial proteases, as well as by classical or alternative pathway activation. Evidence has been presented that such noncomplement enzymes may play a role in the local inflammatory response to nonimmune injury.

Activation of the classical sequence through C3 is required for the enhancement by serum of the phagocytosis of antibody-sensitized erythrocytes or pneumococci. For the latter, maximal enhancement also requires proteins of the alternative pathway. The enhancement of phagocytosis would seem to be one of the most important biological functions of complement and of particular importance for defense against infection by pyogenic bacteria.

A requirement for C3 in the mobilization of leukocytes from bone marrow has been demonstrated experimentally and is suggested by the observation that there is an absence of peripheral leukocytosis during bacterial infection in a patient with hereditary deficiency of C3.

Immune adherence is the property of erythrocytes bearing C4 and/or C3 to attach to primate red cells, mammalian B lymphocytes, macrophages, monocytes, polymorphonuclear cells, and rabbit platelets. Particles other than erythrocytes acted upon by antibody and the first four complement components also exhibit immune adherence. This function of complement is of obvious importance in the clearance from the blood of bacteria and other pathogenic organisms and is a necessary prelude to phagocytosis. It may also be important in the production of humoral antibody to thymus-independent antigens. Because of the normal presence in whole serum of the C3 inactivator which destroys the immune adherence activity, this property is probably short-lived *in vivo*.

IV. Tests Involving Complement

Three main groups of tests involving complement will be considered: (1) those that are designed to measure the concentrations of individual proteins in serum or other body fluids, (2) those that test for complement activity *in vivo*, and (3) those that utilize complement consumption *in vitro* to detect and measure antibodies. The last are commonly referred to as complement-fixation tests.

A. Measures of Complement Concentration

Immunochemical Assays for Complement Proteins. The measurement of complement components as proteins in highly complex mixtures, such as human serum, requires highly specific reagents. This requirement has been satisfied by availability of antibodies against the majority of the complement proteins, most of which precipitate with their respective antigens in whole serum. Quantitative immunochemical techniques are therefore available for the quantitation of complement proteins in serum and other biological fluids.

The most generally applicable, reliable, precise, accurate, and reproducible technique, in our hands at least, is electroimmunoassay. In this method, antibody is incorporated into agarose gel made up in electrophoresis buffer. Wells are cut in a 1-mm film of this gel, and precisely measured volumes of standards and samples are placed in the wells. Electrophoresis is carried out so that rocket-shaped peaks develop to stability and cease to grow. The peak heights of the samples are then related to those of the standards, and antigen concentration in the test samples are thereby established. Practical and theoretical details of the electroimmunoassay technique are discussed by Laurell (1965).

Radial immunodiffusion is a widely used method for the immunochemical measurement of proteins, but it has certain drawbacks compared with electroimmunoassay. In radial immunodiffusion, antibody-containing gel is prepared as described above and wells are cut and filled in a similar manner. Plates are simply incubated until stable sharp rings form. The areas of these rings are then related to a standard curve obtained from measurement of the rings produced by known concentrations of the protein.

A comparison of these two methods as applied to the measurement of C3 is informative. If fresh serum is compared with the same serum stored at 37°C for 3 days (aged serum), in electroimmunoassay peak heights are nearly identical but in radial immunodiffusion the aged serum C3 ring will be considerably larger than the fresh serum ring. The reason for this difference is that the storage conversion product of C3, is smaller than native C3 and diffuses more rapidly into the gel during radial immunodiffusion. In electroimmunoassay, on the other hand, antigen is driven into contact with antibody by electrophoresis so that diffusion is minimal and molecular size is unimportant as a determinant of peak height.

Both the techniques described have a threshold of detection of about 0.25 mg/100 ml (2.5 μg/ml), which can be lowered by "counterstaining" otherwise invisible peaks or rings with a second antibody to the anticomplement antibody. Even further lowering of the threshold can be achieved by the use of radioisotopically labeled antigen or antibody to develop peaks or rings. Thus, virtually all complement proteins can be measured with these methods. For very low concentration proteins, such as properdin, radioimmunoassay is probably most practical.

For the screening of large numbers of samples, a rapid, accurate automated nephelometric method is available. In this technique diluted antiserum is mixed with diluted sample and incubated for 15 minutes, at which time, light scattering by the small antigen–antibody aggregates is read and compared with standard antigen solutions. At present, the automated nephelometric method is limited (among the complement proteins) to the quantitation of C3, C4, C1 inhibitor and factor B.

B. FUNCTIONAL ASSAYS OF COMPLEMENT

The measurement of whole serum hemolytic complement is a useful screening test for the integrity of the complete system. However, decreases in the concentration of individual components to 50% or less of the normal level may have little or no effect in this test. The test is based on the ability of sheep red cells sensitized with rabbit antisheep red cell antibody to be lysed by the complete classical complement sequence. Hemoglobin released by such lysis can be measured spectrophotometrically with great precision, and from this the percentage of cells lysed may be calculated. The dose–response curve is clearly sigmoidal and reflects the complexity of steps involved in the reaction. The slope is steepest around 50% lysis; i.e., small differences in complement input are reflected in large changes in lysis. For this reason, it is conventional to measure hemolytic complement at this end point, and results are thus defined in terms of CH_{50} units. This test must be performed with optimally sensitized red cells under strictly controlled conditions of temperature, ionic strength, pH, Ca^{2+}, Mg^{2+}, and protein concentrations. The standard buffer for dilution is gelatin Veronal-buffer saline of precise formulation. For details and analysis of the test, the reader is referred to Mayer (1961) and Rapp and Borsos (1970).

Hemolytic assays of individual complement components require availability of separate complement components purified to the extent that they are free of the activities of all the other components. All the components except for that being measured are supplied in excess, thus the percent lysis of sensitized sheep erythrocytes is dependent solely on the concentration of the limited component, as described earlier in the discussion of the one-hit theory of immune hemolysis. These measurements are specific, sensitive, and highly reproducible. Individual components can be measured in serum at subnanogram concentrations with an error of no more than ±5%. In the measurement of early-acting components C1, C4, and C2, advantage is taken of the fact that Ca^{2+} is required for the C1 step and Mg^{2+} for the C2 step, but no divalent cation is needed for later steps. Therefore, the terminal components C3 and C5–9 can be supplied as whole serum diluted in EDTA (C-EDTA).

As an example of the functional molecular measurement of a complement component, consider the assay of C1. The cells used for this assay are EAC4, sheep erythrocytes sensitized with relatively large amounts of IgM hemolytic antibody and C4. Portions of a suspension of these cells are mixed with different dilutions of test solution and incubated for the time needed to reach equilibrium. These cells are then exposed to C2 in excess (in other words, adding more C2 would not alter the results) and excess C-EDTA (C3, C5–9) for sufficient time to allow complete reaction. After centrifugation, hemoglobin concentration is determined spectrophotometrically in the supernatant fluid, and from the proportion of cells lysed the number of effective C1 molecules is calculated according to the Poisson distribution.

Quantitative and semiquantitative assays for several other complement-dependent functions have been devised, although none has replaced the hemolytic assay as a primary measure of functional complement component activity, because of a lack of specificity, sensitivity, or ease of performance. For example, a test of immune adherence has been developed that depends on microscopic observation of agglutination of primate erythrocytes in the presence of complement and complement-fixing antigen–antibody complexes. This assay is semiquantitative, at best, and is dependent on the concentration of the first four components; that is, a marked decrease in any of the four will affect the immune adherence assay. Tests of the capacity of sera to generate chemotactic or anaphylactic activities on exposure to zymozan, endotoxin, or antigen–antibody complexes are also dependent on adequate concentrations of multiple components. However, they may be particularly useful, as are assays for opsonic activity, in evaluation of diseases involving primary or secondary deficiencies of complement proteins.

A more complete description of functional assays for individual complement components is given by Rapp and Borsos (1970). This book provides an excellent discussion of both the theoretical bases for these tests and practical details of design and execution of the functional complement assays.

C. TESTS FOR COMPLEMENT ACTIVATION *in Vivo*

The measurement of the serum concentration of complement proteins in patients provides some information about the participation of complement in disease. However, this information, by virtue of its static quality, is somewhat limited. The serum concentrations of all proteins, including those of the complement system, are determined by dynamic equilibrium between synthesis and catabolism. A normal serum level may reflect a balance between abnormally accelerated synthesis and catabolism.

We know that complement activation *in vitro* is characterized by sequential binding of components to antigen–antibody complexes or other activating agents and extensive fluid phase limited proteolytic cleavage of components in the earlier steps. An obvious hallmark, then, of complement activation *in vivo* is the elaboration of cleavage products. Whether or not these are detectable in circulating plasma depends on the rapidity with which these fragments are cleared as well as the rate at which they are produced from native complement proteins. These fragments are usually distinguishable from their parent molecules in molecular size, in electrophoretic mobility, and often in antigenic composition.

The two most common techniques for examining specimens for conversion products are immunoelectrophoresis and antigen–antibody crossed electrophoresis (crossed immunoelectrophoresis). The latter is more sensitive and provides potentially quantitative estimations of conversion. Conditions of collection and storage of specimens are critical since conversion *in vitro* must be avoided. We have found that samples from normal individuals show no evidence of conversion of C3, at least, if (1) the venipuncture is without undue trauma, (2) the first 3–4 ml of blood are discarded, (3) the blood is then collected through the same needle into EDTA, (4) plasma is obtained by centrifugation within 15–30 minutes and immediately frozen in aliquots at −65°C or below. Repeated thawing and freezing of samples induces conversion and is to be avoided. Similar care must be taken in preparation and storage of samples for functional measurements except that EDTA chelation is generally avoided.

Deposition of complement proteins (usually along with immunoglobulins) in tissues such as kidney and skin has been taken as evidence for complement activation in disease. Such deposition is detected by the fluorescent antibody technique, using antibodies to individual proteins such as C3, C4, and properdin. From studies in animals, it is clear that such deposition may result either from filtration and trapping of immune complexes within small blood vessels or from antibody reactive directly with tissue antigens. It is clear, however, that tissue deposition is not an important direct determinant in the lowering of the serum concentration of complement proteins in most diseases. Metabolic studies with radioisotopically labeled purified complement proteins have yielded important information about complement protein metabolism. Although intuitively one might expect that rapid clearance of labeled complement proteins would attend complement activation *in vivo*, that is not necessarily true. It is only the case if fluid-phase conversion products are cleared at a more rapid rate than the native molecule. Such is true of C3b and C4b, which are removed from the circulation at rates five or more times those of the native proteins. No information is yet available for clearance rates of other complement protein fragments.

V. Complement-Fixation Tests

The use of complement "fixation" for detecting the presence of antigens or antibodies has a very long and productive history. This test can be used with soluble or particulate antigen and is based on the loss of hemolytic activity of complement on incubation with antigen–antibody aggregates. This test yields quantitative or semiquantitative data of relative antibody concentrations. Complement fixation is performed in two stages. In the first, the reaction of antigen–antibody in the test sample with a known amount of whole complement is allowed to proceed to completion. In the second step, hemolytic complement is measured to determine the amount consumed. The conditions for the first step are determined by the nature of the antigen and the type of antibody being measured. For example, IgG antibody fixes complement more efficiently at 4°C than at 37°C, whereas the reverse is true of IgM antibodies directed against the same antigen. The conditions for the second step are chosen for optimal detection of the unfixed complement. Suitable controls for "nonspecific" anticomplementary activity must be included for proper interpretation of the test.

Complement-fixation tests can be made quantitative. The most elegant example is the C1 fixation and transfer test (C1FT) of Borsos and Rapp, which is capable of measuring concentrations of either antigen or antibody on a molecular basis. In brief, particulate antigen–antibody complex is mixed with C1 to saturate all C1-fixing sites. The complexes are washed at low ionic strength to remove unbound C1 but preserve C1 bound to the complexes. In the transfer step, the washed antigen–antibody–C1 complex is mixed with indicator cells (EAC4) at physiological ionic strength, which permits the quantitative transfer of the C1 from the complex to EAC4. In the assay step, the number of C1 molecules transferred is determined with the conventional hemolytic assay for C1.

VI. Miscellaneous Tests

The *Treponema pallidum* immobilization test is highly specific for the infectious agent of syphilis. It requires both specific antibody and complement and is used when ordinary tests yield false positive results. Tests for paroxysmal nocturnal hemoglobinuria (PNH) depend upon the unusual susceptibility of red cells in this disease to complement lysis. In the Ham test, the test red cells are incubated in acidified (pH 6.7) fresh serum from an ABO compatible person or from the patient. The minimal complement activation that occurs at somewhat acid pH will produce lysis of PNH cells, but not of normal erythrocytes. The sugar water test for PNH depends upon minimal complement activation probably resulting from euglobulin precipitation.

VII. Complement Abnormalities in Disease

Since the hemolytic activity of complement requires adequate levels of all the classical components, assessment of this activity has provided a useful test for alteration in the concentration of any or all of the complement proteins. As already mentioned, this activity is expressed in CH_{50} units. Hemolytic complement may be unaltered despite considerable changes in the concentration of individual components. For example, isolated reductions in C1, C2, C3, C6, or C7 in human serum to half-normal serum concentrations results in normal or only slightly reduced hemolytic complement levels. In other words, only one or a few components are present in "limiting" concentration with respect to hemolytic activity whereas others are present in excess.

The most common change in hemolytic complement in disease is an increase in association with a wide variety of inflammatory and necrotic disorders as part of the acute-phase plasma protein response. In this circumstance, a substantial rise in serum concentrations of C4, C2, and C3 is noted. Serum hemolytic complement is lowered in a relatively limited group of acquired diseases, such as systemic lupus erythematosus (SLE), acute glomerulonephritis, membranoproliferative glomerulonephritis, acute serum sickness, and other varieties of immune-complex disorders. It is also lowered in advanced hepatic cirrhosis.

As a screening test, the measurement of serum total hemolytic complement for clinical purposes has, in recent years, been supplemented with the immunochemical assay of C3. In general, this protein is reduced in concentration in those disorders in which hemolytic complement activity is reduced, but there is no strict correlation. For example, in SLE, many or all complement components may be reduced in concentration, probably as the result of complement activation *in vivo*, but a decrease in C4 may precede significant changes in C3 concentration. In acute poststreptococcal glomerulonephritis, there is initially a marked fall in all classical complement components, but within 2 or 3 days of the onset of symptoms, most of the components return to normal. The concentrations of C3 and C5, however, remain low for 3–4 weeks. Evidence from metabolic studies with purified ^{125}I-labeled C3 suggests that, in the initial phase, the C3 concentration is lowered as part of activation of the complement system, presumably by antigen–antibody complexes. Circulating conversion products of C3 can sometimes be demonstrated during this initial phase. Studies performed 2 or 3 days after the onset of symptoms suggest that depressed C3 synthesis is responsible for the prolonged lowering of the level of C3 after the initial activation phase.

The situation in membranoproliferative or mesangiocapillary glomerulonephritis (also known previously as chronic hypocomplementemic nephritis) is far less clear. In this disorder, particularly as it occurs in children and adolescents, lowered hemolytic complement is a useful finding. This is almost always the result of markedly reduced levels of C3 and C5 with normal levels of most other complement components. Serum concentrations of properdin factor B are usually normal in these patients or at most slightly reduced. By immunofluorescent techniques using antibodies to immunoglobulins and C3, the latter proteins are demonstrable on the glomeruli in most patients. The serum of some patients with membranoproliferative glomerulonephritis contains circulating C3d and also may contain a protein termed nephritic factor, which, when a normal serum protein (presumably deficient in the nephritic serum) is added, is capable of cleaving C3 *in vitro*. The precise nature of the nephritic factor is uncertain. In any case, the low serum level of C3 in some patients with membranoproliferative glomerulonephritis, including those with nephritic factor, is primarily the result of depressed synthesis.

It appears likely that activation of the classical complement pathway by antigen–antibody aggregates is responsible for the low levels of many complement components in systemic lupus erythematosus and in other kinds of immune complex disease. This has been confirmed in metabolic studies with labeled complement components and by immunofluorescent localization of immunoglobulins and C3 in glomeruli and other tissues of such patients. Recently, evidence for the participation of the properdin pathway has been obtained by the demonstration of properdin in the glomeruli of patients with lupus. The mechanisms by which the properdin system is activated remain unclear.

There is some evidence that complement activation may occur in severe disseminated intravascular coagulation with fibrinolysis. In this clinical situation, it may be that the generated plasmin and possibly also thrombin attack C3 directly. Serum levels of the latter protein may be lowered. The lowered C3 serum concentrations observed in patients with advanced hepatic cirrhosis or other hepatocellular disease may result from associated disseminated intravascular coagulation and fibrinolysis or from interference with C3 synthesis in this organ, which is its site of synthesis. Marked elevations of C3 serum concentration in patients with severe biliary obstruction have been observed. The mechanisms for this elevation are unknown.

Serum concentrations of C1q may be low in patients with agammaglobulinemia, particularly in those with severe combined immunodeficiency. Recent metabolic studies with labeled C1q suggest that this lowering is the result of hypercatabolism rather than decreased synthesis.

In certain cases of acquired hemolytic anemia, C3 is detected on erythrocytes by a Coombs antiglobulin reagent specific for this protein. The presence of C3 on patients' red cells may indicate an antierythrocyte antibody which has "fixed complement," activation of C3 by other means with C3 deposition as part of the innocent bystander reaction, or an unusual abnormality of the red cell membrane making it more "susceptible" to C3 uptake, as in paroxysmal nocturnal hemoglobinuria.

Total serum hemolytic complement and the levels of individual complement proteins are normal or elevated in patients with rheumatoid arthritis, and there is no evidence of complement activation in serum. However, the joint space is relatively sequestered from the circulating plasma, and there is now considerable evidence that complement participates locally in rheumatoid joint inflammation. Hemolytic complement is reduced in joint fluid from patients with rheumatoid arthritis (particularly those with rheumatoid factor and/or with nodules) when compared with joint effusions from patients with other diseases. In rheumatoid joint effusions there is reduction in the relative concentrations of several complement proteins, including C4, C2, C3, and properdin factor B, and conversion products of the latter two proteins are often found. Chemotactic factors, thought to consist of C5a and C567, are found in the majority of rheumatoid joint effusions. By immunofluorescence, C3 and C4 have been identified in the lining cells, blood vessels, and intercellular connective tissue of rheumatoid synovial membranes. It is not clear whether complement activation in joints affected by rheumatoid arthritis results from the presence of complexes of IgG antibody with antigen, of complexes of IgM rheumatoid factor with aggregated γ-globulin, of proteolytic enzymes from leukocytes, or some combination of these factors.

VIII. Inherited Disorders of the Complement System

Hereditary angioneurotic edema was known clinically many decades before it was shown to be the result of an inherited defect in the C1 inhibitor. The tendency to develop episodic attacks of subcutaneous, laryngeal, and gastrointestinal swelling is inherited as an autosomal dominant trait. The subcutaneous swellings are painless, nonerythematous, and nonpruritic. When the lining of the gastrointestinal tract is affected, there is vomiting, abdominal pain, and copious diarrhea; when the respiratory tract is involved, asphyxiation can result. Attacks last 24–96 hours. About 80% of affected families have reduced levels of C1 inhibitor protein whereas, in the remaining 20%, this protein is in normal or elevated concentration but does not function normally to inhibit C1. The clinical picture in these two varieties of the disease is the same. There are probably three or four different mutant genes that produce dysfunctional proteins.

The defect in inhibition of C1 results in a proteolytic attack on C4 and C2, the natural substrates of C1. Serum levels of these proteins are reduced, particularly during attacks, at which time activated C1 ($\overline{C1}$) can be demonstrated in patient's serum. A vasoactive peptide with kinin-like activity has been extracted from the plasma of patients with hereditary angioneurotic edema, but its origin is unknown. It does not appear to derive from either C4 or C2. The fluid-phase activation of the initial part of the complement sequence is relatively inefficient; levels of C3 are within the normal range, and there is only mild elevation in the catabolic rate of C3.

A simple screening test for hereditary angioneurotic edema consists of the immunochemical estimation of C1 inhibitor and C4. If the serum levels of both are normal, the disease is ruled out. If both are low, the patient almost certainly has the disease. If C4 is low but the C1 inhibitor level is normal, the electrophoretic mobility of the C1 inhibitor should be determined. In most cases with dysfunctional proteins, the mobility will be abnormal. The definitive establishment of the diagnosis requires the demonstration of low or undetectable functional C1 inhibitor in the patient's serum.

Hereditary deficiency of C2 has been documented in several families. Affected persons are homozygotes; heterozygotes have 30–50% of the normal level. The level of C2 in serum from homozygotes in different families varies; it ranges from none detectable to 4% of normal. Although abnormalities of complement-mediated functions can be demonstrated in C2-deficient serum, most of the affected individuals are asymptomatic. Recent reports of systemic lupus erythematosus, lupuslike syndromes, and Henoch-Schönlein purpura in C2-deficient individuals may indicate an increased susceptibility to "collagen" disease. However, a meaningful association is far from proved since the populations screened for C2 deficiency consisted largely of patients with known or suspected lupus or glomerulonephritis.

At least three patients homozygous for *C3 deficiency* have been found. In the first of these reported, the clinical history was like that of boys with X-linked agammaglobulinemia; the patient has had numerous serious infections with pyogenic organisms. The level of C3 in her serum is less than 1/1000th the normal, and asymptomatic heterozygotes for the deficiency state have 50% of the normal serum concentration. By means of the inherited structural polymorphism in C3, it has been shown that the deficiency gene (C3⁻) is an allele of normal C3 genes but produces no detectable protein. Complement-mediated functions in the C3-deficient patient's serum are extremely low. Thus, there was no generation of chemotactic activity, no bactericidal activity, and no enhancement of the phagocytosis of antibody-sensitized bacteria. The addition of purified C3 to serum restored these functions. There was furthermore no leukocytosis when one of the patients had severe gram-positive bacterial infection, providing evidence *in vivo* for the importance of the complement system and in particular C3 in the mediation of this function.

Families with *deficiencies of C6 or C7* have recently been found. In homozygous C6 deficiency there is no detectable C6, and heterozygotes have 50% or less of the normal level of this protein. Some C7 is detectable in the serum of the homozygous C7-deficient individual. In neither of these deficiency states are there any important abnormalities of coagulation function although such abnormalities have been described in C6-deficient rabbits. Although affected persons are asymptomatic, hemolytic complement is very low and there is a deficiency of bactericidal activity. Chemotaxis is normal in C6-deficient human serum.

Homozygous *deficiency of the C3 inactivator* resembles C3 deficiency and agammaglobulinemia in its clinical expression in that the patient with this disorder has a markedly increased susceptibility to infection with pyogenic organisms. Deficient complement-mediated functions in his serum are not restorable by the addition of purified C3. No serum C3 inactivator can be detected, and heterozygous family members have approximately half-normal concentrations of C3b inactivator but no other abnormalities. The absence of C3 inactivator results in continuous activation and consumption of the proteins of the alternative pathway *in vivo*. Active factor D is present at all times, factor B is markedly diminished or not detectable, and C3 is markedly diminished, but the properdin level is within the normal range. Circulating C3b is present continuously. It is presumed that C3a is generated *in vivo* since the patient has marked histaminuria and urticaria develops when he takes a shower.

In addition to these disorders, which have well-established inheritance, there are at least three additional abnormalities of the complement system that may have a genetic basis. Marked *deficiency of C1r* with a relative diminution of C1s has been described in two kindred. Affected persons have lupuslike syndromes or nephritis alone. A single patient with low C3, circulating C3c, and a history of life-threatening infections with pyogens has been reported. Studies of her family failed to reveal any abnormality. Complement-mediated functions are grossly abnormal in the patient's serum but were markedly improved by the addition of purified C3. The concentrations of classical and alternative pathway proteins are all normal. Metabolic studies indicated that the patient's low serum C3 concentration is the result of both increased catabolism and decreased synthesis. This defect is found in association with a syndrome of partial lipodystrophy. A familial disorder that may involve a *dysfunctional C5* molecule has been reported in several families. Affected persons have eczema and increased susceptibility to infection with staphylococci and gram-negative bacteria during the first year of life. Their serum exhibits decreased enhancement of phagocytosis of yeast by normal peripheral blood leukocytes. The concentration of C5 is normal by immunochemical estimation and by hemolytic assay. Inheritance patterns are unclear. A true genetic *deficiency of C5* has recently been reported. This is undoubtedly a condition distinct from familial C5 dysfunction and raises questions regarding the role of C5 in yeast phagocytosis since this test is normal using C5-deficient serum. A possible role of human C5 in coagulation has been suggested by studies of C5-deficient plasma.

References

Alper, C. A., and Rosen, F. S. (1971). Genetic aspects of the complement system. *Advan. Immunol.* 14, 252–290.

Austen, K. F. (1974). Symposium on the immunobiology of complement. *Transplant. Proc.* 6, 1–87.

Lachman, P. J., and Lepow, I. H. (1974). Symposium on complement. *In* "Progress in Immunology II" (L. Brent and J. Holborow, eds.), Vol. 1, pp. 171–218. Amer. Elsevier, New York.

Laurell, C.-B. (1965). Antigen-antibody crossed electrophoresis. *Anal. Biochem.* 10, 358.

Mayer, M. M. (1961). Complement and complement fixation. *In* "Experimental Immunochemistry" (E. A. Kabat and M. M. Mayer, eds.), 2nd ed. pp. 133–240. Thomas, Springfield, Illinois.

Müller-Eberhard, H. J. (1975). Complement. *Annu. Rev. Biochem.* 44, 697–724.

Rapp, H. J., and Borsos, T. (1970). "Molecular Basis of Complement Action," p. 160. Appleton, New York.

Detection of Tumor-Associated Antigens in Plasma or Serum[1]

MORTON K. SCHWARTZ

Laboratory of Applied and Diagnostic Biochemistry,
Memorial Sloan-Kettering Cancer Center, New York, New York

I. Introduction

It has been suggested that if the tumor is detected early, 90% of patients with cancer could be cured by presently available therapeutic procedures. The search for a blood constituent useful as an early cancer

[1] Supported in part by U.S. Public Health Service Grant CA-08748 from the National Cancer Institute, National Institutes of Health.

405

diagnostic test has attracted the attention of biochemists for decades. This search has not been successful because the sensitivity of described biochemical procedures does not usually permit detection of tumor-specific material until after metastases have occurred and, in addition, tests have not been cancer specific and have all produced a significant number of "false positives." In recent years a relationship of the cancer cell to an embryonic state has been widely accepted, and analysis of fetal enzymes and antigens in body fluids has been utilized in an effort to detect tumors and to better understand the relationship of fetal macromolecules to the malignant process. The most important developments have been the use of α-fetoprotein (α-FP) at first in evaluating liver tumors and then embryonic tumors; carcinoembryonic antigen (CEA), first as an indicator of colon cancer and then as a nonspecific cancer marker, and placental-type alkaline phosphatase (the Regan isoenzyme) and aldolase, hexokinase, and other fetal isoenzymes in a variety of cancers. It is apparent that the present state of the art, except for α-FP in primary liver cancer, allows the use of these assays in following the course of the disease and the response to therapy, rather than primary diagnosis. The successful use of blood fetal antigen measurements is, in part, due to the development of a powerful analytical tool, the radioimmunoassay, which permits quantitation in the nanogram range. The purpose of this review is to consider the serum determinations of fetal antigens and to discuss the significance of their measurements in the diagnosis of cancer and the evaluation of therapy.

II. α-Fetoprotein

In 1963 Abelev demonstrated the production by hepatomas of an embryonal α-globulin. This fetal protein was then observed in the serum of patients with primary liver cancer. Since these original reports, serum α-FP assays have been widely used as an organ-specific cancer test. With conventional gel double-diffusion technique, Masseyeff has reported only 3 "false positives" out of more than 70,000 tests, and elevations have been observed in about 75% of blacks and 50–60% of Caucasians with primary liver cancer. These percentages have been increased to 85% in the African black population when radioimmunoassays, which are many times more sensitive, were used. The problem in the use of more sensitive procedures is a compromise in the ability of the test to differentiate liver cancer from other forms of liver disease in which small amounts of serum α-FP can be found.

α-FP has also been observed in serum of patients with embryonal malignant teratoblastomas of the testes or ovary, and α-FP assays have become useful in following the progression of these diseases. In addition to evaluation of patients with cancer, measurement of α-FP in maternal serum has been proposed as a marker for the detection of fetal distress and intrauterine death.

During the fetal period, α-FP is produced by the parenchyma of the liver and the yolk sac. In the embryo serum α-FP reaches a maximum concentration at about week 13 of gestation and then rapidly falls so that at 18–22 weeks, it is about 3% of the maximum and at 34–36 weeks, less than 2%. In one fetus at 13 weeks, the serum concentration was 2,790,000 ng/ml. At birth the level is as much as 200,000–300,000 ng/ml and during the first several weeks of life the level decreases with a half-life of about 5 days during the first weeks of life and 3 days after that. The half-life determined by monitoring the fall in serum α-FP after resection of a hepatoma or after injection of purified α-FP, has been reported to be about 6 days.

Early clinical studies of serum α-FP were carried out by Ouchterlony agar gel immunoprecipitation. In an effort to increase sensitivity hemagglutination, immunoradioautography, counter immunoelectrophoresis, and radioimmunoassay have been used. The more sensitive quantitative assays were developed to permit evaluation of disease progression and therapeutic response. The procedures most extensively used are gel double diffusion, immunoelectrophoresis, and radioimmunoassay.

A. PURIFICATION OF α-FETOPROTEIN

α-FP has been precipitated from fetal serum or serum from hepatoma patients with horse anti α-FP antiserum and purified by repeated antigen-antibody precipitation and treatment on Sephadex G-150 or Sepharose columns to separate α-FP from IgG. The procedure used by Hirai *et al.* is as follows:

1. Fetal serum or serum from hepatoma patients is mixed in an optimal immunoprecipitation ratio with horse anti-α-FP antiserum and allowed to stand overnight at 4°C.

2. The precipitate, obtained by centrifugation in the cold at 30,000 rpm for 15 minutes, is washed 3 times with cold 0.15 M NaCl and dissolved in 0 1 M glycine–HCl buffer, pH 1.8.

3. After centrifugation at 10,000 rpm for 15 minutes, the supernatant is neutralized to pH 7.0 with 0.4 M phosphate buffer, kept at 37°C for 60 minutes, and then centrifuged at 3000 rpm for 10 minutes.

4. The α-FP is reprecipitated with antiserum and treated as described above twice more, except that during the last treatment the glycine buffer is not neutralized.

5. The final 0.1 M glycine–HCl buffer (pH 1.8) solution is applied to a Sephadex G-150 column previously equilibrated with the buffer.

6. Elution is carried out with 0.1 M glycine–HCl buffer, pH 1.8. The last of 3 protein fractions contains the α-FP, which is collected, neutralized, placed on a second Sephadex G-150 column, and rechromatographed. The α-FP eluted after this treatment is almost 100% pure on the basis of electrophoresis, ultracentrifugation, and immunoelectrophoresis.

7. α-FP can be crystallized from the purified material by adding saturated $(NH_4)_2SO_4$ to a final concentration of about 2.3 M and keeping of the mixture in the cold for several days.

B. PREPARATION OF ANTISERUM

Although purified α-FP or even antigen–antibody complex can be used for the preparation of antiserum, untreated fetal serum is the antigen source most often used. In the schedule originally used by Abelev in his study of patients, serum from 24-week fetuses (3 ml) was mixed with complete Freund's adjuvant and injected subcutaneously into the abdominal region of rabbits. One and 2 weeks later, additional injections of serum without adjuvant were given to the animals; blood for antiserum was taken on days 7, 14, and 21 after the last injection. Adsorption was carried out with an equal volume of normal adult human serum by incubation at 37°C for 30 minutes and then for 18–20 hours at 4°C.

In other methods rabbits are immunized intramuscularly or in their foot pads with 0.5–1.0 ml of serum from human cord blood or blood from fetuses 20–30 weeks old. The serum is emulsified with an equal volume of complete Freund's adjuvant, and the injection schedule is varied from a single immunization to weekly injections for 3 weeks. Booster injections are given, and antiserum is collected over a period of months. Adsorption is carried out with lyophilized normal human serum. α-FP, purified by electrofocusing, has been used to prepare antiserum in sheep; the antiserum obtained 5 months later is adsorbed with 0.2 mg of lyophilized serum per milliliter or a 1:20 volume of untreated normal human serum. Horses have been used to prepare large volumes of antiserum.

C. METHODS OF α-FP ASSAY

1. Gel Diffusion

a. In the procedure described by Abelev, adsorbed antiserum is poured into the center well of a conventional agar-immunodiffusion plate. Serial nonbuffered dilutions of test serum are placed in the peripheral wells. The greatest dilution of patient serum yielding a visible precipitin line is considered the end point.

b. In the radial immunodiffusion procedure described by Alpert and his associates, 0.1 ml of adsorbed antiserum is used in the central well. In the outside well is placed 0.1 ml of patient sera diluted in 0.9% agar gel buffered at pH 8.2 with sodium barbital–HCl.

2. Counter Immunoelectrophoresis

In this technique, 10 ml of 0.9% agarose in 0.05 M barbital buffer, pH 8.6, are layered on 8 × 10 cm glass plates (Kodak projection slides may be used). After the gel solidifies, double rows of 3–4-mm holes, 1.0 cm apart, are cut. Sera to be assayed (about 12 μl) are placed in one set of holes and the α-FP antiserum in the other. Whatman No. 1 filter paper is used as wicks, and electrophoresis in 0.05 M barbital buffer, pH 8.6, is carried out for 60 minutes (150–180 V, 15–20 mA) with the antiserum wells facing the anode. After electrophoresis the plate is dried and stained with amido black. Under these conditions, α-FP migrates toward the anode and antibodies to α-FP by endosmosis toward the cathode.

In a modification of this technique, lantern slide glasses are covered with a 1-mm layer of 1.25% agar in barbital buffer, and two sample wells are cut adjacent to each other, but each equidistant from a single, anode facing, antiserum well. A positive control (diluted cord blood) in each alternate sample well permits visible observation of a known positive next to the unknown sample. An important consideration in counter electrophoresis is lack of detection and false negative results caused by antigen excess. This point is emphasized because of the fact that serum α-FP levels may range from 2000 ng/ml to 7,000,000 ng/ml.

3. "Sandwich" Counterelectrophoresis

Smith (1970) proposed a more sensitive "sandwich" counterelectrophoresis in which after conventional counterelectrophoresis, the antiserum wells are cleared of liquid by suction and filled with anti IgG antiserum; electrophoresis is reinstituted for 45 minutes.

4. Electroimmunodiffusion

In this technique, 2% agarose in 0.025 M sodium barbital buffer, pH 8.6, is mixed with an equal volume of a 1:16 dilution of α-FP antiserum. Aliquots of the mixture are poured on glass slides (3 × 2 inches) previously coated with agarose and heated to 45°C at the time of pouring. Spacers and a cover are used to maintain the slide thickness at 1 mm. After cooling for 1 hour at 4°C, 32 pairs of 1.6-mm wells are cut with a template. Electrophoresis is performed in 0.05 M barbital buffer, pH 8.6, with gauze wicks held in place with about 2 ml of 1% agarose gel. Capillary pipettes are used to fill the wells, and electrophoresis at 5.2 V/cm is carried out for 2 hours at room temperature. After this time, the slides are washed in barbital buffer for 3 hours, dried at 37°C, and then stained with 1% amido black. The lengths of the precipitin peaks are linearly related to the α-FP concentration, and a standard curve is prepared using fetal serum containing from 350–2700 pg/ml of α-FP. The reproducibility and the linearity of the procedure are excellent.

5. Radioimmunoassay

a. Iodination. The α-FP is labeled by treating α-FP (5 μg) in 1 μl of phosphate buffer, pH 7.0, with 1 mCi of carrier-free Na^{125}I in a volume of 8 μl. Twenty-five microliters of 0.5 M phosphate buffer, pH 7.0, containing 100 μg of chloramine-T is added immediately, followed after 10 seconds' mixing by 100 μl of 0.05 M phosphate buffer containing 240 μg of sodium metabisulfite and 0.2 ml of 2% NaI. The iodinated α-FP is separated from free iodine by gel filtration on a Sephadex G-200, 1.3 × 10 cm column, and the fractions are collected into 0.05% bovine serum albumin. The iodinated antigen can be stored at 4°C for 2 weeks. Incorporation of radioactive iodine ranges from 30 to 52% of the theoretical. Ninety-eight percent of labeled protein can be precipitated by trichloroacetic acid and about 75% by antiserum.

b. Antibody Dilution Curve. An antibody dilution curve is prepared with sequential 5-fold dilutions of antiserum in phosphate buffer containing 0.15 M NaCl and 0.125% bovine serum albumin in a final volume of 0.95 ml. Labeled α-FP is added (2500 cpm in a volume of 100 μl) followed by 50 μl of a 1:85 dilution of normal sheep serum. The antibody bound α-FP is precipitated and the radioactivity in the precipitate counted. An antibody dilution binding 25% of the precipitate counts is selected for the assay. Binding occurs maximally at an antiserum dilution of about 1:25,000, but can be detected at dilutions up to 1:3,000,000.

c. Standard Curve and Assay. The standard inhibition curve is prepared with 0, 0.1, 0.25, 0.5, 1.0, 2.5, 5.0, 10.0, and 25.0 ng of standard α-FP in 0.9 ml of phosphate buffer containing 0.15 M NaCl and 0.125% bovine serum albumin. To these solutions is added 100 μl of a 1:1 dilution of anti α-FP (1:10,000) with normal sheep serum (1:85) and then ^{125}I α-FP as described in the procedure for the antibody dilution curve. In the assay, serum is diluted 1:5 and 1:50 in phosphate buffer containing 0.15 M NaCl and 0.9 ml aliquots assayed as described above.

In another radioimmunoassay 0.1 ml of patient's serum is mixed with 0.7 ml of 0.05 M Tris buffer, pH 7.5, containing 0.075 M NaCl, 0.1 ml of ^{125}I-labeled α-FP (6000 to 8000 cpm) and 0.1 ml of anti-α-FP antiserum (1:30,000 dilution). After incubation for 48 hours at 4°C, 0.1 ml of normal rabbit serum (diluted 1:100) and 0.1 ml of goat antirabbit serum (diluted 1:10) are added and the mixture incubated at 0°C for 24 hours. The solution is centrifuged at 3000 rpm and the radioactivity in the precipitate (bound material) counted. The α-FP concentration is determined from a standard inhibition curve.

D. CLINICAL SIGNIFICANCE AND SENSITIVITY OF THE ASSAYS

It has been estimated that the α-FP radioimmunoassay is about 40,000 times more sensitive than the original immunodiffusion technique. Differences in method sensitivity will obviously affect the reported clinical usefulness of the assay. It is important, when discussing the incidence of elevated α-FP, to state the procedure that was used. In Table I are listed a comparison of the sensitivities of different procedures. In a comparison of cancer specificity of an agar diffusion system and an immunoradioautography method, it was reported that specificity in Africans with hepatocellular cancer increased from 84/118 cases (71%) to 90/118 cases, or 76.3%, and in control group from 10/366 cases (2.7%) to 80/354 cases (22.6%). The increase in positive values in the cancer population is more

TABLE I

SENSITIVITY OF α-FETOPROTEIN PROCEDURES

Method	Detection limit[a] (ng/ml)
Double-gel immunodiffusion	1000–10,000
Immunoelectrophoresis	5000
Counter immunoelectrophoresis	25
Immunoradioautography	10
Radioimmunoassay	0.25

[a] These are approximate values, since the sensitivity of the method will depend in part on the antiserum preparation.

than offset by the increase in the number of "false positives" in the control population.

Nishi and Hirai in 1973 reported a comparison of α-FP assays in the same patients utilizing the conventional gel diffusion technique and a radioimmunoassay. These data are shown in Table II. In this study, α-FP was found in serum of 71% of the hepatoma patients, but in none of the other patients. However, with the radioimmunoassay, elevations were observed in 87% of the hepatoma patients and in 45% of the other patients. Nishioka *et al.* (1973) reported similar findings with elevated α-FP in 33 of 37 patients with the hepatocellular carcinoma. In a collaborative study in which all laboratories used an agarose double-diffusion technique, positive values were observed in 105 of 148 patients with primary liver cancer and in 12 of 555 control patients. In the United States and Europe elevations have been reported in 178 of 331 Caucasian patients. Al-Sarraf (1974) compared a variety of liver function tests in a group of patients with primary liver cancer and found α-FP elevations in 14/19 (74%) of the patients, but alkaline phosphatase elevations in 45/51 (88%), glutamic-oxaloacetic transaminase in 40/51 (78%), lactic dehydrogenase in 34/51 (66%), and glutamic-pyruvic transaminase in 11/32 (34%). Australian antigen was not present in any of 12 patients. Purves *et al.* (1970) has reported that serum α-FP concentrations do not significantly correlate with any other biochemical tests.

α-FP is found in the serum of patients with malignant teratoblastomas of the testes and ovary, but not usually in the serum of patients with other embryonal tumors (seminomas, chorioepitheliomas, neuroblastoma or Wilms's tumor). Using agar gel precipitation, Abelev (1971) found elevations in 17/34 (50%) of the patients, but with an immunoradio-

TABLE II

α-Fetoprotein Determinations by Gel Diffusion and Radioimmunoassay (RIA)

Disease	Gel diffusion		RIA	
	Pts[a]	No. (+)	Pts[a]	No. (+)
Primary liver cancer	56	39	56	49
Hepatitis	43	0	62	28
Cirrhosis	42	0	38	18
Miscellaneous	31	0	35	11
Miscellaneous cancer	58	0	36	3

[a] Number of patients.

autography, 15/20 (76%) of patients had abnormal serum concentrations. Serum α-FP in embryonal cancers appears to be directly related to the size of the tumor and is useful in following the course of the disease. In a typical patient with embryonal carcinoma of the testes, serum α-FP was not detectable during a 2-year clinical remission, but when retroperitoneal metastases occurred the level became positive. When the metastases were surgically removed, the α-FP became negative. Several months later, α-FP was again detected and the patient experienced nonspecific gastrointestinal symptoms. After chemotherapy and surgical removal of a retroperitoneal recurrence, the α-FP concentration decreased. Several months later the patient's clinical condition rapidly deteriorated and the serum α-FP increased precipitously but fell just before the death related to recurrent embryonal carcinoma.

Elevated maternal serum α-FP is associated with the presence of a viable fetus. The assay of serum α-FP and chorionic gonadotropin permits distinction between normal pregnancy and hydatidiform mole or choriocarcinoma, diseases in which α-FP remains within normal levels. A normal α-FP in maternal blood after week 12 of pregnancy indicates the absence of a living fetus.

III. Carcinoembryonic Antigen

Carcinoembryonic antigen (CEA) is the term applied in 1965 by Gold and Freedman to a protein found in intestine, liver, and pancreas of the fetus during the first 6 months of gestation and in human cancerous colon, liver, or pancreas. It was not detected in normal adult human tissues from patients with benign disease of the colon. In 1969, workers (Thompson et al., 1969) used a radioimmunoassay capable of detecting as little as 1 ng of CEA per milliliter of serum and reported values greater than 2.5 ng/ml in 35 of 36 patients with adenocarcinoma of the colon. Values less than this were found in patients with colon cancer who had their tumor removed surgically, patients with other forms of cancer, and all normal persons or those with nonmalignant diseases. Subsequent studies (Booth et al., 1973; Elias et al., 1974; Go et al., 1972; Hansen et al., 1974; Laurence et al., 1972; Sorokin et al., 1974) including a cooperative one encompassing more than 10,000 patients and healthy subjects from 100 institutions, have indicated elevations in about 70% of patients with colon cancer, but elevation in other forms of cancer, particularly lung, pancreas, stomach, and breast, as well as in some patients with benign tumors and patients with emphysema, cirrhosis, and other nonmalignant diseases.

Several radioimmunoassays and a hemagglutination inhibition procedure have been described for the determination of CEA. The radioimmunoassays differ primarily in the method of extraction of CEA from plasma or serum and the procedure for separation of free from antibody-bound antigen.

A. PURIFICATION OF CEA

1. Primary adenocarcinoma of the colon or colon carcinoma metastatic to liver can be used immediately after it is obtained at surgery or at autopsy, or tissue can be frozen at $-30°C$ for at least 6 months.

2. Tissue is trimmed of fat and connective tissue, minced, passed through a commercial meat grinder, suspended in 4 volumes (w/v) of cold distilled water, and homogenized for 60 minutes in a VirTis Chemixer at 15,000 rpm.

3. An equal volume of 2 M perchloric acid is added, the mixture is stirred for 60 minutes and centrifuged at 1732 g at 4°C for 30 minutes, and the supernatant is dialyzed against cold (15°C) running tap water for 24 hours and then deionized water for an equal period.

4. The dialyzed extract is lyophilized to almost dryness, dissolved in water (about 150 ml per 500 gm of original tissue), and centrifuged at 8120 g at 4°C for 20 minutes; the supernatant is passed through a 0.22-μm (average pore diameter) Millipore filter.

5. The solution is lyophilized to dryness, dissolved (50 mg of lyophilized powder per milliliter) in 0.05 M Na_2HPO_4, pH 4.5, containing 0.15 M NaCl applied to 5 × 100 cm column of Sepharose 4B at 4°C and eluted with 0.05 M Na_2HPO_4, pH 4.5, at a rate of 30–40 ml per hour. CEA is monitored in every fifth tube by gel diffusion or radioimmunoassay technique. The fractions with activity are pooled, dialyzed, and lyophilized to dryness.

6. The lyophilized powder is dissolved (3 mg/ml) in 0.05 M Na_2HPO_4, pH 4.5, containing 0.15 M NaCl applied to a 2.5 × 100 cm Sephadex G-200 column, and eluted with the same buffer at a rate of 11 ml per hour.

7. The active fractions are pooled, dialyzed, and lyophilized to dryness. Further purification may be carried out by Sephadex G-25 block electrophoresis. We did not find it necessary. The CEA should be identified by comparison of immunochemical properties with other CEA preparations, as well as analytical ultracentrifugation, immunoelectrophoresis, and physiochemical analysis.

B. Preparation of Antiserum

CEA (2 mg) is emulsified in 2 ml of complete Freund's adjuvant and injected into the rear thigh of a goat. Every 3 weeks 75 ml of blood is removed from the goat to harvest antiserum, and the goat is given a booster injection of 1 mg of CEA emulsified in 1 ml of complete Freund's adjuvant. The antiserum is adsorbed at 37°C for 2 hours with lyophilized normal human serum (50 mg per milliliter of antiserum) and with lyophilized perchloric acid extracts of normal colon and liver. The adsorbed antiserum is centrifuged at 25,000 g for 15 minutes, divided into 3-ml aliquots, and frozen.

C. Methods of CEA Assay

1. Radioimmunoassay

Iodination: Pipette into a beaker immersed in ice, 50 μl of 0.05 M Na_2HPO_4 buffer, pH 7.5, containing 250 μg of purified CEA, 50 μl of $Na^{125}I$ (5 Ci/dl), and 20 μl of 0.05 M Na_2HPO_4, pH 7.5, containing 10 mg/ml of chloramine-T. After the mixture has stood for 5 minutes at 4°C, 250 μg of sodium metabisulfite in a volume of 20 μl is added. The solution is washed with potassium iodide solution (100 gm/liter) onto a 0.5×26 cm Sephadex G-100 column, and 1-ml fractions are eluted with 0.05 M phosphate buffer, pH 7.5, into tubes containing 1 ml of 0.05 M phosphate buffer, pH 7.5, containing 50 mg of bovine serum albumin. The eluents containing the maximum radioactivity (minimum count of 15,000 dpm) are pooled and diluted with normal human serum (diluted 1:100 with 0.50 M borate buffer, pH 8.6) so that 500 μg contains 30,000 dpm. The pooled labeled antigen is divided into 0.5-ml aliquots and frozen at -30°C.

There have been several radioimmunoassays described for the determination of CEA. Three of these will be described. Their basic differences are outlined in Table III.

a. $(NH_4)_2SO_4$–*Perchloric Acid Method* (*Thompson et al.*, 1969).
Step 1. In a centrifuge tube, add with mixing, 5 ml of 2 M perchloric acid to 5 ml of serum.
Step 2. Allow the mixture to stand 10 minutes at room temperature. Centrifuge at 20,000 g for 15 minutes, decant supernatant into dialysis bags, and dialyze against running cold tap water for 48 hours and then distilled water (at least two changes) for 8 hours. Transfer dialyzate to a 16-ml centrifuge tube, and lyophilize to dryness.

TABLE III
RADIOIMMUNOASSAYS FOR CARCINOEMBRYONIC ANTIGEN (DEA)

	Perchloric acid–(NH$_4$)$_2$SO$_4$	Direct-triple isotope	Perchloric acid–zirconyl phosphate gel
Serum (EDTA-plasma)	5.0 ml	0.2 ml	(1.0 ml)
Perchloric acid extraction	+	−	+
Dialysis	2 Days	−	Overnight
Lyophilization	+	−	−
Radiolabeled reagents	CEA-^{125}I	CEA-^{125}I Goat-IgG ^{131}I ^{22}Na	CEA ^{125}I
Goat anti-CEA	+	+	+
Separation	(NH$_4$)$_2$SO$_4$	Horse antigoat IgG	Zirconyl phosphate gel

[a] −, Not included in assay.

Step 3. Completely dissolve the dried material in 500 μl of diluted standardized antiserum, incubate at 37°C for 18 hours, and then add 500 μl of ^{125}I-labeled CEA (about 50,000 dpm) and incubate with shaking for 2 hours at 37°C. The antiserum dilution is that which permits binding of 30–40% of the antigen and is determined by adding 500 μl of diluted (1:100) human normal plasma containing 1.5 ng of ^{125}I-labeled CEA to tubes containing lyophilized perchloric acid extracts of normal human plasma and then incubating the mixture for 18 hours at 37°C. After incubation, the procedure is identical to the assay steps outlined below.

Step 4. Add 1 ml of saturated (NH$_4$)$_2$SO$_4$ to all tubes and incubate with shaking for 30 minutes at 4°C, centrifuge for 12 minutes at 30,000 g, decant the supernatant, and count the radioactivity in the precipitate.

Step 5. The CEA concentration is calculated from a standard inhibition curve prepared with 0, 2.5, 5.0, 10.0, 15.0, 18, 35, and 100 ng of CEA per milliliter.

b. Triple Isotope–Double Antibody Technique (Egan *et al.*, 1972). In this procedure, ^{131}I monitors the precipitation of CEA-goat anti-CEA by horse antigoat IgG, and ^{22}Na is a volume marker for residual supernatant remaining after aspiration of the fluid over the precipitate prior to counting. Goat IgG is labeled with ^{131}I by adding 0.5 ml of goat IgG to 0.1 ml of chloramine-T (60 μg) and then 0.01 ml of Na^{131}I (0.2 Ci). After 3 minutes, 0.1 ml of a solution containing 50 μg of sodium metabisufite is added, and, after 5 minutes at 4°C, the solution is applied to a 0.5 × 25 cm Sephadex G-100 column and carried through the procedure described for the radioactive labeling of CEA. CEA is prepared and labeled as described earlier.

Step 1. In micro test tubes add 20 μl of 0.075 M phosphate buffer, pH 7.2, containing 0.15 M NaCl, 1 mg/ml of rabbit IgG, and about 0.5 ng of ^{125}I-labeled CEA, sufficient ^{22}Na to yield a radioactivity of 50,000 dpm, and enough goat ^{131}I-labeled IgG (about 3 μg) to yield 20,000 dpm.

Step 2. To the tubes add 200 μl of assay serum or CEA dilutions containing 0.0, 2.5, 5.0, 12.5, 25.0, 37.5, and 100 ng/ml for the standard inhibition curve. To each tube add 50 μl of a standard dilution of anti-CEA antiserum. The antiserum dilution is obtained from an antibody titration curve prepared with about 1.2 ng of CEA in each 200-μl sample. A dilution which binds about 40% of the ^{125}I-labeled CEA is used.

Step 3. After incubation for 2 hours at 37°C, 100 μl of horse serum antigoat IgG is added, the solution is incubated for 60 minutes at 37°C, then at -4°C for 15 minutes. The tubes are centrifuged in a microtube centrifuge for 5 minutes at 10,000 g.

Step 4. All but 20 μl of supernatant is aspirated with a needle attached to a vacuum source, and the radioactivity of the residue is counted in a three-channel γ-counter. Focusing the detector crystal and adjusting the gain settings of the instrument are critical steps.

Step 5. Calculation of the counts from each isotope is carried out by use of the following ratios: $R_1 = C_2/C_3$, $R_2 = C_1/C_3$, $R_3 = C_1/C_2$, where $C_1 = {}^{125}$I, $C_2 = {}^{131}$I, $C_3 = {}^{22}$Na.

The radioactivities for each isotope are:

$$^{125}I = C_1 - C_3R_2 - (C_2 - C_3R_1)R_3$$
$$^{131}I = C_2 - C_3R_1$$
$$^{22}Na = C_3$$

c. Zirconyl Phosphate Gel–Perchloric Acid Method (Hansen et al., 1971).

Step 1. Five milliliters of 1.2 M perchloric acid is added to 1.0 ml of EDTA-plasma previously diluted with 4 ml of 0.15 M NaCl. One-milliliter aliquots of pooled normal plasma are used for the standard inhibition curve.

Step 2. After mixing, the solution is centrifuged at 1400 g for 15 minutes, the supernatant is decanted into a 1 $\times$ 10-inch dialysis bag and dialyzed first against 60 volumes of deionized water with five changes during 18 hours and then for about 3 hours with 60 volumes of 0.01 M ammonium acetate buffer, pH 6.4, until the fluid in the dialysis bag has a pH between 6.4 and 6.5.

Step 3. The dialyzates are transferred to 30-ml test tubes; to the tubes to be used in the standard inhibition curve determination is added 0, 2.5, 6.25, 12.5, and 25 ng/ml of CEA.

Step 4. To all tubes is added 100 μl of standard goat anti-CEA anti-serum and then after incubation at 45°C for 30 minutes, 50 μl of ^{125}I-labeled CEA (about 180,000 dpm). The antiserum dilution is previously determined with an antibody-titration curve in which 10 ml of 0.05 M borate buffer, pH 8.3, and 50 μl of ^{125}I-labeled CEA are mixed and treated as in the assay procedure. An antiserum dilution is used which permits 50–70% antigen binding.

Step 5. All tubes are incubated at 45°C and at intervals precisely timed to allow a 30-minute incubation, 5.0 ml of a zirconyl phosphate gel slurry (pH 6.25) is added with quick mixing.

Step 6. At the end of the incubation period the tubes are centrifuged for 10 minutes at 1000 g, the supernatant is decanted, the tubes are drained onto paper toweling, the precipitate is washed with 10 ml of 0.1 mM ammonium acetate buffer, pH 6.25, and the radioactivity in the precipitate is counted. CEA concentrations are calculated by comparison with the standard inhibition curve.

As of December 21, 1973 the Division of Biologics of the Food and Drug Administration has licensed Hoffmann-La Roche, Inc. to market the reagents necessary for this CEA assay. It has been our experience that the three described radioimmunoassays yield similar clinical information, but that the zirconyl phosphate gel method is the most convenient for clinical use. The precision is good, and the quality control of frozen aliquots assayed daily over 1 month was 5.4 ng/ml (SD = 0.97) and 3.0 ng/ml (SD = 1.6).

There have been several published modifications of these radioimmuno-assay procedures. Laurence and his associates (1972) have used the double antibody procedure, but have eliminated the addition of ^{22}Na and thereby mandated critical control of the pipetting steps if good precision is to be obtained. Go and his associates (1972) have used the zirconyl phosphate methods, but have eliminated plasma extraction and dialysis steps. Their reaction volume was reduced to 1.0 ml (0.1 ml plasma), and the mixture was incubated overnight at 4°C rather than at 45°C for 60 minutes.

2. Hemagglutination Inhibition Procedure (Lange et al., 1971)

Five milliliters of serum is extracted with 5 ml of 1.1 M perchloric acid for 20 minutes. After centrifugation the supernatant is dialyzed, then lyophilized and reconstituted to 500 μl. For the hemagglutination in-hibition assay, 25 μl are serially diluted and assayed by use of human "O" indicator erythrocytes coupled to CEA. This method appears to be sensitive to CEA levels as low as 2–5 ng/ml.

D. CLINICAL SIGNIFICANCE OF CEA

The original report of Thompson and his associates (1969) that abnormal plasma CEA values were observed in 97% of patients with adenocarcinoma of the colon has not been substantiated by other workers, and elevations in colon cancer have been shown to be related to the extent of the disease, with elevations in patients with many other forms of cancer, as well as in patients with benign tumors and nonmalignant disease.

The most complete study is a collaborative effort by Hansen *et al.* (1974) using the perchloric acid extract–zirconyl phosphate gel procedure. In this study over 35,000 samples from more than 10,000 patients and healthy subjects were analyzed. Levels less than 2.5 ng/ml were observed in 88.5% of 1425 healthy subjects, and values less than 5.0 ng/ml in 98.7% of these persons. In 2107 other healthy subjects in whom a smoking history was obtained, 865 of 892 nonsmokers, 592 of 620 smokers, and 219 of 235 former smokers had levels less than 2.5 ng/ml. In Table IV are listed the CEA elevations in the patients with cancer and other diseases included in this study. Of 576 patients without clinical evidence of cancer who underwent barium enema examination, 23 were found to have colon cancer, and of these, CEA values greater than 2.5 ng/ml were detected in 18 and greater than 5.0 ng/ml in 15. Forty-six other patients with positive CEA values had acute inflammatory disease

TABLE IV

PLASMA CARCINOEMBRYONIC ANTIGEN IN PATIENTS WITH DISEASE

Disease	Number of patients	Percent of patients with values less than	
		2.5 ng/ml	5.0 ng/ml
Cancer			
Colon-rectal	544	28	51
Lung	181	24	49
Pancreas	55	9	40
Stomach	79	39	71
Breast	125	55	73
Leukemia-lymphoma sarcoma	150	66	24
Pulmonary emphysema	49	43	90
Alcoholic cirrhosis	120	30	77
Ulcerative colitis	146	69	87
Pancreatitis	95	47	78

of the colon or a variety of metabolic diseases. An important observation was that in a third of the "false" positive group, normal values were obtained upon assay of a second sample.

A major use of CEA is serial assays of CEA in assessing the status of the patient during therapy. Persistent elevations may be indicative of therapeutic failure whereas following successful surgery or chemotherapy the levels will fall toward normal levels and remain at that level until a recrudescence of the disease occurs. In a prospective study of 102 patients who had no clinically detectable disease following colorectal surgery, CEA levels became elevated in 12 patients. Six of these developed recurrent cancer 0 to 29 months after the elevated CEA was detected. The other 6 patients did not develop a recurrence, and in 2 patients recurrence was observed despite normal CEA. Most workers now agree that the role of CEA is an adjuvant to other diagnostic procedures (endoscopy, radiology, and cytology) or in following the course of disease, but not as a screening test to detect cancer in the general population.

The assay of CEA in urine, feces, and colon washings is now under investigation and may become useful in the management of patients with certain forms of cancer. In a study of urinary CEA, 75% of patients with carcinoma of the bladder had elevated values which returned to normal when the tumor was removed. Elevations were not observed in urine from patients with prostatic carcinoma or hypernephroma. High levels were observed in patients with urinary infections and in 5 men who had no evidence of bladder carcinoma. This latter finding was attributed to the fact that seminal fluid contains relatively high concentrations of CEA-like material.

IV. Other Antigens, Antibodies

A. Polypeptide Antigen

Björklund (1973) and his associates have extracted a "cancer-specific" polypeptide from human tumors and from placenta. They have used a hemagglutination inhibition reaction and detected the antigen in serum of 58/80 patients with metastatic carcinoma, 51/95 patients with untreated primary carcinoma, or a total of 109/175 (62%) of patients with cancer. Elevations were observed in 1% of 760 normal blood donors, 41% of 46 patients with hepatitis, 14% of 165 patients with lower respiratory infections, 23% of 104 patients with urinary tract infections, and 3–8% of patients with skin, gastrointestinal, or other infections.

1. Preparation of Polypeptide Antigen and Antiserum

The antigen is prepared from a pool of human cancer tissue of various types. Frozen tissue is homogenized in water (10 ml per gram of tissue), and lipid and other ether-soluble material is extracted by shaking with ethyl ether for 60 minutes and centrifugation for 5 minutes at 1000 g. The powder obtained by shell freezing, lyophilization, and ball-mill grinding is reextracted with ethyl ether, and the sediment is dried *in vacuo*. The crude tissue powder is suspended at neutral pH in 500 ml of 0.15 M NaCl, homogenized, stirred at 0°C for 30 minutes and then centrifuged at 1000 g for 40 minutes at 0°C. This is repeated and the material lyophilized. The powder (10 mg/ml) is extracted in water and adjusted to pH 9 with NaOH; the active material is precipitated at pH 4.8. The precipitate is dissolved in one-tenth of the original homogenization volume and then maintained at 98°C for 5 minutes. The antigen was further purified by adsorption with BioGel P_{30}.

Antiserum was prepared in horses or rabbits and absorption was with tissue powder prepared from normal tissue or plasma.

2. Preparation of Antigen-Tagged Red Cells

Sheep red cells are treated with tannic acid by mixing 1 volume of red cells previously washed with Alsever's solution and suspended in phosphate buffer, pH 6.8 (10^9 cells/ml) with an equal volume of buffer containing tannic acid (18 μg/ml). After standing for 5 minutes at 0°C, the tannic acid-treated cells are washed twice in phosphate buffer, pH 7.5, and then suspended in the buffer (10^9 cells/ml). One volume of the treated red cells is added with stirring to an equal volume of phosphate buffer, pH 7.5, containing per milliliter 3 μg of polypeptide antigen and 200 μg of human serum albumin. The mixture is allowed to stand at 0°C for 10 minutes, and then the red cells are removed by centrifugation and resuspended in phosphate buffer, pH 7.5, containing 1.25% pooled inactivated human serum previously absorbed with packed sheep red cells. The tagged cells are standardized to a concentration of 1.60×10^8 cells/ml.

3. Polypeptide Antigen Assay

Serum is inactivated at 56°C for 30 minutes and then adsorbed overnight with an equal volume of packed sheep erythrocytes. In two wells of a plastic hemagglutination tray is pipetted 25 μl of adsorbed sample and then in wells 3–8, 25 μl of phosphate buffer, pH 7.5, containing

1.25% inert human serum. Serial dilutions of sample are then made by sequentially pipetting and transferring 25-μl aliquots from wells 2 through 8 and discarding the final 25-μl aliquot removed from well 8. To all wells is added 25 μl of antiserum previously diluted so that it can precipitate 90% of 50 μl of erythrocytes (8×10^6 cells). The trays are kept at $0°-1°C$, and 50 μl of polypeptide antigen-labeled red cells are added. After standing in the cold overnight, the plate is read for the minimum dilution which inhibits hemagglutination and compared with a similar set of wells containing 0.03, 0.06, 0.13, 0.25, 0.50, 1.0, and 2.0 μg of polypeptide antigen per milliliter of inert pooled human serum. Serum from normal persons contains no more than 0.09 μg/ml of the antigen.

4. Clinical Significance of Polypeptide Antigen

Björklund (1973) and his associates reported their experience with this assay through May 30, 1973. Elevations of polypeptide antigen were observed in 109 of 175 (62%) patients with metastasizing cancer of un-treated primary disease. The percentage elevation was 73% in the pa-tients with metastases and 54% in the patients with untreated primary cancer. Elevations were observed in only 8 of 760 (1%) normal blood donors. Elevations were observed in more than 70% of the patients with cancer of colon-rectum (27/32), pancreas (8/8), and breast (16/22). Elevations were also found in 41% of 46 patients with hepatitis, 19% of 165 patients with lower respiratory infections, 23% of 104 patients with urinary tract infections, and 3–11% of patients with other viral or bac-terial infections. These elevations are no longer detected when the in-fection has disappeared.

B. T-GLOBULIN

In 1970 Tal and Halperin proposed the assay of serum "T-globulin" as a cancer diagnostic procedure. The test is based on the assumption that the cancer cell produces a unique glycolipid which serves as a hapten to produce a cancer-specific protein antibody (T-globulin).

Antigen is prepared from pooled serum from cancer patients by precipitation of α-globulins with a half-volume of saturated $(NH_4)_2SO_4$ and then separation by agar gel electrophoresis. The relatively slow migration of T-globulin in agar gel permits removal of most of the con-taminating proteins. The material in agar disks cut from the electro-phoresis plate near the anode (T-globulin) is mixed with Freund's adjuvant and injected subcutaneously into the abdominal wall and thigh of rabbits. Antiserum is obtained by heart puncture 10 days after antigen injection on days 1, 3, 5, 14, 17, and 22. In the assay, serum is treated with a half-volume of saturated $(NH_4)_2SO_4$ and the precipitated globulin dissolved in sterile 0.15 M NaCl (the precipitate from 10 ml of serum is dissolved in 2 ml of solution). The samples are dialyzed to remove sulfate and centrifuged; the protein in the solution was determined. Dilutions of the sample are made to yield preparations with 20 mg and 10 mg of protein per milliliter, and these specimens were subjected to immunoelectrophoresis for 1 hour on 75 × 50-mm glass slides covered with a 4 mm layer of 2% Nobel agar dissolved in 0.1 M sodium barbital buffer, pH 8.6, with 0.05 M buffer in the electrophoresis bath. A positive result was defined as a precipitin line at both sample dilutions. In the original study of 520 patients, negative results were obtained in 163 of 164 patients without cancer and positive results in 337 of 350 cases of cancer.

C. Pancreatic Oncofetal Antigen

Using two-dimensional immunoelectrophoresis in agarose gel, Banwo et al. have demonstrated a characteristic antigen in serum from 36 of 37 patients with carcinoma of the pancreas. The antigen was not observed in serum from patients who had colon cancer and abnormal concentrations of CEA, nor in serum from patients with hepatoma and detectable α-FP. The antigen was also not found in serum of persons with pancreatitis or jaundice. The antiserum was prepared in rabbits using homogenates of human fetal pancreas emulsified with an equal quantity of complete Freund's adjuvant. The antiserum was adsorbed using homogenates of adult pancreas and human serum albumin. The clinical role and significance of this assay has yet to be determined.

V. Conclusion

The introduction of a powerful analytical tool, the radioimmunoassay, has made possible quantitation of tumor-associated antigens in serum and plasma. The current interest in α-FP and CEA will undoubtedly lead to evaluation of a large series of different antigens. The success of the search for cancer-specific antigens will be a function of the ability to separate and purify individual antigens in sufficient amounts for use in sophisticated analytical procedures. Regrettably, the view of Maugh (1974) accurately presents the present state of the art that serum antigen assays are not yet available for screening purposes, that FDA requirements may delay for years any introduction of any new antigen assay, and that certain antigen assays now available have limited use in assessing therapy.

References

General

Berlin, N. (1974). Early diagnosis of cancer. *Prev. Med.* 3, 185.
Bodansky, O. (1974). Reflection on biochemical aspects of human cancer. *Cancer* 33, 364.
Maugh, T. H. (1974). Fetal antigens: A biochemical assay for cancer? *Science* 184, 147.
Schwartz, M. K. (1973). Enzymes in cancer. *Clin. Chem.* 19, 10.

α-Fetoprotein

Abelev, G. I., Perova, S., Khramkova, Z., and Irlin, I. (1963). Production of embryonal α-globulin by transplantable mouse hepatoma. *Transplantation* 1, 174.
Abelev, G. I. (1971). Alpha-fetoprotein in ontogenesis and its association with malignant tumors. *Advan. Cancer Res.* 14, 295.
Alpert, E. (1972). Alpha-1-fetoprotein: Serologic marker of human hepatoma and embryonal carcinoma. *Nat. Cancer Inst., Monogr.* 35, 4152.
Alpert, E. (1974). Alpha-fetoprotein: Need for quantitative assays. *N. Engl. J. Med.* 290, 568.
Alpert, E., Hershberg, R., Schur, P. H., and Isselbacher, K. J. (1971). α-Fetoprotein in human hepatoma: Improved detection in serum, and quantitative studies using a new sensitive technique. *Gastroenterology* 61, 137.
Alpert, M. E., Uriel, J., and de Nechaud, B. (1968). Alpha fetoglobulin in the diagnosis of human hepatoma. *N. Engl. J. Med.* 278, 984.
Al-Sarraf, M., Go, T. S., Kithier, K., and Vaitkericius, V. K. (1974). Primary liver cancer. A review of the clinical features, blood groups, serum enzymes, therapy, and survival of 65 cases. *Cancer* 33, 574.
Elgort, D. A., Abelev, G. I., and O'Conor, G. T. (1972). Dependence of the specificity of the serologic test for primary liver cancer in different areas of the world on sensitivity of the method used for detecting alpha-fetoprotein. *Int. J. Cancer* 10, 331.
Gitlin, D., and Boesman, M. (1966). Serum α-fetoprotein, albumin, and γG-globulin in the human conceptus. *J. Clin. Invest.* 45, 1826.
Hirai, H., and Toru, M., eds. (1973). "Alpha-Fetoprotein and Hepatoma," No. 14. University Park Press, Tokyo.
Kohn, J. (1971). Method for the detection and identification of alpha-fetoprotein in serum. *J. Clin. Pathol.* 24, 733.
Nishi, S., and Hirai, H. (1973). Radioimmunoassay of α-fetoprotein in hepatoma,

other liver diseases, and pregnancy. In "Alpha-Fetoprotein and Hepatoma" (H. Hirai and M. Toru, eds.), No. 14, pp. 79–87. University Park Press, Tokyo.

Nishioka, M., Okita, K., Okamoto, Y., Kodama, T., and Fujita, T. (1972). Comparison of various precipitin tests in the detection of α-fetoprotein in serum. Digestion 6, 205.

Nishioka, M., Okamoto, Y., Shigeta, K., Hironaga, K., and Fujita, T. (1973). Further observation on α-fetoprotein in the diagnosis of diseases of the digestive tract. Digestion 8, 396.

O'Connor, G. T., Tatarinov, Y. S., Abelev, G. I., and Uriel, J. (1970). A collaborative study for the evaluation of a serologic test for primary liver cancer. Cancer 25, 1091.

Purves, L. R., Bersohn, I., and Geddes, E. W. (1970). Serum alpha-fetoprotein and primary cancer of the liver in man. Cancer 25, 1261.

Rowe, D. S. (1970). Method for increasing the sensitivity of radial-immunodiffusion assay. Lancet 1, 1340.

Ruoslahti, E., and Seppälä, M. (1971). Studies of carcinofetal proteins. III. Development of a radioimmunoassay for α-fetoprotein. Demonstration of α-Fetoprotein in serum of healthy human adults. Int. J. Cancer 8, 374.

Ruoslahti, E., Seppälä, M., Vuopio, P., Saksela, E., and Peltokallio, P. (1972). Radioimmunoassay of alpha-fetoprotein in primary and secondary cancer of the liver. J. Nat. Cancer Inst. 49, 623.

Ruoslahti, E., Salaspuro, M., Pihko, H., Anderson, L., and Seppälä, M. (1974). Serum α-fetoprotein: Diagnostic significance in liver disease. Brit. Med. J. 2, 527.

Seppälä, M., Bagshawe, K. D., and Ruoslahti, E. (1972). Radioimmunoassay of alpha-fetoprotein: A contribution to the diagnosis of choriocarcinoma and hydatidiform mole. Int. J. Cancer 10, 478.

Smith, J. B. (1970). Alpha-fetoprotein: Occurrence in certain malignant diseases and review of clinical applications. Med. Clin. N. Amer. 54, 79.

Smith, J. B. (1971). Alpha-fetoprotein in neoplastic and nonneoplastic conditions. Proc. Conf. Workshop Embryonic Fetal Antigens Cancer, 1st, 1971 p. 305.

Carcinoembryonic Antigen

Booth, S. N., King, J., Leonard, J. P., and Dykes, P. W. (1973). Serum CEA in normal individuals and in clinical disorders. Ann. Immunol. (Paris) 124C, 631.

Egan, M. L., Latenschleger, J. T., Coligan, J. E., and Todd, C. (1972). Radioimmune assay of carcinoembryonic antigen. Immunochemistry 9, 617.

Elias, E. G., Holyoke, E. P., and Chu, T. M. (1974). Carcinoembryonic antigen in feces and plasma of normal subjects and patients with colorectal carcinoma. Dis. Colon Rectum 17, 38.

Fleisher, M., Oettgen, H. F., Besenfelder, E., and Schwartz, M. K. (1973). Measurement of carcinoembryonic antigen. Clin. Chem. 19, 1214.

Go, V. L. W., Schutt, A. J., Moertel, C. G., Summerskill, W. H. J. and Butt, H. R. (1972). Radioimmunoassay of carcinoembryonic antigen (CEA). A modified method and a clinical evaluation. Gastroenterology 62, 754.

Gold, P., and Freedman, S. O. (1965). Demonstration of tumor-specific antigens in human colon carcinomata by immunological tolerance and absorption techniques. J. Exp. Med. 122, 467.

Hansen, H. J., Lance, K. P., and Krupey, J. (1971). Demonstration of an ion sensitive antigenic site on carcinoembryonic antigen using zirconyl phosphate gel. *Clin. Res.* 19, 143.

Hansen, H. J., Snyder, J. J., Miller, E., Vandevoorder, J. P., Miller, O. N., Hines, L. R., and Burns, J. J. (1974). Carcinoembryonic antigen (CEA) assay. A laboratory adjunct in the diagnosis and management of cancer. *Hum. Pathol.* 5, 139.

Kupchik, H. Z., Hansen, J. J., Sorokin, J. J., and Zamcheek, N. (1972). Comparison of radioimmunoassays for carcinoembryonic antigens. *Proc. Conf. Workshop Embryonic Fetal Antigens Cancer, 2nd, 1972* p. 261.

Lange, R. D., Chernoff, A. I., Jordan, T. A., and Collmann, I. R. (1971). Experience with a hemagglutination inhibition test for carcinoembryonic antigen: Preliminary report. *Proc. Conf. Workshop Embryonic Fetal Antigen Cancer, 1st, 1971* p. 379.

Laurence, D. J. R., Stevens, V., Bettleheim, R., Darcy, D., Leese, C., Turberville, C., Alexander, P., Johns, E. W., and Neville, A. M. (1972). Role of plasma carcinoembryonic antigen in diagnosis of gastrointestinal, mammary and bronchial carcinoma. *Brit. Med. J.* 3, 605.

McPherson, T. A., Band, P. R., Grace, M., Hyde, H. A. and Patwardhan, V. C. (1973). Carcinoembryonic antigen (CEA): Comparison of the Farr and solid-phase methods for detection of CEA. *Int. J. Cancer* 12, 42.

Sorokin, J. J., Sugarhaker, P. H., Zamcheck, N., Pisick, M., Kupchik, H. Z., and Moore, F. P. (1974). Serial carcinoembryonic antigen assays. *J. Amer. Med. Ass.* 228, 49.

Thompson, P., Krupey, J., Freedman, S., and Gold, P. (1969). The radioimmunoassay of circulating carcinoembryonic antigen of the human digestive system. *Proc. Nat. Acad. Sci. U.S.* 64, 161.

Other Antigen-Antibodies

Banwo, O., Versey, J., and Hobbs, J. R. (1974). New oncofetal antigen for human pancreas. *Lancet* 1, 643.

Björklund, B., ed. (1973). "Immunological Techniques for Detection of Cancer," *Proc. Folksam Symp.*, 1972. Bonniers, Stockholm, Sweden.

Tal, C., and Halperin, M. (1970). Presence of serologically distinct protein in serum of cancer patients and pregnant women. *Isr. J. Med. Sci.* 6, 708.

Neutrophil Function

MICHAEL E. MILLER

Department of Pediatrics, University of California, Los Angeles, School of Medicine at the Harbor General Hospital, Los Angeles, California

I. Introduction

Interest in phagocytic function has increased markedly in recent years. Of the many factors contributing to this, two have played major roles. The first of these was the discovery by Holmes and co-workers, in 1966, of an inborn error of polymorphonuclear leukocyte (PMN) function in which PMNs from afflicted subjects failed to kill bacteria intracellularly after phagocytosis. The recognition of a basic defect of PMN function

427

in this genetically determined entity, known as chronic granulomatous disease (CGD), proved of major interest to scientists of many disciplines. It was soon apparent that other PMN functions, such as phagocytosis and movement, might, if deficient, also lead to recurrent infections in an afflicted subject. Consequently, the development of methods for the evaluation of these phagocytic functions has been intimately involved with the increasing recognition of clinical disorders involving abnormalities of phagocytes. [It is interesting to note in passing that the recognition of such disorders was predicted by Metchnikoff (1893) in his classic papers before the turn of the century.]

Second, increasing knowledge of the significant interactions between T and B cells and "effector" cells of the immune response has prompted the need for more precise methodology in the understanding of the role of phagocytes in many aspects of the immune response.

Predictably, these interests have led to numerous assays for the study of phagocytic function. Equally predictable has been the intensity of claims and counterclaims of superiority by supporters of a particular assay. Through this controversy three general points emerge:

1. There are no "standard assays" for any of the phagocytic functions of ingestion (phagocytosis), movement, or bactericidal activities. Multiple variables, as discussed below, make it virtually impossible for a single assay to satisfy all requirements. A particular problem in the study of PMN function is the fact that neutrophils maintain complete functional integrity for a very short period of time after removal from the body. Unlike lymphocytes, therefore, they are not well studied in relatively long-term *in vitro* assays. Repeated and time-consuming attempts at purification to the range of 95–100% pure PMN suspensions may not, therefore, be appropriate. The potential functional artifacts introduced thereby must be weighed against the disadvantages of other cell types present in relatively unpurified suspensions.

2. Most, if not all, phagocyte functions involve both humoral and cellular components. Progress in the understanding of these interactions was hampered by a 20–30 year debate during which the relative importance of humoral and cellular factors were argued. Prior to the turn of the century, Metchnikoff stressed the importance of cellular phagocytes, or "microphages" in body defenses. Wright and Douglas (1903) and also Neufeld and Rimpeau observed shortly thereafter that humoral factors, or "opsonin" played a critical role in phagocytosis. It is now clear that the process of phagocytosis, as well as other PMN functions are dependent upon a complex set of humoral and cellular interactions, each of which may have a significant affect upon a particular assay.

3. The applicability of an *in vitro* assay to *in vivo* disorders characterized by recurrent infections, or to a precise role in the immune-inflammatory response is not always readily determined. This is due to several factors. First, the conditions of most *in vitro* phagocyte assays differ substantially from what is believed to be actual *in vivo* conditions under which they function. Second, current information on the interactions and relative importance of individual components of the inflammatory response is limited.

It is, therefore, often difficult to ascribe an etiologic role to a particular *in vitro* defect in the cause of recurrent infections or impaired immunity in a given patient. This is particularly true in those situations in which combined defects involving movement, ingestion, and/or killing are demonstrated.

Despite the limitations raised in these introductory comments, it would be unfortunate to leave the impression that the current "state of the art" in the study of phagocyte functions has been unrewarding. Few fields have yielded such a varied and consistently useful store of information contributing to the understanding of the normal and abnormal immune-inflammatory responses.

This chapter summarizes the types of assays and methodologic limitations of PMN ingestion (phagocytosis), bactericidal activities, and movement [directed (chemotaxis) and passive]. The review is basically concerned with PMNs.

II. Phagocytosis

Methods for study of phagocytosis are many and varied. In recent years, more sophisticated techniques have been introduced. Despite the superiority claimed by their supporters, however, there is presently no conclusive evidence that they more accurately or precisely measure the phagocytic process. Their utility may lie more in the study of specific aspects of the cellular mechanisms involved in phagocytosis.

Assays for phagocytosis fall into four general categories.

A. Quantitative Assays that Count the Number of Particles Ingested by a Cell

Assays that directly quantitate uptake have the obvious merit of directly measuring the phagocytic process. In theory, at least, they correlate the best of all the assays with *in vivo* activities.

Many particles and agents have been utilized for counting in such systems. They fall into three general areas: (1) Direct quantitation by light microscopy (examples of particles that have been used in such systems are India ink, rice starch, yeast, and various bacteria). Indirect quantitation of ingested materials can be obtained by (2) measurement of radioactivity of phagocytosed radiolabeled particles, such as bacteria or immune complexes, or (3) extraction in soluble form of ingested particles—for example, dioxane extraction of starch, or of an easily stained lipid, such as oil red O.

Quantitative assays have been criticized for their cumbersome nature and their relative imprecision. Neither of these limitations is necessarily present, however, and these types of assay are utilized by many workers in the field.

B. Assays that Measure the Removal of the Test Particle from the Fluid Medium Surrounding the Cells

In principle, such assays differ little from the above group, the only difference being that phagocytosis is measured by determining disappearance of the particles from the extracellular medium rather than intracellular uptake. Such measurements can also be made either by direct quantitation or by indirect measurement. For example, quantitative count can be made of the bacteria remaining in the extracellular medium after phagocytosis. The difficulty of most such assays, however, is to separate bacteria that are attached to the cell membrane from those that have actually been ingested. Also, such bacterial assays often fail to achieve suitable reproducibility. The role of serum in killing bacteria is also hard to correct for in such measurements. Other assays employing a similar principle use such particles as complement-sensitized sheep or human erythrocytes (number of erythrocytes not phagocytized assayed spectrophotometrically) or polystyrene particles (number of polystyrene particles not phagocytized measured turbidimetrically).

C. Assays that Measure Metabolic Change Occurring during Phagocytosis

A number of assays have been described in which phagocytosis is correlated with the increment of a particular metabolic change involved in the process. Such assays assume that a sensitive and precise relationship exists between quantitative uptake and the particular metabolic event being measured. Unfortunately, very few such assays have adequately compared the relationship between particle uptake and metabolic increment in all ranges of uptake. Further, recent data suggest that intracellular events associated with the phagocytic process may be triggered by contact of the particle to be ingested with the cell membrane. Thus, a number of metabolic assays may fail to differentiate particle adherence and particle ingestion.

Metabolic assays may be direct or indirect. An example of the former is the measurement of glycolysis and/or hexose monophosphate shunt activity occurring during phagocytosis. An example of the latter is the reduction of a dye, nitroblue tetrazolium (NBT) to blue formazan by hydrogen ion transfer during phagocytosis.

D. OTHER METHODS

A variety of other methods have been employed in the study of PMN phagocytosis. Of these, one of the more promising is that of chemiluminescence. Allen, Stjernholm, and Steele have demonstrated that PMNs emit flashes of luminescence during phagocytosis of bacteria, and that the luminescence correlates with activity of the hexose monophosphate shunt in these cells. This chemiluminescence can be quantitated in a liquid scintillation spectrometer. Although the precise relationship between chemiluminescence and number of particles ingested requires definition, the method holds significant promise as a relatively simple, inexpensive, rapid and reproducible assay of phagocytosis.

While the study of phagocytosis would best be served by the adoption of a "standard" method, it is apparent that no single assay satisfies all parameters. In selecting the most appropriate assay for a given set of experiments, the following general considerations should be borne in mind.

1. Humoral components and cellular components of the phagocytic process should be measured by an assay, both separately and in combination. For example, an assay that simply mixes a test particle with whole blood offers little opportunity for characterization of the defect.

2. Reproducibility is obviously important. While it is often difficult to completely standardize a phagocytic assay between laboratories, one can at least work with a system that gives highly reproducible results within a given laboratory. Among the variables that make quantitative assays difficult to standardize are failure to control variables such as PMN count, particle count, conditions of incubation, and precise determination of the optimal conditions for a particular assay.

3. Ease of count. Many particles have been utilized in phagocytic systems. The particle chosen depends, in part, upon how easily it is visualized within the phagocyte after ingestion. In direct counting sys-

tems, obvious fragmenting and variability of staining characteristics inside of the phagocyte make it difficult, if not impossible, to obtain accurate results.

4. Humoral factors. The source of humoral factors, or opsonins, involved in a phagocytic system, will have a major effect upon results. For screening of patients, whole serum or plasma is generally used. While such media should contain all factors necessary for maximum uptake of a test particle, they often contain acute phase proteins and other abnormal factors that may affect the *in vitro* assay. It is optimal if one knows the precise humoral requirements for a maximum uptake of a given particle, for then the investigator need add only those materials. Such work is painstaking, however, and has seldom been accomplished.

Not only do different bacteria require different antibodies, but it is now evident that the complement requirements differ for optimal phagocytosis of various particles.

5. Random exposure of the particles and phagocytosis is essential. Systems in which, for example, the particles and phagocytes are mixed by inverting and then allowing them to stand during the period of phagocytosis are not likely to give consistent results. It appears essential for constant mixing to take place throughout the experiment.

6. Ratio of particles being phagocytized to cells (phagocytes) is critical for any assay and should be determined prior to the institution of a phagocytic assay.

7. Relationship of indirect systems to phagocytosis. Those systems which measure phagocytosis by an indirect method, such as NBT reduction, are accurate only as far as increments of metabolic change and/or NBT reduction can be shown by precise experiments to correlate with numbers of bacteria or particles ingested. To date, few such studies have been reported.

8. Correlation of *in vitro* with *in vivo* results. This is obviously vital, and it represents the entire basis upon which a phagocytic assay is deemed useful in the study of the normal and abnormal inflammatory response in humans. At present, our understanding of the inflammatory process precludes accuracy in this area and tests of phagocytosis, as well as those of killing and movement (next two sections) must be viewed as supportive, not diagnostic.

III. Bactericidal Assays of Neutrophils

As above, numerous methods exist for the study of postphagocytic killing of bacteria within neutrophils. Those methods based upon survival rate of ingested bacteria within PMNs seem most direct, and regardless of the initial method employed (such as metabolic or NBT, see below), should be performed before concluding that any patient has a defect of neutrophil bactericidal activity.

A. Assays that Directly Measure Intraleukocyte Bacterial Killing

The most frequently used type of assay is that of Quie and co-workers, in which viable intracellular bacteria are separated from nonphagocytized bacteria. This system was utilized in the first demonstration of a bactericidal defect of PMNs, i.e., chronic granulomatous disease (CGD). Many modifications of this method have been described. For example, extracellular bacteria may be killed with antibiotics or other agents instead of being separated by differential centrifugation. Such systems assume that antibiotics do not penetrate the PMN, a point upon which not all workers agree.

B. Nitroblue Tetrazolium Tests

Several variations of this test exist, all of which are based upon the increased metabolic activity generated during PMN-bacteria ingestion and/or killing. The test identifies leukocytes with oxidase activity. NBT is colorless in the oxidized form but can be detected in the reduced state of blue formazan. While this test has been utilized in the *screening* of patients for CGD, demonstration of defective intracellular bactericidal activity is essential for the definitive diagnosis of CGD.

Three basic NBT tests have been described. (1) Slide tests: In these tests, resting PMNs are simply mixed with NBT, incubated, and the percentage of PMNs containing formazan granules is determined microscopically. Such tests have been utilized for the differentiation of bacterial from nonbacterial infections, but much controversy exists as to their actual utility for this purpose. (2) Tube tests: PMNs, autologous plasma, latex particles, and NBT are incubated. With normal PMNs, the supernatant changes to gray or purple. This is a rapid and simple *screening* test for CGD. (3) Quantitative test: This is the most accurate and most difficult of the three procedures to apply to clinical testing. In this assay, reduced NBT is extracted with pyridine and measured spectrophotometrically at 515 nm. The accuracy of this procedure permits detection of carriers (heterozygotes) of the X-linked form of CGD.

C. Metabolic Assays for PMN Killing

Of the various assays in this category, the bacterial iodination test has been most utilized for patient screening. Inorganic iodide is fixed to bacteria (or a yeast particle) by myeloperoxidase in the presence of hydrogen peroxide (the latter generated within a normal PMN following phagocytosis). The *in vitro* assay employs radioactive inorganic iodide, isolated leukocytes, zymosan or bacteria, and serum; it can be used to detect CGD, CGD heterozygotes, or myeloperoxidase deficiency. The iodination is defective when there is a failure in peroxide production.

IV. Assays of Neutrophil Movement

Although the recognition of disorders of neutrophil movement is more recent than that of phagocytic and bactericidal activities, the field has grown rapidly and has now reached the point of considerable complexity. Unfortunately, all the problems discussed in the areas of phagocytosis and killing also plague the field of cell movement, in some cases to an even greater degree. Two clinically significant types of cell movement are now recognized—*directed* locomotion (chemotaxis) and *random* or passive locomotion.

A. Measurement of Directed Locomotion (Chemotaxis)

The period prior to the early 1960s was characterized by much controversy in methodology. In 1962, Stephen Boyden described an assay for measurement of chemotaxis which offered fair reproducibility and ease of performance. It was thus possible to run multiple experiments at the same time. While the Boyden assay has produced significant controversy (see below), significant increases in our understanding of the chemotactic process have occurred through its use. Several products of the serum complement system have been shown to have chemotactic activity, including molecular fragments of the third and fifth components (C3a and C5a) and a trimolecular complex $C\overline{567}$. More recently, chemotactic activity has also been associated with Hageman-factor activation, kallikrein, and plasminogen activator.

There are many modifications of the Boyden assay, but all employ the same general principle: Cells to be chemotaxed are placed in the upper portion of a double chamber and separated from a source of chemo-tactically active material(s) on the bottom by a small-pore filter. After incubation, usually for 3 hours at 37°C, the filter is removed, cleared, and stained, and the number of cells that have migrated through the filter is determined microscopically. Some of the more common problems of this assay are discussed below.

1. Filter variability. This variability plagues all who work in the field. Filters may vary significantly, not only from lot to lot, but, not infrequently, even within the same box. There has been no way to standardize these filters so that any two investigators can be sure of starting with the same materials. Until this problem is solved, a substantial compromise is effected upon the reliability of data derived from such chemotactic assays.

2. Objectivity. Variations in microscopic counting are considerable, even among investigators in the same laboratory. It is difficult to get two observers to agree upon which layer is actually that of farthest migration and, upon what represents a reasonable "focusing distance." Such variability must be taken into account in the interpretation of data from different laboratories.

3. Cells dropping off the filter. This is a highly controversial point. Some observers report substantial difficulty with cells dropping off the filter into the lower chamber, but others do not encounter this problem.

4. Standardization of cell number. It is essential that the same concentration of cells be utilized in all preparations if results are to be comparable. The minimum concentration found necessary to measure directed migration is in the range of 2.3×10^6/ml. Below this concentration, one may only be measuring passive locomotion (see below). In the same study, Patten and co-workers determined the limiting concentrations of various anticoagulants for chemotactic preparations.

5. Addition of fetal calf serum. One of the most disturbing factors of these assays is the need to add fetal calf serum or similar material to the chamber in order to get consistent results. Although the fetal calf serum is heat inactivated and placed in both portions of the chamber, the presence of such a foreign protein is obviously undesirable. Despite many studies, the mechanism(s) by which fetal calf serum works is unknown.

Other Chemotactic Assays

In an attempt to avoid some of the problems noted above, a number of other methods for cellular chemotaxis have been described. Among the most promising of these are (1) direct observation of cells moving in fluid medium toward a chemotactic source, as described by Zigmond and

Hirsch: and (2) the use of ^{51}Cr-labeled PMNs and counting the radio-activity in a double filter system. The major advantage of the radioactive counting systems is the large number of preparations that can be counted at one time. They may have particular utility in the study of the kinetics of chemotaxis. Filter variability, although less troublesome than in the Boyden assay, is still a problem. Further, there is an unresolved question as to the comparative sensitivity of radiolabeled assays to the Boyden counting assays. Finally, the use of a Boyden-type assay is still required for the characterization of cell type as, for example, in the study of eosinophil or basophil chemotaxis.

A newer technique which may have utility is the measurement of membrane deformability (Miller, 1975).

B. MEASUREMENT OF PASSIVE OR RANDOM LOCOMOTION

The clinical importance of separating passive locomotion from chemotaxis is emphasized by the recognition of clinical disorders in which the two processes are independently involved (Miller, 1975).

Two methods have most commonly been employed for the study of passive locomotion. The first of these is a modification of the Boyden method. The essential differences are that no chemotactic gradient is present and a large pore filter is used. The determination of passive locomotion by this method can be difficult and may be masked by simultaneously occurring chemotaxis.

The second method utilized in a study of passive locomotion is the capillary tube assay, a number of modifications of which exist. PMNs are placed in microhematocrit tubes and placed in a vertical position on the microscope stage as in a sedimentation rate preparation. At hourly intervals, the distance of migration from the top of the buffy coat layer to the farthest group (two or more cells) is measured with an ocular eyepiece. Optics of the system may be substantially improved by placing the tubes in a specially constructed chamber from two microscope slides sandwiched around capillary tubes and embedding them in adhesive clay placed in the bottom. The chamber is filled with immersion oil. The entire chamber, including the capillary tubes, is then examined.

Recent observations have suggested that *both* assays of passive locomotion should be performed in patients suspected of disorders of leukocyte movement. Although the mechanisms by which these assays operate is not well understood, it is clear that they each have value in the characterization of host defects.

References

Baehner, R. L., and Nathan, D. G. (1962). Quantitative nitroblue tetrazolium test in chronic granulomatous disease. *N. Engl. J. Med.* **278**, 971.

Harris, H. (1954). Role of chemotaxis in inflammation. *Physiol. Rev.* **54**, 529.

Holmes, B., Quie, P. G., Windhorst, D. B., and Good, R. A. (1966). Fatal granulomatous disease of childhood. An inborn abnormality of phagocytic function. *Lancet* **1**, 1225.

Klebanoff, S. J. (1971). Intraleukocyte microbicidal defects. *Annu. Rev. Med.* **22**, 39.

Metchnikoff, E. (1893). "Lectures on the Comparative Pathology of Inflammation" (transl. by F. A. Starling and E. H. Starling) Kegan, Paul, Trench, Truber & Co., London.

Miller, M. E. (1975). Pathology chemotaxis and random mobility. *Semin. Hematol.* **12**, 59.

Newsome, J. (1967). Phagocytosis by human neutrophils. *Nature (London)* **214**, 1092.

Quie, P. G. (1972). Disorders of phagocyte function. *In* "Current Problems in Pediatrics," Vol. II, No. 11. Yearbook Publ., Chicago, Illinois.

Ward, P. A. (1972). Insubstantial leukotaxis. *J. Lab. Clin. Med.* **79**, 873.

Wright, A. E., and Douglas, S. R. (1903). An experimental investigation of the role of the blood fluids in connection with phagocytosis. *Proc. Roy. Soc., London* **72**, 357.

Subject Index

R

Reticuloendothelial system
cellular studies
Küpffer cells, 298
monocytes, 299–302
pulmonary macrophages, 296–298
splenic macrophages, 298
tissue macrophages, 299
clearance testing, 290–295
Rebuck skin windows, 295–296
Rheumatoid factors
clinical significance, 367–371
commonly used tests, 371–373
general test procedures, 366–367

T

Thrombocytes
autoantibodies against, 355–356

results and significance of tests,
358–359
tests for, 356–358
Tumor-associated antigens
carcinoembryonic antigen, 413–414
assay methods, 415–418
clinical significance, 419–420
preparation of antiserum, 415
purification, 414
α-fetoprotein, 406–407
assay methods, 408–411
clinical significance and sensitivity of
assay methods, 411–413
preparation of antiserum, 408
purification, 407–408
pancreatic oncofetal antigen, 423
polypeptide antigen, 420–422
T-globulin, 422–423